The Perception of Illusory Contours

Susan Petry and Glenn E. Meyer

Editors

The Perception
of Illusory Contours

With 279 Illustrations, 7 in Full Color

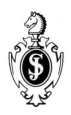

Springer-Verlag
New York Berlin Heidelberg
London Paris Tokyo

Susan Petry
Department of Psychology
Adelphi University
Garden City, New York 11530
USA

Glenn E. Meyer
Department of Psychology
Lewis and Clark College
Portland, Oregon 97219
USA

Library of Congress Cataloging-in-Publication Data
The perception of illusory contours.
    Includes index.
    1. Visual perception.   2. Optical illusions.
I. Petry, Susan Jane.   II. Meyer, Glenn E.
BF241.P435   1987   153.7′4   87-4572

Typeset by TCSystems, Shippensburg, Pennsylvania.
Printed and bound by Arcata Graphics/Halliday, West Hanover, Massachusetts.
Printed in the United States of America.

9 8 7 6 5 4 3 2 1

ISBN 0-387-96518-1 Springer-Verlag New York Berlin Heidelberg
ISBN 3-540-96518-1 Springer-Verlag Berlin Heidelberg New York

Acknowledgment

The idea for a book on illusory contours grew out of a conference on the topic, which we organized and which took place at Adelphi University in November 1985 (Petry & Meyer, 1986). While not a proceedings, much of the material presented in the individual chapters originated with ideas presented and exchanged at that conference. Although an exceedingly popular research topic, illusory contours have never been the sole topic of a book before. We believed that their time had come.

We undertook the project of editing a book on illusory contours for a variety of reasons and with a variety of emotions. It frequently seems that the major thing one learns when undertaking a project of this magnitude is never to do it again. Although we wish to reserve judgment on this point, we can say that the experience has been unforgettable.

It has been a pleasure and an honor to work with the distinguished groups of researchers who are the contributors to the book. To them, first and foremost, we give heartfelt thanks.

Four contributors deserve special acknowledgment. Anne Hogg translated both the Schumann (1900) and Ehrenstein (1941) articles, a time-consuming and arduous task. Walter Gerbino graciously and painstakingly translated the Kanizsa (1955a) article. Ross Day served as keynote speaker at the conference, and has been a source of inspiration for us. Finally, Nick Wade provided an intriguing artistic conclusion to the book.

Additional thanks for their help in various aspects of the book go to Lothar Spillman, Walter Ehrenstein, John Tagney, and Marc Seabrechts. We would also like to extend our thanks to the faculty, staff, and students at Adelphi University and Lewis and Clark College for all their help, in particular to the graduate students in the Perceptual Organization II Seminar, who read and commented on the chapters in manuscript form, and to our hardworking and underpaid secretaries—Eleanor Shaw, Pat Carey, Karen Thompson, Susan Masotti, and Marge McKenna.

Partial funding for this project came from the U.S. Air Force Office on Scientific Research Grant (#86-0028), and we are extremely grateful for this.

We would also like to thank the people at Springer-Verlag, for their helpful and timely information, encouragement, and support.

Finally, we would like to thank our families—Wayne Martin, Melanie Anne Meyer, and Courtney, Ross, and Owen Martin—for everything.

Susan Petry
Glenn E. Meyer

Contents

Contributors

John Beckner
Department of Psychology, University of Cincinnati, Cincinnati, Ohio 45221, USA

Melanie Bishop
Department of Psychology, University of Keele, Keele, Staffordshire ST5 5BG, England

Drake R. Bradley
Department of Psychology, Bates College, Lewiston, Maine 04240, USA

James M. Brown
Department of Psychology, State University of New York at Buffalo, Buffalo, New York 14260, USA

Nicola Bruno
Department of Psychology, Cornell University, Ithaca, New York 14850, USA

Stanley Coren
Department of Psychology, University of British Columbia, Vancouver, British Columbia V6T 1W5, Canada

Ross H. Day
Department of Psychology, Monash University, Victoria 316B, Australia

William N. Dember
Department of Psychology, University of Cincinnati, Cincinnati, Ohio 45221, USA

Charles M. M. de Weert
Psychological Laboratory, Catholic University, Montessorilaan 3, Postbus 9104, 6500 HE Nijmegen, The Netherlands

David Fish
Department of Psychology, Lewis and Clark College, Portland, Oregon 97219, USA

Robert Gannon
Department of Psychology, Adelphi University, Garden City, New York 11530, USA

Angus Gellatly
Department of Psychology, University of Keele, Keele, Staffordshire ST5 5BG, England

Walter Gerbino
Istituto di Psicologia, Universita di Trieste, Trieste, Italy

Barbara Gillam
School of Psychology, University of New South Wales, Kensington, New South Wales 2033, Australia

Arthur P. Ginsburg
Vistech Consultants Inc., Dayton, Ohio 45432, USA

James Gordon
Department of Psychology, City University of New York, Hunter College, and Department of Psychology, Rockefeller University, New York, New York 10021, USA

Richard L. Gregory
MRC, Brain and Perception Laboratory, Department of Anatomy, The Medical School, University of Bristol, Bristol SB8 1TD, England

Stephen Grossberg
Center for Adaptive Systems, Boston University, Boston, Massachusetts 02215, USA

Diane F. Halpern
Department of Psychology, California State University–San Bernardino, San Bernardino, California 92407, USA

Anne Hogg
Neurologisches-Universitats Klinik, University of Freiburg, 7800 Freiburg, West Germany

Scott Jones
Department of Psychology, University of Cincinnati, Cincinnati, Ohio 54221, USA

Maxwell K. Jory
Department of Applied Psychology, Chisholm Institute of Technology, Caulfield Campus, Caulfield, East Victoria 3145, Australia

Gaetano Kaniza
Institute of Psychology, University of Trieste, Trieste, Italy

Victor Klymenko
Department of Psychology, Park Hall, State University of New York at Buffalo, Amherst, New York 14260, USA

Phillip J. Kellman
Department of Psychology, Swarthmore College, Swarthmore, Pennsylvania 19081, USA

John M. Kennedy
Department of Psychology, Scarborough College, West Hill, Ontario MIC 1A4, Canada

Martha G. Loukides
Department of Psychology, Swarthmore College, Swarthmore, Pennsylvania 19081, USA

William M. Maguire
Department of Psychology, St. John's University, Jamaica, New York 11437, USA

Glenn E. Meyer
Department of Psychology, Lewis and Clark College, Portland, Oregon 97219, USA

Ennio Mingolla
Center for Adaptive Systems, Boston University, Boston, Massachusetts 02215, USA

Gian Franco Minguzzi†
Department of Philosophy, University of Bologna, Bologna, Italy

Robert A. Padich
Department of Psychology, University of Cincinnati, Cincinnati, Ohio 45221, USA

Theodore E. Parks
Department of Psychology, University of California–Davis, Davis, California 95616, USA

Susan Petry
Department of Psychology, Adelphi University, Garden City, New York 11530, USA

Clare Porac
Department of Psychology, University of Victoria, Victoria, British Columbia V8W 2Y2, Canada

V. S. Ramachandran
Department of Psychology, University of California–San Diego, La Jolla, California 92093, USA

Irvin Rock
Department of Psychology, University of California at Berkeley, Berkeley, California 94720, USA

Marco Sambin
Departimento di Psicologia Generale, Universita Delgi Studi di Padova, Padova, Italy

Robert Shapley
Department of Psychology, New York University, New York, New York 10003, USA

Leonard H. Theodor
Department of Psychology, York University, Downsview, Ontario, Canada

Noud A. W. H. van Kruysbergen
Psychological Laboratory, Catholic University, Montessorilaan 3, Postbus 9104, 6500 HE Nijmegen, The Netherlands

Nicholas Wade
Department of Psychology, University of Dundee, Dundee DDI 4HN, Scotland

Joel S. Warm
Department of Psychology, University of Cincinnati, Cincinnati, Ohio 54221, USA

Naomi Weisstein
Department of Psychology, Park Hall, State University of New York at Buffalo, Amherst, New York 14260, USA

† Deceased.

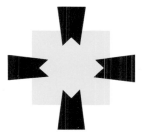

FIGURE 4.14. For a discussion of this figure, see page 45.

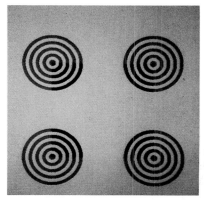

FIGURE 17.1 f. The assimilation of the dark lines in the inner square makes conditions optimal for color induction in the center due to outer lines. For further discussion, see page 167.

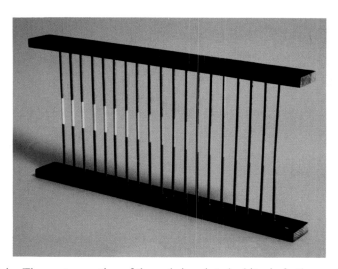

FIGURE 28.5. Misty Strip. The center portion of the rods is painted white, in farther regions, or gray, in nearer regions. Subjects see a Misty Strip join the painted bands. The gradations in the central white strips on each bar cannot readily be reproduced here, but the idea should be clear, and some of the effects should be present for the viewer. Construction by Colin Ware. For further discussion, see page 256.

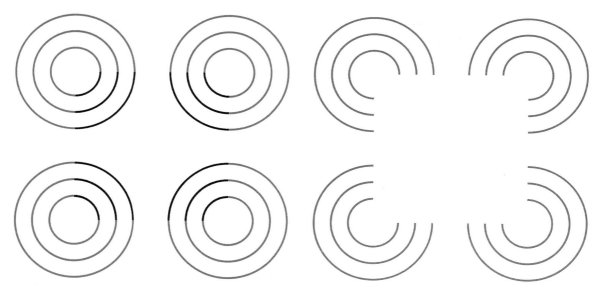

FIGURE 27.5. A reddish square in a greenish surrounding. Contrast or assimilation, or both? For further discussion, see page 250.

FIGURE 27.6. Line endings produce intensive contrast, but no chromatic induction. For further discussion, see page 250.

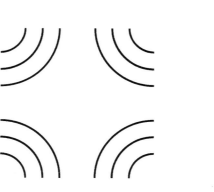

FIGURE 27.7. Chromatic assimilation within the central square. For further discussion, see page 250.

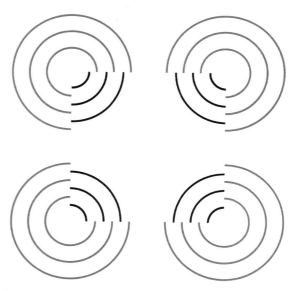

FIGURE 27.8. The central square is brighter than in Figure 27.7 because of intensive contrast induced by green line endings. For further discussion, see page 251.

SECTION I

Introductory and Historical Material

Chapter 1, the introduction by Petry and Meyer, presents a somewhat lighthearted overview on the topic of illusory contours. It is descriptive rather than evaluative, and focuses on the types of illusory contours, the history of research on the topic, their use in nonperceptual fields, and a brief discussion of theoretical positions.

Chapters 2, 3, and 4, which are historical material, consist of translations of three articles. Schumann's 1900 article, in addition to being the first to describe and print a figure of what is now referred to as an illusory contour, is one of the most widely referenced articles in the field of form vision and perceptual organization. Next, Ehrenstein's 1941 article presents one of the first and most influential sets of parametric observations of the phenomenon. Finally, Kanizsa's 1955 article represents the first of the modern era and has given rise to an extraordinary number of studies on the form of illusory contour which bears his name.

Top-Down and Bottom-Up: The Illusory Contour as a Microcosm of Issues in Perception

Glenn E. Meyer and Susan Petry

Stealth bombers, invisible men, ghosts, phantoms, phantom contours, illusions, Scheinkanten, illusory contours, subjective contours, virtual contours, cognitive contours, anomalous contours, contours without gradients, 'magini quasi percettivi' (quasi-perceptual contours).

From the terrors of the real world, to the terrors of childhood and superstition, we can see one common trend. The question is, what determines reality? Is it our senses? Are our senses reliable? These questions have been the center of speculation probably from the beginning of our species' self-awareness. Some of our religions regard the world itself as illusion. We are most frightened by the possibility that something is there, sees us, but we cannot see it.

However, we are fascinated by other possibilities. Can we be tricked into seeing when there is nothing there, no physical stimulus? In dreams, hallucinations, and images, we experience worlds that are not real but these experiences do not have an objective referent. For vision researchers and artists, there are other options to explore the fragile nature of reality. By putting pigment to paper or electrons to phosphors, we can make you see that which does not exist. This is the topic of this book and the referent of the terms in our list above.

Psychology has been fascinated by the problem of illusion. Our perceptions do not always mirror reality. No student has passed through introductory psychology without seeing the Mueller-Lyer illusion (at least, they're supposed to see it). Most of us have wondered why the moon looks bigger at the horizon. Those of us who have studied the literature on the phenomenon still wonder why the moon looks big-

ger at the horizon. Many types of illusions have been studied. Coren and Girgus in 1978 reported that at least 1,000 articles have been written on the subject. However, most of this literature refers to the classic or geometric illusions, such as distortions of length, angle, and curvature; underestimations and overestimations of size or length; or displacements of position due to frames of reference. In all these examples something is there but it is altered.

Here, we are going to deal with a different situation. It is the problem of seeing lines, borders, surfaces, hues, and textures which are not there. Of course, we are familiar with things like this. Our archetypal introductory psychology student has seen negative afterimages. However, we are going to be dealing with something different: an image of a surface produced by some simple inducing elements. Consider Figure 1.1.

Most of us see a whiter than white triangle (Fig. 1.1a) and a blacker than black triangle (Fig. 1.1b). The triangle isn't real. There are just some pacmen with their mouths aligned. There has been much controversy in modern perceptual research regarding the relative contributions of low-level versus higher-level processes in perceptual experience and the utility for theorists of the study of illusions (Uttal, 1981). One phenomenon is an exquisite example of this conflict: illusory contours (we'll use this term for now and discuss definitional issues below).

With this book, we hope to gain some insight into these issues by enabling a large number of the major researchers in this field to present their current ideas on this topic. Illusory con-

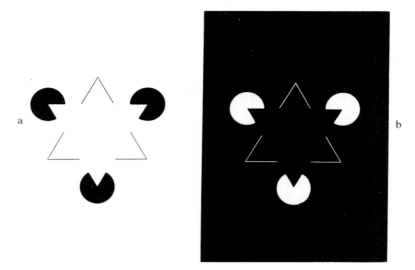

FIGURE 1.1. a and b, Kanisza triangles in black and white.

tours have generated an enormous amount of interest in the psychological, physiological, and artificial intelligence communities. They are not regarded as an isolated but interesting visual "toy." Rather, current theory suggests that comprehending the illusory contour will be crucial to our understanding of normal vision, e.g., since our retinal image is so subject to interruptions in pattern by retinal blood vessels and so much of real-world image is interrupted by the overlap of objects (see Grossberg & Mingolla, 1985a & b; Waldrop, 1984, p. 1227; Marr, 1982, for analyses). It is evident that no theory of human perception would be acceptable if it could not handle an illusory contour configuration, nor would any artificial intelligence effort at real-world pattern recognition.

Thus, we thought the time was right for a conference and subsequent book which would allow the discussion of these issues. Invitations were sent for a conference to be held at Adelphi University (November 24–26, 1985—see Petry & Meyer, 1986). Although not a compilation of proceedings, some of this book is based on the discussions of the participants at the conference.

History

Illusory contours were not created out of thin air by perceptual psychologists. The compelling nature of this illusion led to its use and discov-ery many times in the arts, as we will discuss later. In scientific literature, however, illusory contours seem to have been first displayed and discussed by Frederich Schumann in 1900. The great master Helmholtz presented two clear examples of illusory contours in Volume 3 of his *Treatise* (1866, Figs. 26 and 27, p. 193). The first is an illusory circle over a set of radiating lines (what we would now call a modified Ehrenstein figure) and the second is an illusory triangle defined by the ends of lines. However, Helmholtz seems to have taken no notice of the phenomenal appearance of these figures. Schumann was different. Starting in 1900, he wrote a series of monographs on the topic of form perception which were used in defense of the newly formed field of experimental psychology, which we could call *phenomenalistic psychophysics* ("systematic practice in introspection"). These were collected and reprinted in 1904 (the first monograph of this important work is translated and presented as Chapter 2 of this volume). In a discussion of the stimulus conditions which gave rise to the perception of figures and contours, Schumann presented his Figure 7 (see Fig. 2.7 in this volume), in which the observer perceives a "white rectangle with sharply defined contours . . . that are objectively not present." Thus, both the edge and the surface quality (brightness enhancement) were described or alluded to by Schumann. Of the two, the edge feature seems to be the more important one for Schumann. Schumann's series of articles were well received. Of course, the question of form perception became a major focus of Gestalt psychology.

Other important examples followed, such as Prandtl (1927), who found that if grids of lines contained interruptions, bright illusory contours could be seen bounded by the intersection points. He noted that they could be seen with colored inducers and in afterimages. The latter finding suggested they were not due to eye movements. Matthaei (1929, Fig. 1, p. 13) presented an illusory white bar superimposed over the words "Bonn/Rh." in a manner similar to Kanizsa's (chap. 4, Fig. 4.18) "Roma." A little bit of metropolitan chauvinism! Matthaei emphasized the special quality of the subjective band—that it was lighter than the background or the white space enclosed by the curved parts of the letters, and that it seemed to be in front of the letter segments, which seem like ground and have a sense of completion behind the white band. He also pointed out that an analytical attitude would lead to letter fragments not being seen and there would be no perception of the illusory band. Hartmann (1935, Fig. 21, p. 121) reproduced the Matthaei display and also gave a quite cogent description of the illusory contour. Interesting examples of illusory squares and circles were produced also by Koffka (1935, Fig. 20, p.145, see Fig. 5.2) and Ehrenstein (1941; see chap. 3). Koffka related his figure to the filling-in process found in the blind spot and the need to consider internal organizational events when examining the psychophysical field.

While the phenomena of illusory contours were known to the psychological community and even presented in texts (Gibson, 1950; Hartmann, 1935; Osgood, 1953; Woodworth, 1938) our ghostly squares, circles, and triangles languished in obscurity, perhaps trapped in the miasma of the Behaviorist paradigm which so slowed the progress of perceptual theory in the United States. They were perhaps a victim of the decline of the Gestaltists. However, this situation was to change. In 1955 the Gestalt psychologist Gaetano Kanizsa (see chap. 4) published what was to become one of the most widely referenced articles on illusory contours. While there was earlier work, this one was seminal as it contained a quite complete description of illusory contours and stunning examples with a compelling artistic and aesthetic quality that

went far beyond the early displays. Kanizsa emphasized the enhancement of brightness, sharp apparent edge, and finally, the depth segregation effects in his figures, which were also related to phenomena of motion-induced contours and transparency effects. This work was brought to the forefront of the perceptual community's attention by Coren's (1972) and Gregory's (1972) theoretical articles and Kanizsa's (1976) *Scientific American* article, which is much more than a popularization. With this start the game was afoot and there was a massive explosion of interest and literature. However, little did we know that the game was to be PACMAN.

Definitions

What determines the label to be used for our topic of discussion? Should illusory contour or subjective contour be used? There are many different versions of such displays in the literature and it seems reasonable to have some common label and a set of defining characteristics. First, we will examine some terminology, then we will look for commonalities among the display types.

Many terms have been suggested, and the choice of terms sometimes implies a theoretical bias. As pointed out above, Schumann (1900) brought the phenomena to the attention of the perceptual community. He referred to them as *Scheinkanten,* which may be translated as "false or illusory contours," but this German phrase did not have the staying power of terms like *ganzfeld* or *prägnanz.* Certainly the later works did not use it. However, he did note that the contours were not "objectively present." Other effects such as those discovered by Prandtl (1927), Ehrenstein (1941) and Koffka (1935) are usually referred to by their discoverers' names.

In the current wave of literature we find many different names. As Kanizsa was the key figure in the modern literature, his terminology is of importance. In his early work (1955a, 1955b) he used *quasi-perceptive contours* but abandoned this for the more common usage of *subjective contours* (1976, 1979). This term was made popular by Coren's (1972) important review and is found in use as early as 1938 in Woodworth's description of Schumann's pattern, which he labeled as subjective contour (Woodworth, 1938, Fig. 191, p. 637) and described as "figures . . . in which a contour is subjectively completed" (Woodworth, p. 636). Woodworth also suggested the term *tied image,* but this has not been found in common usage. Osgood (1953) also used *subjective contour* but seems not to be the term's progenitor as some have suggested.

While *subjective contour* seems a winner, there are other major alternatives. Kanizsa (1979) prefers the term *anomalous contours and surfaces,* which was suggested by Lawon and Gulick (1967), or alternatively *contours without gradients.* Kanizsa finds these terms preferable since the contours occur in the absence of the normal conditions for contour perception, cannot be explained by the usual models of visual perception, and the terms are theoretically neutral. While the terminology seems reasonable, some of our theorists might object to the rationale. Quite a few might regard the illusory contour phenomena as being a normal part of vision. Similarly, the use of *cognitive contour* as proposed by Gregory (1972) is too theoretically loaded for most. *Virtual contour* has been used by Goldstein and Weintraub (1972). The term seems neutral although Kanizsa regards virtual lines as not having a visible presence. Similarly, Tynan and Sekuler's (1975) use of *phantom contours* seems to be restricted to their movement-based effect. Ghostly contours or spectral triangles seem not to have been suggested.

The term we are using for this book is *illusory contour,* although we find our authors using most of the possible terms and we might also slip. It is a most common usage and seems to pass the neutrality test. Kennedy (chap. 28) might object, as he feels illusions convey a sense of reality even though it is distorted. One can easily tell you that some configurations contain lines which are not real. A more serious issue is what determines when one has an illusory contour and is the use of the term *contour* adequate?

Defining Characteristics

Many authors have attempted to describe the phenomena (as seen in this volume and the reviews which are referenced). It seems to us that there are three major determinants of the presence of the illusion. They are described below.

1. There is the sense of a bounded surface which has some property which differentiates it from an abutting or surrounding surface. At the conference, it was suggested that the term *illusory surfaces* might be more descriptive than *illusory contours* (Petry & Meyer, 1986). The surface quality is most typically one of brightness enhancement. However, changes of hue, texture, and depth have been produced. The sense of surface is most important as it eliminates other phenomena from consideration, such as the Hermann (1870) grid's little spots, Motokawa grids, Mach bands, or Springer lines (see Lindsay & Norman, 1977). The phenomena we are discussing are not linelike or pointlike but have noticeable extent. Some might disagree with this distinction, but the line must be drawn somewhere, although the boundary we have chosen may in itself be illusory.

2. There is a sense of a boundary or edge around this surface. The edge may be sharp or diffuse but we are not looking at a spread of a surface quality of undetermined extent. Inducing a nonveridical brightness or hue change in a ganzfeld would not qualify, nor would similar phenomena found with afterimages or stabilized images. Thus the brightness spread of the Craik–O'Brian–Cornsweet illusion or its analogs with hue and stereopsis (see Uttal, 1981 for review) would not qualify. We find that the older literature emphasized the illusory brightness changes in the early examples of illusory contours (Woodworth, 1938; Hartmann, 1935). We must thank Kanizsa for emphasizing the property of contour induction, which is so important to modern theory. A new approach to this issue is found in Chapter 5 by Day.

3. A crucial property is that the edge and surface connect or continue through discontinuities of the inducing patterns. This eliminates from consideration the typical brightness contrast demonstration where one area is completely surrounded by another and the surround induces a surface change. There are no edges or contours added in this situation. In the Kanizsa triangle, contours based on edge-stopping, motion-induced contours, or sparse random dot stereograms, we find edges that connect the in-

ducing elements and bound the illusory surface in areas where there are no physical changes in the display.

At this point, one might puzzle at our not mentioning the necessity of there being a depth stratification, sense of interposition, or amodal completion in the display. These certainly occur in many of the illusory contours. However, there is some controversy as to their being necessary. Examples exist where contours and abutting surfaces can be seen but the sense of overlay is weak (see Day & Kasperczk, 1983a, 1983b; Kennedy, 1978a, 1978b) or the surface that is produced would be physically impossible if based on an overlay or depth interpretation (see Gerbino & Kanizsa, chap. 27). In textural displays, there are contours and surfaces but not the necessity of depth stratification (Julesz, 1980, 1981a & b; Treisman and Gelade, 1980). Thus we did not include depth stratification as a necessary part of the definitional properties.

This is not to deny, however, that occlusion or amodal completion has a role. Discussion of this role may be seen in the chapters by Gillam (30), Gregory (9), Kellman and Loukides (16), Minguzzi (7), and Rock (6).

It is also quite important not to make the naive assumption that all the properties mentioned in our definition are perfectly correlated. Petry, Harbeck, Conway, and Levey (1983) have convincingly demonstrated the need for separating these factors and making a careful examination of their interactions.

The Common Types of Illusory Contours

When examining the literature one finds many different examples of illusory contours which we hope will fit under our definition. We would like to describe some of the basic configurations now in order to establish a background for the chapters in this book. It is not our purpose to be encyclopedic and list every study done with a particular technique or describe every possible variant. We hope to map out the major configurations and point to reasonable examples of these in the literature. Also, we will point out configurations which are combinations of basic types.

The Kanizsa Triangle or Pacman Configurations

One of the most compelling illusory triangle configurations is that of the Kanizsa triangle, where three pacmen (now the common usage among the cognoscenti for inducing elements—and much more piquant a term than "sectored inducing disc-like elements") produced a clear illusory triangle (Fig. 1.1). The phenomenon is not confined to triangles but can be made to yield squares, curves, and other shapes. The defining characteristic is that a solid element (a circle or other element) seems overlain by a part of a shape. Ullman (1976) has presented an interesting model of this curve-fitting process. These types of contours produce a clear depth segregation for most people. While the common configuration is that of an object in front of the inducing elements, they can be arranged such that the elements produce the illusion of a hole in the page (Kanizsa, 1979) or such that the inducing elements take on the aspect of the holes in a slice of Swiss cheese. This latter illusion has some import as to the role of depth segregation in the illusory contour (Bradley & Petry, 1977; Meyer & Dougherty, 1987; Pradzny, 1985; Ramachandran, 1985, chap. 10). Also of importance is the shape of the inducing elements. While circles and squares are most common, some shapes (Geneva crosses, spiked elements) have varying degrees of inducing power, which is quite important to many theories (Coren, Porac, & Theodor, chap. 26).

The other characteristics of the inducing pacmen (hue, texture, depth, temporal modulation) are discussed in later sections. However, one interesting variant occurs when the polarity of the contrast of the inducing elements is altered. The typical Kanizsa figure has black elements on white or vice versa. Some researchers have presented figures composed of both white and black pacmen on middle grey backgrounds and analyzed the results in terms of the implications for brightness contrast models of illusory contours (see Shapley and Gordon, chap. 11). Also important are the effects of luminance (Bradley & Dumais, 1984; Dumais & Bradley, 1976; Parks & Marks, 1985; Warm, Dember, Padich, Beckner, & Jones, chap. 19).

Shadow Writing

Shadow writing may be an interesting version of the Kanizsa configuration where illusory letters overlap their own hypothetical shadow or other shaded sides. Such type fonts can be found in standard art and graphics references (Solo, 1982). Some are illustrated in Figure 1.2.

These fonts seem to have first appeared in the 1700s in France, went out of fashion in the nineteenth century, but had a modern revival in the 1910s–1920s in France and Germany (Berry, Johnson, & Jaspert, 1962). Many different illusory contour type faces were developed in the 1930s. They seem almost to be a natural extension of dropped shadow or shaded lettering, where the shadow is used to convey a strong sense of raised lettering and then the letter is eliminated leaving only the shadow. However, the letter is still seen. One wonders if the designers of those times appreciated the illusion or if it seemed natural to them (Kennedy, chap. 28). Who knows what letters lurk in the minds of men—the Shadows know! Although they are presented in reviews of the illusory contour literature, not much research has been done on these interesting figures, although it has been noted that inverting the letters will weaken the illusion (Coren, 1972). One might predict a re-

surgence of interest as shadowing is a crucial part of computer graphics display techniques and is regarded as an important part of scene segregation in the machine vision community.

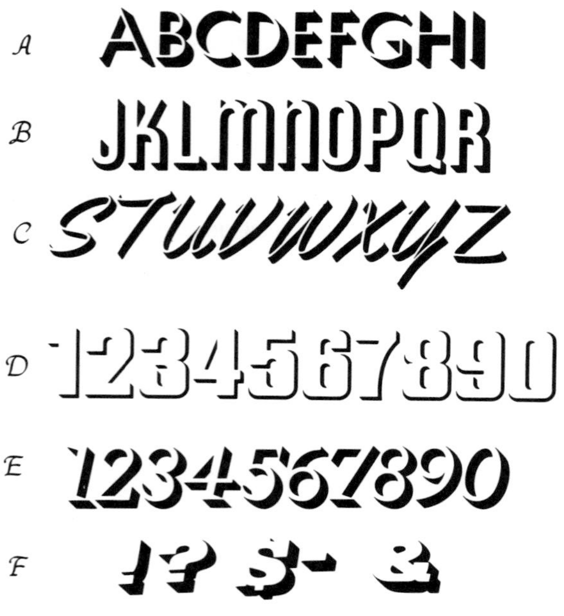

Edge-Stopping Illusory Contours

So far we have discussed configurations where the inducing elements have been solid figures. Another set of equally strong contours can be generated using inducing elements composed of line segments. These contours are important theoretically as they address the role of inducing area and brightness contrast. One would expect from the literature (Uttal, 1981) that larger inducing areas would produce stronger illusory contours if the phenomenon is similar to standard brightness contrast (note that brightness contrast itself is not so simply related to area, e.g., the Benary cross—Kanizsa, 1979). Since line-based illusory contours are quite powerful, this must be explained by a theory to be acceptable. There are three basic configurations using these elements. The first configuration is arranged such that the elements are similar to the Kanizsa solid element configuration. The solid pacman is replaced by a series of concentric circles (or concentric whatever the element is) with a corner, sector, or wedge of curved element removed. For an example see Figure 5.6a.

This produces a contour which has an appearance of overlay and is phenomenologically similar to the original Kanizsa figure. The pacmen can also be composed of an area of dense dots with a sector removed (Frisby & Clatworthy, 1975; Kennedy & Ware, 1978). The similarity of the edge-stopped versions to be solid paceman types is under some study and debate (Halpern, 1981; Warm et al., chap. 19).

The second edge-based variant also has the appearance of overlay. An interrupted set of radiating or even random (Gillam, chap. 30) lines gives rise to the appearance of an occluding surface over the line set. This is an important configuration historically as the Ehrenstein and Koffka (1935) illusions belong to this class. This configuration is used by Kennedy (1976a, 1976b, 1978a, 1978b) to produce contours with diffuse edges. It is also possible to pull sharp edges into curves with appropriate spacing of the elements (Day & Jory, 1980; Day, chap. 5). The strength of the resultant illusory contour is

FIGURE 1.2. A variety of illusory contour type fonts (from Solo, 1982; with permission).

dependent on the configuration, density, spacing, and thickness of these elements as well as their effective contrast and the angle of the inducing element relative to the tangent of the illusory contour at that point (deviations from 90° weaken the contour). The appearance of the illusory contour is quite powerfully determined by these factors (Petry et al., 1983; Spillman, Fuld, & Gerrits, 1976; Sambin, chap. 14).

A third variant of illusory contours induced by lines consists of displays in which line segments abut in a manner similar to that used when testing vernier acuity (Jory, chap. 20). This generates a sharp curved or straight edge between the misaligned line segments and there may be a sense of two adjoining surfaces. However, the role of depth stratification in such displays is of theoretical interest: Is it a necessary part of the effect or a by-product of the process of edge production (see Day & Kasperczyk, 1983a, 1983b)?

Finally, in the domain of spatial Fourier analysis, illusory contours can be generated by changes in any three of the following fundamental sine wave grating parameters: phase, orientation, and spatial frequency as shown in the square wave heads of Figure 1.3.

It is also possible to create contours in which the inducing lines are not broken, but rather bent or curved (see Wade, chap. 31). These latter contours are of some importance to the analysis of texture gradients seen in the work of the Gibsonians (Gibson, 1950).

Interestingly, Ware and Kennedy (1978) have constructed three-dimensional versions of these configurations and produced illusory volumes perceived to lie in between the rods and boards of the inducing sculpture. There is no report to our knowledge of any other solid versions of illusory contours in the literature.

The configurations mentioned above have been historically the most popular of the illusory contours. The remaining types are variants or combinations of these configurations. They are growing in popularity and many offer new insights into illusory contour theory.

Illusory Contours Based on Hue, Assimilation of Brightness, and Transparency

In the illusory contours described above the inducing elements are usually achromatic. They consist of black and white elements. If the elements have some color to them (as the phosphors on a display), the chroma is of no importance to the situation. The illusory surface that is formed is typically black or white, the opposite of the inducing elements but the same as the background except for the brightness enhancement effect, such as the blacker than black or whiter than white Kanizsa triangle.

There are, however, illusory contours that produce, as Parks (1984) describes it, an impression of filled extent. There is a film of transparent or translucent gray or of some color that starts at the inducing elements and spreads through the illusory contour area. The illusion is usually generated by filling in the empty area of a typical illusory contour-inducing element

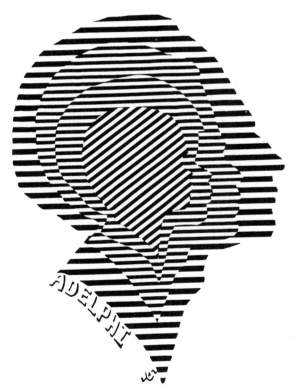

FIGURE 1.3. Illusory contour heads. This figure, used as the logo for the Illusory Contour Conference, is composed of four overlapping square wave silhouettes that vary in orientation, phase, and fundamental spatial frequency. These parameters (plus contrast or amplitude) completely specify a stimulus (in a Fourier analysis framework), and any parameter alone is sufficient to generate an illusory contour.

with a chroma or value. This leads to the perceived extention of that chroma or value across the illusory surface. However, the spread of complementary colors is possible (DeWeert & vanKruysbergen, chap. 17; Gerbino and Kanizsa, chap. 27), and the necessary conditions to determine the nature of illusory filling have not been fully determined. Examples of achromatic translucent illusory surfaces can be found in Kanizsa, 1976, 1979, and in Figure 5.6c.

Chromatic versions can be seen in Varin (1971), Ware (1980), and Meyer and Senecal (1983). A particularly strong version of this effect is referred to as the neon illusion, where a latticework of lines can take on the aspect of an impressive color film (Van Tuijl, 1975). Redies and Spillman (1981a, 1981b) and Redies, Spillman, and Kunz (1984) have demonstrated these phenomena with the Ehrenstein and Prandtl configurations. Edge-stopped variants are also possible (Gerbino & Kanizsa, chap. 27). The effects are sometimes related to transparency theory (DeWeert & vanKruysbergen, chap. 17; Maguire & Brown, chap. 23), physiological mechanisms (Grossberg & Mingolla, 1985a, 1985b; chap. 12; Redies et al., 1984), structural information measures (Van Tuijl & Leeuwenberg, 1979), assimilation (Ware, 1980), or direct modes of perception (Gerbino & Kanizsa, chap. 27).

There are several other points of interest. First, the impression of an area of noticeable hue would rule out illusory contours as being the result of a strictly scotopic process. Second, isoluminant patterns in which the inducing elements and background differ only in chroma have not produced strong contours (e.g., Frisby, 1980; Gregory, 1977). Last, these color effects are sometimes classified as different from the usual subjective contour as the illusion is one of color or brightness assimilation (Ware, 1980) rather than one of contrast. This may be an inappropriate distinction. While the typical Kanizsa configuration seems to be the result of contrast induction, it could be related to assimilation in which the contrast-induced brightness or hue in the mouth of the pacman spreads by assimilation across the whole region. Crucial to this would be the perception that the pacman is a circle overlayed by a corner of a triangle.

Stereopsis and the Illusory Contour

Stereopsis is phenomenologically fascinating and a major problem for any theory of vision (Marr, 1982). It can be related to illusory contours in several respects. The question first is a definitional issue: Does the contour produced in a random dot sterogram meet our criteria for being considered a subjective contour? We feel the answer must be yes. If you think of the classic random dot stereogram (Julesz, 1971), there is a densely packed region of elements seen to be clearly in front or in back of the plane of the screen or book page. There really are not any gaps in the stereoscopic-induced edge. This seems a violation of our third criterion. However, this problem is easily remedied. Julesz (1971) and Frisby (1980) present very sparse random dot stereograms where a set of dots cover only a small percentage of a surface. When the dots seem to rise off the page, they also seem to pull that surface up off the page and produce a boundary to that surface that continues through areas of nonexistent physical gradients. Thus stereoscopically induced depth of random dot elements will enable these scattered dots to act as an inducing set of elements and produce an illusory contour.

The second question concerns the role of stereopsis in the formation of other kinds of illusory contours. Using Kanizsa type displays some researchers (Gregory & Harris, 1974; Harris & Gregory, 1973; Lawson, Cowan, Gibbs, & Whitmore, 1974; Whitmore, Lawson, & Kozora, 1976) found that stereoscopically induced depth of the inducing elements or the illusion itself can affect an illusory contour depending on whether or not the direction of depth is in agreement with the stratification "implied" by illusory contour. Hamsher (1978) found a relationship between local and global stereopsis and Kanizsa figure perception and suggests all these processes share spatial localization processes. Prazdny (1985) reported transparent "glass sheet" subjective surfaces were possible if congruent with stereoscopically induced depth. Similarly, Gellatly (1982) demonstrated that a colored subjective cross was made visible when depth stratification was added by stereopsis. Also, the "Swiss cheese" appearance has been reported with stereoscopic Kanizsa figures (Pradzny, 1985). Interestingly, Smith (1984) found that a subject with visual agnosia who was unable to see interposition cues in two-dimensional displays could not see illusory contours unless stereoscopic cues were also provided. Whether producing pacmen with random dot stereograms alone will produce illusory contours is under debate (Mustillo & Fox, 1986; Prazdny, 1985).

Motion-Induced Illusory Contours

One possible factor in the induction of illusory contours can be the motion of the display elements. There are several well-defined movement-based illusory contours. However, there is some debate as to the uniqueness of the motion cue: Is motion just a supplementary form of information to the contour-inducing process such that movement-induced illusory contours are a subset of the general phenomenon, or are they in some way unique?

It has been found that standard subjective contour configurations can be used to create apparent motion. Thus the illusory figure seems to leap between the contour-inducing elements (Ramachandran & Anstis 1983; Ramachandran, chap. 10; Von Grunau, 1979). Interestingly, Ramachandran reports that the moving illusory surface will carry with it the surface texture of the background. Moreover, rotary apparent motion of pacman figures or radiating lines can greatly enhance stationary illusory contour strength (Petry & Gannon, chap. 21; see also Kellman & Loukides, chap. 16).

In the above demonstrations, there was an illusory contour visible even in stationary displays. However, it is possible to produce illusory contours which are made visible only when the figure is in motion. There seem to be four major demonstrations that claim this.

First, if a pattern of dots or other elements is moved such that the pattern seems to pass under an edge, there is a clear sense of a contour at the border. This kinetic optical occlusion (Andersen & Braunstein, 1983; Kellman & Loukides, chap. 16) can be very powerful. Without motion the dots give no sense of contour. Random dots are also used in kinematograms (Julesz, 1971), in which a correlated area of dots is seen to leap around against a background of dots. As in our discussion of stereopsis, this bounded area would seem to qualify as an illusory contour, and in this case the motion is the sole inducer as disparity previously was. Another interesting percept can be created by flickering a section of a uniform texture of dots (Wong & Weisstein, 1983). In this case the flickered region becomes background and the nonflickering region becomes foreground. These bounded regions seem to meet our three criteria and might be justifiably called illusory contours and surfaces. Their relation to other illusory contours is just being analyzed (Meyer & Dougherty, in press).

Motion also defines contour in a second situation. Kellman and Cohen (1984) presented a stimulus in which the contours of the illusory triangle are seen as rotating in front of inducing circles. At any one time, not all three of the apices of the triangle were present. However, the illusory triangle was seen as complete. This meant that one apex had to persist in an area where there was no stationary cue for that apex. Similar studies by Bradley and Lee (1982) and Bradley (chap. 22) found an illusory triangle to persist when the rotating configuration did not contain any physical cues for the apices of the illusory triangle. Illusory contour inducement seems dependent on an analysis of motion.

A third example is the motion-induced contour. Klymenko and Weisstein (1981, 1983; chap. 15) report that moving chervons that are perceived as the top and bottom surfaces of a cube will cause the appearance of an illusory edge joining the corners of the two surfaces. This contour was considered to be separate from the ordinary type of subjective contour and only visible with the appropriate kind of movement. Interestingly, a similar phenomenon was reported by Purdy (1936) and illustrated by Osgood (1953). Purdy's illusory edge also seems to be visible only with certain types of movement. However, Klymenko and Weisstein's pattern uses only two angles to define the upper and lower surfaces of the rotating cube. As stationary chervon patterns with many elements do produce strong illusory edges, it may be the case that in the reduced situation, motion is only enhancing rather than producing the edge.

The fourth motion-based illusory contour is referred to as the visual phantom. Tynan and Sekuler (1975) found that "fields of gratings flanking and moving parallel to a central spatially homogeneous region induce the perception of phantom gratings moving through the central region" (Mulvanny, Macarthur, & Sekuler, 1982, p. 35). Mulvanny et al. also cite an earlier report of a similar effect by Rosenbach (1902). Since similar spread of pattern is sometimes seen in stationary patterns, motion may act only as an enhancer. Maguire and Brown (chap. 23) discuss this and the relation of phantoms to other illusory contours.

Texture-Based Illusory Contours

Apparent textural qualities of a surface can be manipulated by illusory contour inducers, producing apparent magnification or change (Kanizsa, 1979; Kennedy & Lee, 1976; Parks, 1986). However, differences in textural qualities can also be used to induce the perception of a border or a surface. Recently, there has also been a resurgence of interest in texture segregation as this task has been related to preattentive visual processing, statistical properties of the patterns, and physiological mechanisms (Julesz, 1980, 1981a, 1981b; Julesz & Bergen, 1983; Treisman & Gelade, 1980). The basic task is to determine whether some elements in a stimulus array stand out easily (or without the need for focal attention) from the rest of the stimulus or whether the element difference can be seen only with close scrutiny (see Figs. 10.16 and 25.4). In texture segregation displays one can have the impression of a bounded area and see an edge surrounding the textured patch. Thus, these displays seem to qualify as illusory contours (for further discussion see Meyer & Fish, chap. 25). However, unlike traditional illusory contours, texture segregation has been characterized as being fast, preattentive, and not drawing on capacity pools (Julesz & Bergen, 1983; Treisman & Gelade, 1980). This may not be the case for subjective contours, and the situation also may be more complicated than originally thought for textures (Enns, 1986). There are also cases where the texture displays contain standard illusory contours

which define the edges of the texture (Beck, 1983; Nothdurft, 1985). Here, it is important to note that these illusory surfaces do not necessarily produce a sense of depth segregation or overlay.

Reversible Illusory Contours

The last illusory contour we present is not produced by new methods of induction. However, it is theoretically an interesting variant. All psychologists with normal vision have experienced the Necker cube, and Escher's drawings and woodcuts are now quite popular. Similar perceptual instability can be found in the world of illusory contours. The issue is of importance as ambiguous figures may imply the role of higher order processing in perception as subjects seem to have the ability to initiate organizational changes by volition.

Ambiguous Kanizsa figures have been designed by Bradley and Dumais (1975) and Scrivener (1983). In these, superimposed spokes, wheels, and Kanizsa triangles come and go and merge into complex figures such as six-pointed stars (see Bradley, chap. 22, Figs. 22.4b and 22.6). A most impressive demonstration is found in Bradley and Petry's (1977) illusory version of the Necker cube (chap. 22, Fig. 22.8), which demonstrates that illusory contours can generate ambiguous objects and is a prime example of the ambiguous configuration now starting to be known as the Swiss cheese effect. New reversible illusory figures are presented by Sambin (chap. 14).

Reversible figures are also possible with line- and edge-based stimuli. One common configuration is that of concentric squares (see Fig. 1.4a). It reverses organizations between wedges of vertical and horizontal gratings with an illusory boundary between them and concentric squares where the segmentation into separate surfaces and the boundary is lost (see Jenkins & Ross, 1977; Wade, 1978). Similarly, edge-stopped stimuli can be used to construct versions of the Rubin faces/vase figure where one can see the alternation of the figure-ground with the areas being outlined in illusory contours (see Wade, chap. 31). Meyer and Phillips (1980) combine both effects and produce an illusory Rubin (1921) vase/faces figure that alternates between concentric squares, faces and vases

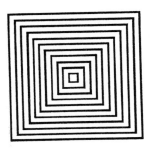

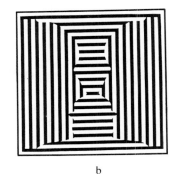

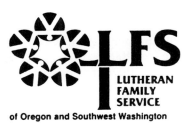

a   b   c

FIGURE 1.4. A variety of reversible illusory contours. a. A set of concentric squares which can be seen as wedges with strong illusory borders or as squares with the disappearance of the edges. b. Rubin face/vase from Meyer and Phillips (1980). It alternates between a vase, two faces, and concentric squares. In the latter case, the illusory curves disappear. c. The logo of the Lutheran Family Service of Oregon and Southwest Washington. First, it demonstrates the appeal of the illusory contour in graphic design. Second, it has several reversible illusory contour interpretations. One can see an illusory pentagon. One can see the human figures, losing the pentagon, but causing the unfilled segments of the circles to complete. One can see the black-filled pentagon as figures, in which case, there is the impression of a thin black edge crossing the necks of the human figures' heads. Also, there is a thin white line running across their bodies at armpit level.

(see Fig. 1.4b). A most impressive illusory contour logo which is also reversible again demonstrates the appeal of the illusory contour (see Fig. 1.4c).

Texture-based versions of reversible figures are also possible (Julesz, 1971, Fig. 2.8-2 for a Rubin face/vase) as are ambiguous random dot stereograms (Julesz, 1971; Kontsevich, 1986).

Illusory Contours, Art, and Graphic Design

As seen in the work referenced above, illusory contours can be perceptually very compelling. It would be surprising if they were unique to the field of perception. For example, one of us (Meyer) has seen the Neon illusion lurking as a chromatic mist in the logo stamped on the strings of his daughter's tennis racket. One obvious use of illusory contours derives from their ability to enhance brightness without physical gradient. This seems a perfect technique for so many artistic problems, as Halpern (chap. 18) points out. She has found such enhancements used in the letters of illuminated manuscripts and prayer books 900 years old and in an edition of the *Canterbury Tales* from the 1500s.

We have found illustrative examples from the same period. Illusory suns, moons, and halos can be seen in Medieval and Renaissance woodcuts (Jacobi, 1951). An illusory sun similar to the Ehrenstein illusion shines over the scene in a 2-ducat gold coin minted in 1682, celebrating the 1100th aniversary of the Salzburg Archbishopric on the Austro-Bavarian frontier (Krause & Mishler, 1986, p.55). The same type of sun or radiant halos based on edge-stopping can be found later in the 1825–1837 gold coins of the Central American Republic and more recently on a 1972 Brazilian 300-cruzeiros piece (Krause & Mishler, p. 84) or on the reverse of the American $20 Liberty gold piece (p. 603). Kennedy's diffuse sun which has been of much theoretical importance shines over a building on the reverse of a 1971 Malaysian Ringgit coin (p. 423). Of course, this list is not comprehensive. It would seem that when working with monochromatic media such as the metal of coin or a black-and-white woodcut, subtleties of lighting may easily be portrayed by illusory contours, and art preceded the science of perception.

Many of the illusory contour types can also be found in Japanese art (Neuer, Liberston, & Yoshida, 1981). In Japanese woodcut production techniques (ukiyo-e), dating from the 1600s, and in the artwork's deliberate use of empty space to create an illusion of filled space, illusory contours seem almost necessary to their artistic paradigm. Neuer et al. (pp. 50–51) present a fascinating demonstration of how one polychromatic print was assembled from separate woodblock prints, each in a separate color. Each of the different prints glows with illusory contours as the areas of the picture not in that color are now suggested by illusory components. It seems that the artisans must have had an appreciation of the nature of such contours as they prepared their woodcuts.

In the finished art, we find many examples of what seem to us the classic illusory contours. Edge-stopping illusions define the hair of men and women and the feathers of birds in innumerable prints. Ehrenstein (chap. 3) and Kennedy (chap. 29) figures become cherry blossoms and chrysanthemums (pp. 84, 176, 181). Kanizsa's (1979, Fig. 12.14, p. 206) figure of an illusory chain is found as the design of a short kimono in a print of two actors from 1794 (p. 249). A 1796 portrait (Kanizsa, 1929, p. 138) of a female impersonator (males played females in the Japanese theater) has the sleeves of the black kimono suggested by the apparent overlay found in so many of Kanizsa's figures (p. 178, Fig. 10.10). Since the artists could not use continuous variations in pigments because of the limitations of woodcuts, their choices would be to outline (often done) or use illusory contours. Similarly, transparency-based illusory contours were used to generate the perception of overlap and filled extent (Neuer et al., p. 279).

Illusory contours have some aesthetic appeal in more recent times. We see this in the development of many subjective type fonts. Contours leap at us from trucks and industrial logos. United Technologies uses a modified Ehrenstein illusion as a logo; the logo on Adelphi's printer (Primage, Inc.) consists of an edge-stopped "globe" counterphase with its background. We have seen subjective panda bears in advertisements for our children's toys and on sweaters that our students wear to perception class. The local ambulance company uses a subjective Geneva cross on its vehicle, and a furniture mover uses subjective contour wheels. We have even seen a four-element Ehrenstein figure resembling a Coptic cross used in a newspaper advertisement offering to bring one closer to God with the caption "Do you see the light?" This appeal is well docu-

mented in the work of one of our contributors (Wade, chap. 31). Similarly, an examination of work in computer graphics finds many of our illusions dancing across CRTs in both commercial graphics and artistic presentations. At the 1985 meeting of the National Computer Graphics Association, there were edges based on kinetic occlusion in several displays, Klymenko and Weisstein's corner floated through an Evans and Sunderland demonstration, and a transparent subjective contour defined an illusory dancer who pranced around Mick Jagger in a music video.

If one looks at television, one can see Max Headroom in front of a corner that could be from Day and Kasperczyk (1983a, 1983b). Schumann's figure composes the label of Wakaebisu brand sake (Kondo, 1984, p. 87). In a somewhat eerie coincidence, Kondo describes this brand of beverage as "superficially simple but mysteriously subtle." What better way to describe both pleasurable stimuli!

Some artwork is clearly created by individuals with extensive background knowledge of perception and perceptual principles and offers insight to the visual scientist. A discussion of the pictorial and representational nature of illusory contours can be found in Parks (chap. 8). These principles are very important in the work of Albers (for example, in his 1975 revised edition of his earlier 1963 work). Conversely, his analysis of transparency and color are of major importance to illusory contour design and theory. Albers (1975, plate XIII-1) presents a clear subjective contour, comments on its enhanced lightness, and relates it to assimilation of brightness and the work of Bezold in the 1870s. At the time, Albers stated (p. 33) that "there is so far no clear recognition of the optical-perceptual conditions involved."

In any case, an excellent review of the interaction of modern visual science and art is found in Vitz and Glimcher (1984). In their work, for example (Figs. 7.13–7.14, p. 202), they point to the work of Vasarely, where illusory contours of many types form a central emphasis of his art. Vitz and Glimcher make several important points which are relevant to both art and theories of perception. Modern art stressed reductionist principles, as the purity and simplicity underlying form was trying to be expressed. The reductionist view was clearly influenced by the same trend in science. This reductionist tendency in viewing form may in part constitute the appeal of illusory contours as we try to find the minimal stimulus which will create an elegance of form, where the object springs forth in perceptual clarity from a hint in the stimulus. A brief discussion of the philosophy underlying this point may be found in Petry and Gannon (chap. 21). In this sense we are taking more of the reductionist view of the Gestalt psychologists, whose powerful principles of organization were the primitives of perception (see Hatfield & Epstein, 1985). As Arnheim (1986, p.821) points out, the Gestaltists felt their demonstrations contained the pure embodiment of essence as well as clarity, simplicity, and integrity. *Pragnant* did not just mean simplification but "distinguished, most perfect structural states" (p. 823).

Thus, it is natural to conclude that illusory contours are not the exclusive property of perceptual psychologists. Most convincing of this to us was the finding of clear examples of edge-stopped illusory contours, defining the bodies of bison in Paleolithic cave drawings between 10,000 and 30,000 years old (Leroi-Gourhan, 1967). As these representations were not unsophisticated in some cases, the sense and appeal of the illusory contour seems universal.

Theories of Illusory Contours

As many of our authors will have much to say about the various theories of illusory contours, it would be redundant for us to present an extensive literature review of this area. Rather, our goal will be to illustrate the major positions in the field, to look at their differences and at current attempts to combine disparate ideas.

A reasonable approach to this endeavor is suggested by Uttal's (1981) analysis of the role of macrotheories in perception and Bourassa's (1986) review of the history of models of sensation and perception. Basically, macrotheoretical approaches spell out a global way that perceptual processes occur (Uttal, 1981). As we will see, many of the macrotheoretical approaches have been applied to illusory contours (unless they officially are uninterested in illusions), such that the debates that rage over this stimulus type contain a microcosm of the major issues in perception.

Uttal (1981) suggests that perceptual theories can be characterized by how they stand on three major axes. These axes can be characterized by three major questions:

1. Is perception mainly innate or learned?
2. Is perception direct or mediated by inferential processes?
3. Is the overall configuration the main influence in perception or are the individual stimulus parts more important to the resulting percept?

The following discussion of theories will focus on these issues.

Bottom-Up Theories Based on Neuroreductionism

One major view characterizes illusory contours as an easily explainable by-product of our visual neurophysiology. This may be referred to as the neurophysiological-reductionistic approach. Another popular term is *bottom-up* theories. Within this position, we find several variants at the microtheoretical level. Thus, in a single-cell type theory a line detector in the cortex is deceived by the pacman alignments or arrangement of stopped edges, etc., producing the illusory contour. This theory is supported by demonstrations both of stimulus contingent aftereffects with illusory contour stimuli (Smith & Over, 1975, 1976, 1979) and of the oblique effect (Vogels & Orban, 1985). However, this position is regarded by most as too simplistic. Curved subjective contours are easily seen but single-cell detection of curvature does not seem to be the strategy of the cortex (Ullman, 1976). Other models based on straightforward applications of simultaneous contrast have been attempted but contrast alone is not much in favor today. However, an interesting approach to the interactions of such factors is found in Jory (chap. 20).

Currently popular neurally based theories are much more sophisticated and use spatial filtering approaches (Ginsburg, chap. 13) or intricate nets of neural functioning, such as the work of Grossberg and Mingolla (chap. 12), Shapley and Gordon (chap. 11), and the hypercomplex based cell theories of Redies and Spillman (Redies & Spillman, 1981; Redies, Spillman, &

Kunz, 1984). Also, some of the newer models are much more interactive, including higher level processes (Ginsburg, chap. 13; Grossberg & Mingolla, chap. 12). This makes some of them more difficult to pigeonhole. Moreover, higher level theorists reach down into neural substrates more, as the neuronal modeling is now so much more sophisticated than it once was.

Direct tests of neuronal responses to illusory contours have just started to appear. Issues which must be considered in evaluating this kind of work are: type of stimulus, animal used, cell classification, and site in the visual system being tested (Teller, 1984). Various models use different cell responses. Finally, theorizing in the past seemed restricted to properties of striate cortex which were most well explored by neurophysiologists. Given the plethora of visual areas with different properties (Van Essen, 1979), this is dangerous habit. Also to be avoided is a tendency to look at the visual system in a linear manner (see Shapley & Gordon, chap. 11, for a discussion). Feedback loops between the areas are extensive (Van Essen, 1979), and to deal with one in isolation seems inadequate.

Direct recording has had some recent impact on the field. The most influential study is that of von der Heydt, Peterhans, and Baumgartner (1984). Primate cells in area 18 were found to be responsive to a Kanizsa type illusory bar. Area 17 cells did not respond. However cell type was not differentiated. Similarly, Gregory (1985; chap. 9) reports that he and his co-workers did not find responses to illusory contour stimuli from units in cat area 17. However, Redies, Crook, and Creutzfeldt (1986) tested in lateral geniculate nucleus, striate cortex, and area 18 of cat and found that C cells in 17 and 18 would respond to a phase shift (edge-stopped) illusory border. Other illusory contour types have been tried. In cat, Hammond and MacKay (1977) found striate complex cells did respond to texture differences. However, Nothdurft and Li (1985) report cat striate cells of various types respond to luminance differences at texture borders but such cells failed to encode the illusory contour boundaries contained in their stimuli. They feel their data are in accord with von der Heydt et al. (1984). Also tested have been random dot stereograms by Poggio, Mot-

ter, Squatrito, and Trotter (1985). Nearly all the complex cells in V1 and V2 in monkey were responsive.

Although there are obviously few data from humans, there are reports that brain damage can lead to an overproduction of illusory edges (Purdy, 1936) or a lack of their appreciation (Smith, 1983). Visual evoked potentials to Kanizsa triangles (Brandeis, Lehmann, & Mueller, 1985) and textures (Victor, 1985) have been reported. Wasserstein, Zappulla, Rosen and Gerstman (1987) & Hamsher (1978) have suggested there is right-hemisphere involvement in illusory contour perception. However, such reports can only be suggestive. Thus, there is some controversy as to cortical responsiveness to illusory figures.

Top-Down or Cognitive Theories

A major competitor of the neural theories is one of Uttal's (1981) modern rationalisms: Constructionism. With ideas perhaps dating back at least to Helmholtz (1866), the constructionist theorist would have the illusory contour viewer using some process of inference, usually unconscious, to produce the illusory contour. This orientation is sometimes referred to as top-down processing. The contour is suggested by the stimulus configuration and formed as a perceptual hypothesis. The illusory contours and surface are completed on the basis of this analysis. Early analyses of illusory contours seem to be compatible with this view. Zigler (1920) demonstrated that contours developed as subjects appreciated the meaning of the figure (see Coren et al., chap. 26). Similarly, Purdy (1936) quotes Muller in 1923 as saying that an illusory contour filling-in occurs only when the figure is apprehended as an incomplete square. Woodworth (1938) echoes these sentiments when he presents the Schumann figure as an example of how central factors enhance and complete contours.

There are several modern variants as to how this process is implemented and the most important type of stimulus information for the inference problem. Depth stratification has been suggested as having a major role (Coren, 1972). In 1972, Gregory proposed that the illusory contour is the solution to a puzzling stimulus array. In his chapter (chap. 9), he presents a new and intriguing approach to the problem. Rock and Anson (1979) and Rock (chap. 6) have described and elaborated some of the details of the inference problem, suggesting that the normal figure ground segregation of the inducing elements on the background is interpreted as reversed and the possibility of the subjective contour is then tested in a second stage of the process. Obviously, many other theorists have used versions of this approach, as will be seen in this volume. One major problem with top-down theories is the interaction of these with neural theories. There is a risk of being too exclusive, and many of the authors in this volume see the need for a consideration of the various levels of processing and possible feedback systems.

Gestalt Theories

Is the Gestalt view of the illusory contour simply a subset of the top-down viewpoint? This depends on the rigor of the interpretation of Gestalt concepts. Gestalt psychology proposed a set of principles which led to an organization of the field. In common usage, many assume that it led to a sense of "goodness," which meant the simplest interpretation of the stimulus given the entire configuration of the display's components. One should not assume that the use of organizational principles in Gestalt psychology assumes an inferential process with a great use of computational or cognitive problem-solving resources. As Uttal (1981) and Hatfield and Epstein (1985) point out, the Gestalt organizational principles can be looked at as basic perceptual primitives which operate without what we normally consider to be cognitive or inferential mediation. They are usually viewed as innate by the Gestalt theorists. In this sense, these principles are reductionistic. Today, whether or not the organizational principles are learned or developed through natural selection is controversial. As Hatfield and Epstein (1985) point out, the use of a minimalist principle in a perceptual theory which entails a computation of the "simplest" interpretation of the figure may face a combinatorial explosion of possibilities. Thus, the search for the simplest configuration may demand too much resource allocation. This would suggest that applications of information metrics such as coding theory to predict illusory contours might not be productive (Van Tuijl & Leeuwenberg, 1982). However, in Gestalt theory some configurations flow as a natural consequence of the physical situation and do not require computation.

Gestalt views suggest that the illusory contour is a consequence of organizational principles rather than being actively computed (Bruno & Gerbino, chap. 24; Gerbino & Kanizsa, chap. 27; Kanizsa, 1979, chap. 4; Minguizzi, chap. 7; Sambin, chap. 14). There is a subtle difference in the use of organizational principles in Gestalt and cognitive models, and a different use of reductionism in Gestalt and neural models (Arheim, 1986; Gronit, 1977; Uttal, 1981). It remains to be seen whether tests can be devised to separate out inferential and cognitively based organizations from the Gestalt ones and if such tests can be applied to illusory contours. Certainly, illusory contour perception takes appreciable amounts of time (Petry & Gannon, chap. 21). It would seem that reaction time analyses might be appropriate (Bruno & Gerbino, chap. 24; Meyer & Fish, chap. 25).

Behavioristic Theories and Empiricist Concerns

A macrotheoretical level analysis would have to touch on Behaviorism and the importance of nativist versus empiricist issues. As is well known, Behaviorism's rejection of mentalisms and experiential reports had a chilling effect on perceptual research (Bourassa, 1986; Uttal, 1981). When considered, analyses by theorists such as Hull (1952) found perception explainable as conditioned responses due to stimulus generalization of past responses. There have been conditioning models of some currently popular perceptual phenomena like the McCollough effect (see Skowbo, 1984, for a critical review). So far, such views seemed not to have been applied to illusory contours. One might propose that the pacmen act as a CS to a real triangle's US such that the illusory contour is the CR. Before one blanches with horror, recall most modern learning theorists happily use our concepts in explaining the "classical learning phenomena" (for example, Dawson, Schnell, Beers, & Kelly, 1982).

Animal training techniques are useful in nonhuman and infant psychophysics, demonstrating phenomena such as the McCollough effect (Maguire, Meyer, & Baizer, 1980). While there has been some use of these techniques with illusory contours in infants (see below), we are unaware of any behavioral research with animals and illusory contours although texture segmentation has been demonstrated in cats (Wilkinson, 1986). It is also clear that learning and practice are important to illusory contour perception (see Coren et al., chap. 26), and Gellatly's skills analysis (chap. 29) is certainly intriguing.

Relatively little is known about illusory contour perception in infants and children. Salapatek (1975) has reported evidence for texture segregation in 2-month-olds. Berenthal, Campos, and Haith (1980) demonstrated a consistent selectivity for Kanizsa square illusory contours in 7-month-olds. Shimojo, Birch, Gwiazda, and Held (1986) used a vernier acuity pattern which produces a strong subjective contour in adults and found discrimination in 3-month-olds. Kinetically defined contours also seem to be visible between 3 and 7 months (Fox & McDaniel, 1982; Granrud, Yonas, Smith, Arterburry, Glicksman, & Sorknes, 1984; Kaufmann-Hayoz, Kaufmann, & Stucki, 1986). Similarly, random dot stereograms may be appreciated at 4 months (Fox, 1981). Some work has been done with older children, who seem to have shown perception of Kanizsa triangles (Abravanel, 1982) between 3 and 5 years of age, of Ehrenstein figures at 5 years (Soubitez, 1982), and of the illusory contour Rubin faces and vase pattern at 6 years (Meyer, Coleman, Dwyer, & Lehman, 1982). Kennedy (chap. 28) reports on young children's judgment of the phenomenal reality of subjective contours.

While these are exciting findings, the development of illusory contour perception is still an open area for study. We know how various conditions such as strabismus can alter visual functions but it would be interesting to test illusory contour perception in such conditions. Similarly, Gellatly and Bishop (chap. 29) compare illusory contour perception to the development of reading skill. Just as sophisticated psychophysical and neurophysiological models have been applied recently to reading deficits (Lovegrove, Martin, & Slaghuis, 1986; Williams and Bologna, 1985), perhaps illusory contours might serve some diagnostic purpose for visual problems in children.

Direct Realism and Other Gibsonian Variants

One could not study perception and not be aware of the impact that J. J. Gibson has had on the field. Illusions, per se, were not of major importance to Gibson and we do not find illusory contours to be a major topic of discussion in his work even though some examples can be found in his writing (1950, 1966). Usually, these displays are part of discussions of texture, depth, or occlusion. Rather than constructive process, Gibson emphasized the direct detection of invariants in the visual field (Kelley, 1986). This approach had been most applied to problems of movement (Klymenko & Weisstein, chap. 15). There is little discussion of Gibson's views in the illusory contour literature but the Gibsonian approach has been influential in the computational theories of vision (Marr, 1982; McArthur, 1982), and these theories do consider the problems of illusory contours (Marr, 1982; Ullman, 1976).

Computational Vision and Illusory Contours

No one can deny the excitement generated by the work of Marr (1982) and others in the area of computational vision. This approach seeks to understand the complex processing of visual information on three levels: (1) computational theory—the goals, strategy, and logic of the process; (2) representation and algorithm—the data structures, algorithms, their inputs and outputs; and (3) hardware implementation—the "wetware" or physical reality of the system. Marr emphasizes that physiological analyses are not totally explanatory or useful without the other levels. He also stresses that appeals to higher order or more "cognitive" mechanisms should not be done until algorithmic approaches have been exhausted. There is no reason to assume from sheer intuition that some process must be behind an impenetrable barrier of "cognitive inference" until algorithms are tested. (See Gregory, chapter 9, for a new discussion of this issue.) We find in Ullman (1976) an attempt to apply this approach to the perception of curved subjective contours. Certainly, the work of Grossberg and Mingolla (chap. 12) can be seen in this light as their theory attempts to specify the segmentation processes and boundary and surface interactions that lead to illusory contours as well as other phenomena. Ramachandran (chap. 10) offers an interesting perspective with his "utilitarian" theory of perception which postulates that there exists a special-purpose set of tricks for visual perception, which are derived through natural selection and which do not entail sophisticated computational or cognitive models. This seems to echo some of the Gibsonian and Gestalt insights. Pure "cognitive" models must be careful to demonstrate that some algorithm would not predict a seemingly inferential result. Also physiological models need to contain more than a reference to a cell which might have a nice property for illusory contour perception. The linking hypotheses need to be explicit. However, there may be more commonality in these viewpoints then a categorization seems to suggest (McArthur, 1982).

The Plan of the Book

The book is organized into six major sections, and a summary of the chapters is found at the beginning of each section. However, ideas, positions, and phenomena cannot be so easily classified. There is much overlap, and true organization is not unidimensional. We follow the lead of other recent volumes and include a matrix of authors by important topic for the clarification and use of the readers in finding subjects of their choice (Tables 1.1 and 1.2).

TABLE 1.1. The chapters in the book classified by research emphasis and theoretical orientation.

Major emphasis in research or discussion.

Author and chapter	Color[1]	Brightness	Edge	Depth[2]	Texture[3]	Configuration[4]	Time/Motion/RT
Bradley (22)	X	X	X	X		X	X
Bruno & Gerbino (24)				X		X	X
Coren et al. (26)		X	X			X	
Day (5)	X	X	X	X			
deWeert & van Kruysbergen (17)	X	X				X	
Ehrenstein (3) trans. Hogg		X	X			X	
Gellatly & Bishop (29)						X	
Gerbino & Kanizsa (27)	X	X		X			
Gillam (30)			X	X	X	X	
Ginsburg (13)		X	X			X	
Gregory (9)				X			
Grossberg & Mingolla (12)		X	X	X	X		
Halpern (18)		X				X	
Jory (20)		X	X				
Kanizsa (4) trans. Gerbino	X	X	X	X		X	
Kellman & Loukides (16)		X	X			X	X
Kennedy (28)			X	X		X	
Klymenko & Weisstein (15)			X	X			X
Maguire & Brown (23)	X		X				X
Meyer & Fish (25)			X		X		X
Meyer & Petry (1)	X	X	X	X	X	X	X
Minguzzi (7)				X		X	X
Parks (8)	X						
Petry & Gannon (21)		X	X			X	X
Ramachandran (10)	X			X	X	X	X
Rock (6)		X	X			X	
Sambin (14)		X	X			X	
Shapley & Gordon (11)	X	X	X	X			
Schumann (2) trans. Hogg			X			X	
Warm et al. (19)		X	X				
Wade (31)		X	X	X	X	X	

[1] Includes appearance of hue in illusory contours, use of chromatic inducing elements, and induction of translucent film-like surfaces of both chromatic an achromatic appearance.
[2] Includes depth stratification, interposition, amodal completion, and steropsis.
[3] Includes texture segregation, texture-based boundaries, and perceptual grouping phenomena.
[4] A significant concern with the arrangement of inducing elements and how this influences various illusory contour phenomena.

TABLE 1.2. The chapters in the book classified by research emphasis and theoretical orientatation.

Author and chapter	Historical review	Art	Major theoretical orientation or discussion		
			Physiological	Perceptual (Gestalt/ecol.)	Cognitive combined
Bradley (22)					x
Bruno & Gerbino (24)				x	
Coren et al (26)	x				x
Day (5)	x			x	x
DeWeert & Van Kruysbergen (17)				x	
Ehrenstein (3) trans. Hogg	x		x		
Gellatly & Bishop (29)					x
Gerbino & Kanizsa (27)				x	
Gillam (30)				x	
Ginsburg (13)			x		
Gregory (9)	x		x	x	x x
Grossberg & Mingolla (12)				x	x x
Halpern (18)	x	x			
Jory (20)				x	
Kanizsa (4) trans. Gerbino	x			x	
Kellman & Loukides (16)				x	
Kennedy (28)			x	x	
Klymenko & Weisstein (15)				x	
Maguire & Brown (23)			x		
Meyer & Fish (25)				x	x x
Meyer & Petry (1)	x	x	x	x	x x
Minguzzi (7)				x	
Parks (8)		x			x x
Petry & Gannon (21)				x	x
Ramachandran (10)			x		x
Rock (6)					x
Sambin (14)				x	
Shapley & Gordon (11)			x		
Schumann (2) trans. Hogg	x			x	
Warm et al. (19)					x
Wade (31)		x			x

This endeavor has been most enjoyable to the editors. We cannot adequately express our admiration and gratitude to our contributors and publishers. Thank you all.

Acknowledgments. The authors would like to thank Dr. Frank Chance for suggesting some of the references from the art literature. We would like to thank Lynn Fulton of Lutheran Family Services of Oregon and Southwest Washington for enabling us to reproduce their logo. Also appreciated is the help of Dr. Jan Bender with some of the German language work referenced in this article. Finally, we would like to thank Stephen Nyberg for drawing our attention to the ad using the illusory contour cross.

CHAPTER 2

Contributions to the Analysis of Visual Perception—First Paper: Some Observations on the Combination of Visual Impressions into Units*

F. Schumann (Translated by Anne Hogg)

Introduction

Without a doubt, the view is now commonly held that there is only one source of knowledge in psychology: experience. And naturally, it is primarily a question of inner experience or introspection. It is known, however, that in comparison to outer perception, inner perception is so unreliable that only few of the facts obtained by this method can really be stated with confidence. If we look at the data from different experimenters of today, there are very few results of introspection that are even to some extent in agreement. Because of this, introspection alone as it is normally practiced does not give a solid enough foundation for developing the science of psychology. In fact, the scientists who try to discover comprehensive laws that rule mental events also use numerous hypothetical assumptions, so that the reliability of their claims naturally suffers considerably.

A strong impetus towards a more precise treatment of the psyche has recently been given, on the one hand, by pathological experiences (amnestic aphasia, word blindness and word deafness, psychic blindness, etc.) and, on the other hand, by accurate experiments in sensory physiology. From the large success obtained in both these fields emerged the attempt to found an experimental psychology that would start with sensations but would gradually also try to treat the higher mental processes more precisely, especially by making them more accessible to counting and measurement.

There are two main reasons why experimental psychology has not been able to convince even those who are not directly concerned with our science of the great significance of the results obtained up to now. First, one must think that setting up the science of experimental psychology can be compared in a certain sense with erecting a large building on marshy ground. In such a case, the ground must first be made safe enough by work which cannot be seen afterwards by the observer (driving in piles, etc.). Similarly, experimental psychology requires a comprehensive preparatory work before it can start with the real problems. But these preparations have by now already reached quite extraordinary proportions. The number of detailed experiments on problems of sensory physiology, on measuring just noticeable differences, on duration of mental events, on the reconstruction of mental images and memory deficits has grown so enormously that one experimenter has trouble working through them all with the necessary critical care. Thus, in addition to a diverse knowledge and a wide experimental experience, much care and very precise thinking are necessary, if one wants to really have a command of these experiments,

---

* Translated from Beitrage zur Analyse der Gesichtswahrnehmungen. Erste Abhandlung. Einige Beobachtungen über die Zusammenfassung von Gesichtseindrucken zu Einheiten, by F. Schumann, 1900. *Zeitschrift für Psychologie und Physiologie der Sinnesorgane* **23**:1–32. Copyright 1900 by Verlag von Johann Ambrosius Barth. Translated with permission.

and not merely to learn about them from the superficial treatment of a textbook.

Nevertheless, now that the preliminary work is considerably advanced, it is time for experimental psychology to turn determinedly to its main task, the study of mental phenomena. However, here, as a second large obstacle, the same imperfection of introspection again appears, which to begin with disturbs the experimenter in the same way as it does the nonexperimenting psychologist. He cannot dispense with it, because the experimental series of measurements cover such complex mental dimensions, about which not nearly enough is known, that analysis through the obtained data alone cannot be accomplished. For example, the blending of consonant tones is a fundamental fact, which could hardly have been stated without introspection.

At the same time, this example shows that in some cases introspection can be reliable to a great extent. It was only received as generally correct after Stumpf pointed out the long overlooked fact of tone blending. This raises the question as to whether there is a special reason for the relatively high reliability in this case. And I believe that, in fact, one simple reason exists. One can produce consonances and dissonances easily using any musical instrument, so that numerous observations of consonant intervals and numerous comparisons of these with dissonant intervals are possible. My opinion is that by using this method a greater reliability than usual is possible, because as a rule, psychologists have limited themselves mostly to observations which are used in everyday life. This, however, does not lead to a large reliability because these effects are mostly of a transient nature and the observation of the faded images that remain are known to be a source of errors.

My opinion is further supported by the recent success of repeated observations in another two cases, which make available conscious facts of inner perception that are important for the description of the laws ruling mental phenomena. Stumpf, namely, once showed that the judgment of the clarity or unclarity of intervals is dependent upon mood. In addition, I myself have shown that in judging small simple sounds of a certain length, apart from the sensation of sound, specific contents appear in awareness which play a fundamental role in the judgment itself.

For this reason, I see that one of the main advantages of using experiments in psychology is that in this way, it is possible to produce events within us as often as we like, and to compare them, as often as we like, with other more or less different events. And I am sure that through systematic practice in introspection at the moment, more will be reached in many areas than through quantitative experiments. Thus, I have shown, especially in the judgment of small time intervals, that a series of quantitative experiments can often only be set up in a purposeful way because of the results of the judgment process from inner perception, and that only on the basis of these results is it possible to understand the results found experimentally.

Certainly, a lot of practice and critical diligence are required if one wants to learn the difficult art of introspection correctly. Recently a psychologist has shown that a certain event in the field of tone sensitivity could be easily demonstrated on the piano, and two years later he thought he could prove the opposite easily using introspection. To make the results of one's own introspection more reliable, it is best to give them to another competent person for examination. Here, psychologists from this field are best suited as they have many years of experience. But because, for obvious reasons, they are not often available, a professor of psychology must mainly rely on his students. However, one must make a careful choice, because many have little aptitude for introspection. Whereas one perhaps does not have the ability to analyze at all, because for him only the outside world is interesting, others are susceptible to self-deception. If one has the chance to have practice experiments, however, one can relatively easily recognize whether someone is a good and reliable observer. When one has found a good observer who has repeatedly shown himself to be trustworthy, he is an especially valuable subject for further experiments. Unfortunately, the number of such people always remains very limited because only few are prepared for the high demands placed on their endurance by the laborious investigations of experimental psychology.

Eventually, if a series of experimental facts

can be explained without the additional help of introspection, a relatively high degree of reliability has been reached.

Naturally, it is not to be expected that with the most complicated mental phenomena, introspection will be shown to be trustworthy immediately. On the contrary, for the present, only the simplest diagrams can be used. In the first place, one must look at the procedures that occur unmediated after the sensation: comprehension, comparison, differentiation, cognition, recognition, judgment. And I hope to show in a series of experiments that much can be reached by using introspection carefully to obtain a closer knowledge about these events.

So, in the following contribution, the problem of spatial perception will be thoroughly investigated. There are many experiments by excellent researchers concerning this problem, but nevertheless, there are still a large number of complicated questions to be solved. So, for the time being, the effect of the outer stimulus will be followed only to the retina. The further physiological processes that lie between retina and perception are still completely veiled in obscurity and we are dependent on very dubious hypotheses—at least as regards the properties of those processes that are directly related to the spatial properties of visual perception. There are also so many arguments against the hypothesis of muscle sensation that a considerable contamination by such sensations in spatial perception seems to be excluded. But it is high time that we make a determined attempt to enter this unknown field, because the development of an accurate theory of the cognitive events that follow visual perception, is considerably dependent upon the success of these experiments. There are also a large number of conspicuous though not yet explained facts, which drive one on to further experimentation. In some later contributions to this series of publications, I will, therefore attempt to do such experiments. However, I do not immediately expect to be able to completely explain the events intervening between retinal excitation and perception because they are certainly too complicated. Moreover, to begin with I hope to deal only with some general hypotheses and to develop them slowly with other experimental studies, as it is known that a hypothesis, even when it does not correspond completely to the truth, is still of use, in that it leads to new questions for experimental investigation.

I

1. If I intend to count the number of lines on a printed page (e.g., the one at hand), I normally proceed by concentrating on the ends of the first three lines, which thus become more prominent; then I mark the space between the third and fourth lines with the point of a pencil, so that the next three lines stand out, and so on. I proceed in the same way when I want to count tuning fork movements that are recorded on charcoal paper. However, I can hardly make the ends of more than three lines or three waves prominent.

Similarly, without effort, I can make only three elements of a row of small figures (spots, lines, circles, squares, etc.) prominent, if they are spaced equally apart.

By asking a large number of people, it was shown that by concentrating in this way, many can easily isolate four or five elements.

With lines, something else unusual takes place (see Fig. 2.1). Each pair of lines quite easily join together to form a group, so that each white area lying between the two lines builds up a complete whole with the lines, which then phenomenally emerge. On the contrary, the white areas between groups recede and appear quite different. One has the impression that one sees a fence made of wooden planks. It also often occurs that the planks of the fence stand out (i.e., are conspicuous), not only in awareness, but also out of the plane of

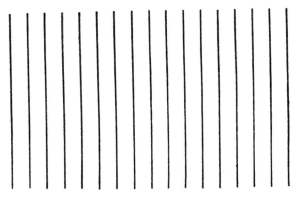

FIGURE 2.1.

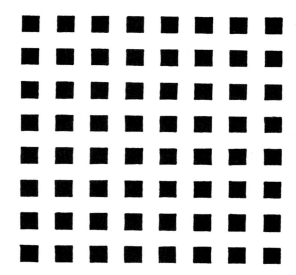

FIGURE 2.2.

the paper. When the lines have formed such groups, I can once more easily isolate three such groups from the rest, using attention, apparently because each group, as it were, forms an element again.

When using spots, squares, etc. that are only arranged in a row next to each other, grouping is less easy; on the contrary it appears convincingly when many rows are arranged equally spaced apart. Thus, by observing Figure 2.2, I can see quite involuntarily, the black squares arranged in groups of four and certainly I see the whole board arranged in such groups during free viewing, where a new group always appears in my awareness. Voluntarily, I can, by concentrating, also make a larger square consisting of three-by-three small squares stand out, and I can also divide this group again into various subdivisions. Either one unit is then always formed of three squares in a horizontal row (or three vertical) or I divide the nine again into one of five and one of four, in which I separate out as five, the four corner squares plus that lying in the middle, from the other four small squares. Further, by concentrating, I can also isolate a larger group of four-by-four small areas, which, however, very easily divides into four smaller groups of two-by-two each. Indeed, if I look at the center, I can even divide the whole figure into four subgroups, each of four-by-four small areas, where, of course, the single elements are quite indistinct. Lastly, I

can even make other groups stand out, e.g., the squares which lie on both diagonals of the figure.

Another special phenomenon sometimes appears along with the last described observation. The white stripe, which divides one complete group from the neighbouring black areas, often appears vividly in awareness, whereas the stripes between the elements of the group seem to remain in the background. At the same time, the white stripes which are prominent appear broader than the other, objectively equally broad stripes that remain in the background. Some subjects can even voluntarily become aware of the white cross which is made from the middle vertical and the middle horizontal stripes and which divides the four larger squares, each of 16 elements. Both of the stripes forming the cross appear to them as broader than the remaining ones, and the illusion appears more clearly, the more conspicuous the cross.

If the elements are arranged equidistantly, the grouping depends totally on choice and changes extraordinarily easily. By grading the size of the space, a specific grouping always appears at first involuntarily and only changes after a great deal of effort, as is shown in Figure 2.3. Here, at first, four small areas form a group, and then four such groups form one unit of the next level. Further, one will easily notice that the broader white stripes emerge perceptually.

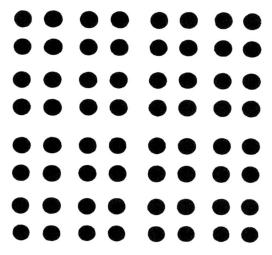

FIGURE 2.3.

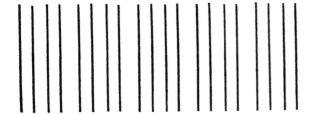

FIGURE 2.4.

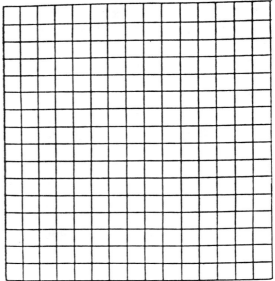

FIGURE 2.5.

Instead of black circular areas, one can also take other colored or other shaped elements (spots, squares, lines, etc.): by varying the spacing, one always obtains a specific grouping and the larger spaces always emerge perceptually. Figure 2.4 serves as another example.

Indeed, it is not even necessary for the elements to be the same as each other. If one observes, e.g., this printed page, the letters of each word are joined into one unit and the distances between the words are always larger than the distance between letters. In addition, it is very noticeable that when reading, the small distances between letters totally recede perceptually, while, on the other hand, the larger distances between words are conspicuous.

In the section above, if I have spoken about lines, spaces, etc. emerging perceptually, I naturally do not mean that they stand out spatially, but only that they become conspicuous perceptually. Sometimes, it appears that the spaces, etc. also spatially stand out (from the level of the paper), but this is in no case the rule.

2. We can observe similar phenomena when we divide a large square by straight lines into small squares (see Fig. 2.5). Here one can easily make a large square comprised of three-by-three small ones stand out. At the same time, the four dividing lines of these larger squares also stand out, or for a moment, the two vertical or two horizontal lines stand out on their own. In the first case, all nine small squares are distinct and I am aware that I see all nine all of the time. If I go further, and get four-by-four small squares to emerge as a square, this reduces normally into four smaller ones, each of which again contains two-by-two elements. After some practice I often succeed in bringing together more small squares into a larger one with seven-by-seven or even with nine-by-nine elements. However, with three-by-three element

squares, I have all the elements distinctly in front of me, while with five-by-five elements only the dividing lines of the whole stand out and everything within these dividing lines is indistinct. Also, I am no longer aware of the number of elements that are included in the larger square.

In addition, I can join the elements into large rectangles or crosses, etc. instead of squares.

If one tries to find out through introspection in what way the lines, areas, etc. that stand out differ from the others, one notices immediately that the former appear blacker and have sharper borders.

3. The lines so far used to present the phenomena in the preceding paragraph were not really contours (i.e., lines dividing different colored areas) but only very narrow black areas on a white background. Now, it is interesting that quite analagous phenomena are produced when one takes real contours instead of black lines. Accordingly, by observing Figure 2.6, one can easily combine a number of small black and white areas into larger triangles or squares and, in doing so, notice that the border lines that differentiate the group from the other elements become more prominent. Because one becomes aware of a contour which is relatively segregated from the areas between which it lies, and because it joins together other similar elements

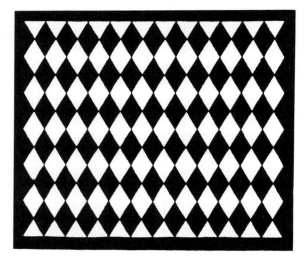

FIGURE 2.6.

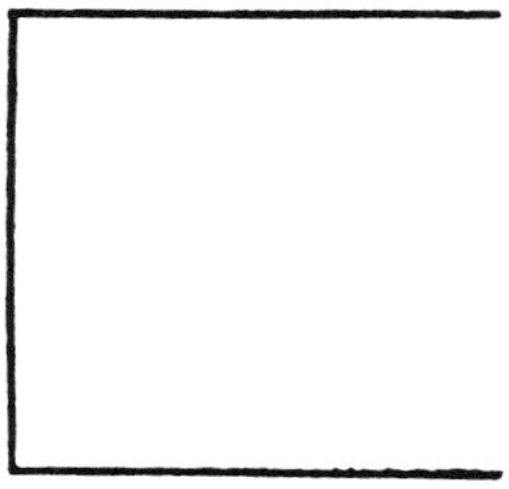

FIGURE 2.8.

into units, it is a relatively independent element of awareness.

Such contours do not only appear when two different colored areas come together. On the contrary, one can see them appear, under the appropriate conditions, in areas that are objectively quite uniformly colored. Thus, by observing Figure 2.7 one can see that in the middle, a white rectangle with sharply defined contours (border lines) appears, which objectively are not there. However, under the appropriate conditions, I have only succeeded in inducing straight lines and never regularly curved ones.

Further, if one draws two identical horizontally parallel lines, which are not too far apart from one another, one can easily see dividing lines appear, which join the ends of the parallel lines lying under one another. The ability to see such contours is, by the way, not equally devel-

oped in all subjects, so that not all people fill in the missing dividing line in the square in Figure 2.8. The subjects who succeeded in doing this saw, at the same time, that the white area inside the square was somewhat differently colored than that outside. While on this subject, one should also mention a similar phenomenon. When observing two small horizontal lines (see Fig. 2.9) that lie in one horizontal plane and are not too far apart, many see a joining line; and this subjective line appeared to some of my subjects as a somewhat pale, very small stripe that was whiter than the background, whereas others reported that the mental image appeared as a black line. The brighter line is perhaps only a contrast image that occurs because the eye moves from one side to the other.

Subjective lines also appear when observing the two parallel lines in Figure 2.10, which I can see in two ways. First, I have the impression of a parallelogram, so that subjective contours appear, which join on the one hand both lower ends of the parallel lines, and on the other hand both upper ends. Second, I can also see the lines as a step, in which the lower end of one line is joined to the upper end of the other. Several subjects reported that in the latter case, they actually had the mental image of a line. I cannot maintain the same. I have the impression of a step clearly, but cannot confirm the imaginary line by introspection.

One subject reported that she drew with an inkless pen an imaginary letter on paper, and shortly afterwards, really believed she could see it, and it was with lines that were brighter than the white background.

4. We take four small squares and arrange them so that the corners form an (imaginary)

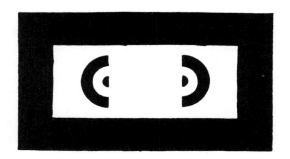

FIGURE 2.7.

FIGURE 2.9.

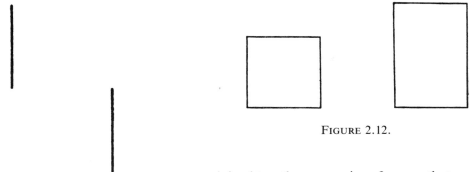

FIGURE 2.12.

FIGURE 2.10.

joined together, assuming of course that we also have the subjective impression of a square and the vertical sides are not overestimated.

It has often been assumed that during the inspection of an oblong, a special comparative event must take place, which first reckons the difference between the sides. But, in fact, inner perception knows nothing about such a special processes, and on the contrary, we recognize an oblong as such, at first sight. The same applies to the square. It will be shown in more detail in the next paper that the alleged properties of both figures (after their property of possessing four right angles) are really influential for their interpretation.

In addition to the longer side of an oblong becoming more prominent, something else often occurs: we often traverse these sides with our attention so that its parts become successively prominent. Of course, my glance crosses the one or the other side of the square, but in doing this, the single parts in general do not stand out successively—assuming that the square does not exceed a certain size. The line in question is really caught as a whole by attention and is as a whole clearly before me. In such a case, one indeed talks of attention wandering, but it is really only a wandering of the fixation point. Thus, the part lying near the fixation point does have a sharp contour for a certain time, but the reason for this is purely physiological. It is clearer to see the single parts becoming successively prominent when observing two parallel lines that are not too short. Only after my attention has wandered does the whole stand clearly before me for a minute. The next paper shows some cases in which this successive standing out is especially clear.

If we turn a square, whose sides initially are horizontal and vertical, by 45°, it looks quite different (see Fig. 2.13). Mach was the first to

oblong whose sides are vertical (see Fig. 2.11). At first sight, they form groups of two, and the space between the two squares lying under one another becomes more prominent, whereas the space between two squares lying next to one another recedes. On the contrary, if four small squares form the corners of a larger square, every small square is as closely joined to that below (or above) as to the one lying next to it. In addition, none of the spaces between the squares stands out. Of course, it is better to make the horizontal distances somewhat larger than the vertical, because in general the latter is somewhat overestimated.

In a similar way, we can characterize squares and oblongs when they are limited by lines. At first sight the two longer sides of an oblong (see Fig. 2.12), on the one hand, and the two short sides, on the other hand, each combine immediately into one unit. Further, the longer lines are more closely joined together and emerge perceptually. One can indeed say that this is a primary characteristic of the figure. With a square, on the contrary, all four sides are quite equally

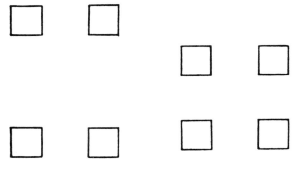

FIGURE 2.11.

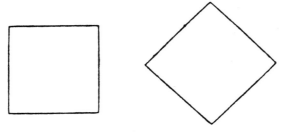

FIGURE 2.13.

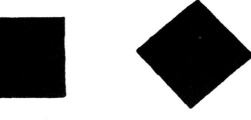

FIGURE 2.15.

point out this phenomenon (Beiträge zur Anal-yse der Empfindungen, p. 44). Without mechan-ical and intellectual operations, he says, one would never recognize that the two squares are identical.

The intellectual operation by which one im-mediately recognizes both figures as identical is of a very simple nature. If one concentrates on one side of the square on the right and thus isolates it if possible, the square becomes more similar to the other one. Involuntarily, both pairs of sloping lines, lying symmetrical to the vertical diagonal, are pushed into our aware-ness at the same time: they build one complete whole. Of course, the sides of the square lying on the left also form one complete whole, but they are more equally joined together, whereas the four sides of the other square form two pairs which are especially closely joined together. On the contrary, one can see the square on the left as being similar to the other. One needs only to concentrate on one corner, then the lines that come together at that corner join together into one unit.

The close relationship between each pair of lines forming one unit, however, is not the only distinctive property of the square on the right. In addition, the distance between opposite cor-ners (the diagonals) plays a role in awareness, which in general is not the case with other squares. This conspicuousness of the diagonal is shown perhaps even more clearly if we take

an acute-angled parallelogram with sides of equal length instead of a square (see Fig. 2.14).

The real borders of areas behave in the same way as the black lines, as is shown in Figure 2.15.

One can see the mentioned relationships even more clearly if one takes four small circles and arranges them so that they form the corners of a square (see Fig. 2.16). Of the four circles on the right, each pair lying on a diagonal easily form one unit and the space between them becomes prominent. If we voluntarily bring two circles which lie on one side of the imaginary square to join into one unit, it becomes clear immediately that both complexes are exactly congruent.

Further, if we draw a cross from simple lines, with arms of equal length, on the one hand lying and on the other hand standing, an immediate difference is shown in the interpretation (Fig. 2.17). In the first case, both halves of each are combined into one unit, and in the other case, two vertical or horizontally lying symmetrical halves form a unit.

If we turn now from a square to a rhombus (Fig. 2.14), we can likewise say again that all sides are equally joined to each other, when the two parallel sides lie horizontally, and that when one diagonal lies vertically, both sides about the vertical are especially closely joined together. As I mentioned before, in the last case, the diagonals play a role in awareness, and the longer diagonals are always more prom-

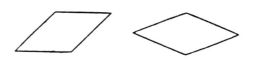

FIGURE 2.14.

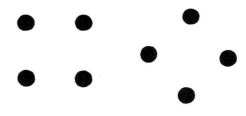

FIGURE 2.16.

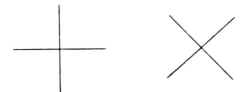

FIGURE 2.17.

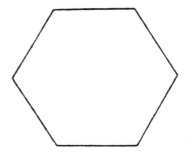

FIGURE 2.19.

inent than the shorter. Further, the parallelogram with sides of different lengths differs from a rhombus in the same way that the oblong differs from the square.

With changing orientation in the plane, the irregular triangle with different lengths of sides can be seen in three different ways. One obtains them when one gradually turns Figure 2.18 always in the same direction, until it returns to its original position. One can easily see that the horizontally lying side is always isolated, whereas the other two are more closely joined together and are really characteristic for the triangle. I can also see the three views at will, without changing its position, by trying to concentrate my attention on each pair of lines that come together in a corner.

Further, the combination of different lines into units leads to different views of the regular hexagon. I can think of Figure 2.19 as an upper and a lower half placed together: then the three upper lines are especially closely joined together, as are the three lower ones. On the other hand, I can also think of the six lines as being divided into three groups, in which I join the upper and lower horizontals, the two sloping lines on the left and the two on the right. The latter view is the most common when the figure is rotated by 90°.

If one observes the regular octagon (Fig. 2.20), a very characteristic grouping of the eight

lines appears. If one thinks of the lines as being numbered 1–8, on the one hand sides 1,3,5,7, join into a group, and on the other hand, sides 2,4,6,8. When one of the group emerges, the other recedes. Moreover, one can obtain even other groups at will.

If the number of sides increases even further, the figures become too complex.

Finally, the difference between a circle and an ellipse (Fig. 2.21) can be characterized in a similar way as the difference between a square and an oblong. When a square is lying on its side, no line becomes prominent and when standing on a corner, neither of the two diagonals stands out more than the other. Similarly with a circle, no diamter (direction) becomes prominent. On the other hand, the ellipse has a main direction, as do the oblong and the rhombus that stands on a corner.

5. Two similar lines that come together at one point and which lie symmetrical about the vertical, are joined together especially closely, as we have seen with the square standing on a corner and in other figures (rhombus, hexagon, octagon, etc.), and also as we can easily see with

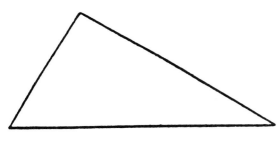

FIGURE 2.18.

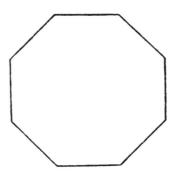

FIGURE 2.20.

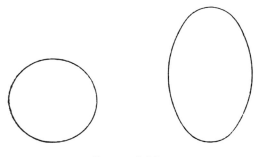

FIGURE 2.21.

two isolated lines. The same holds when straight lines are replaced by curved ones.

Furthermore, if we take a figure built from a larger complex of lines where the vertical is a symmetrical axis, we can say in general that each pair of lines that lie symmetrical about the vertical are joined together especially closely. Because of this, the two halves of the figure are joined into a special single whole, which we can easily observe, e.g., when we look at the two hexagons in Figure 2.22. The hexagon built symmetrical to the vertical is a whole in itself, whereas the other divides into two halves and the more extended half becomes more prominent. The latter hexagon can also be interpreted in a special way, thus avoiding the division into halves. One only needs to direct attention to the three longer sides on the left and to join them into one unit. Then, as soon as one turns the figure 90° so that the three longer sides build up the lower half, it appears that they stand out on their own.

II

6. As we saw, the black lines and circular areas that emerge from the background differ from those that remain in the background in that they appear blacker and more sharply defined. Such differences often occur because the eye is more accommodated to certain lines than to others. However, if a pattern like that below (see Fig. 2.23) stands out from the large group of squares in Figure 2.5, the acute sharpness of such a complex of lines cannot originate in accommodation. Further, the lack of clarity in indirect vision cannot be used to any great extent as an explanation, because indirectly viewed lines often stand out, while at the same time the directly seen ones recede. Thus, we must consider central factors as the main cause of the illusion.

However, I believe that the lines, areas, etc. that emerge are differentiated from the others, not only in that they are blacker and more sharply defined, but also because of another specific unique factor. Others have maintained (see Külpe, Zur Lehre von der Aufmerksamkeit, Zeitschr. f. Philos. Vol. 110, p. 31) that the clarity (or lack of clarity) which follows attention and the blurred image, which is an effect of inattention, portray two opposing conditions of awareness. I do not want to discuss whether or not this view portrays the truth accurately. At least it appears to me that it comes close to the truth.

Further, it should be mentioned that the elements that stand out isolate themselves from

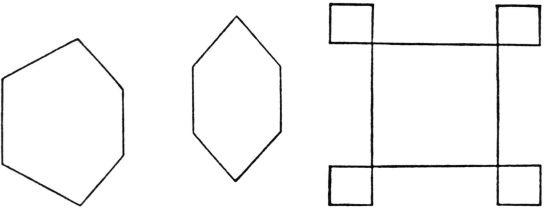

FIGURE 2.22.   FIGURE 2.23.

the others and normally form a complete whole. From this, however, we cannot conclude that the combination of elements is a function which simply coincides with the function of that of standing out, because as we saw above, a group of elements that stands out can be divided into different subgroups (e.g., nine into a five and a four).

7. In the above discussion, I have been using the term *unit* (Einheit) without defining it further. As Lipps recently quite rightly emphasized (Tonverwandtschaft und Tonverschmelzung, Zeitschr. f. Psych., Vol. 19, p. 3), this is a term which has so many meanings that one should always explain exactly what is meant by it.

If we look first for analogies in other sensory areas, we find that tones can also combine, more or less closely into units. Stumpf has proved convincingly that two simultaneous consonant tones form one unit and that the complex is even more homogeneous, the larger the consonance. What is meant by this, is that both tones appear more like one single auditory impression in our awareness.

Analogously, we can speak of the unity of sensory impressions. If we observe Figure 2.2 (above), then assuming that no voluntary or involuntary division into subgroups takes place, one single mass of elements is presented to us. On the other hand, by observing Figure 2.3 we see four smaller masses, which divide even further into four even smaller masses. We can also say that the view that the first figure offers gives more the impression of a large square area, made up of many squares plus the spaces between them: in contrast to this, the second figure is made up of 16 small isolated square areas, where each four build another complex that is similar to one black square.

Or, let us draw a long row of similar spots, first next to one another in a straight line so that all the spaces are the same, and in a second case, always in groups of, e.g., five spots, spaced a larger distance apart. We can then say that in the first case we have an impression that is more like a straight line than in the second case.

In addition, we can speak of a second meaning of unity. If one turns one's attention to one element of a uniform whole, the other elements also intrude in one's attention at the same time.

In fact, if one observes Figure 2.4 above, one must take a lot of trouble to isolate a single line from one group. Further, if one turns one's attention to a group of two lines, the relevant group in the next higher order of the complex stands out along with it (although less strongly). The same phenomenon is shown when one observes the small circles in Figure 2.3. Even in the larger complex of squares, shown in Figure 2.2, all small squares are generally forced on me at the same time, and an involuntary grouping first occurs after I have given some trouble to form groups at will. On the other hand, if I observe a board on which there are as many different colored squares as possible (or different shaped areas), the single elements do not behave equivalently in my awareness. A disturbance enters and soon every element enters my awareness.

Lastly, we can speak of unity in a third way: Each group works as a whole on the mental image. Three small black areas, spaced equally apart and arranged next to each other, immediately evoke in me the number 3. If I see two such rows arranged under each other, the number 6 is evoked, etc. Complexes that are made of more than 16 elements no longer evoke in me an immediate numerical image.

If we now turn to the square lying on its side, we can say that it is a numerical unit (similar to one impression), as well as working as a whole, because I am aware at first sight that I see a square, without a special comparison process taking place that determines the equality of the sides. However, I can also say regarding these two properties that every square forms a single whole. The square and the rhombus are excellent to the extent that all four sides become equally prominent in awareness. They differ from a rectangle, whose sides are not all the same length, in a similar way that an area arranged regularly with the same element differs from a second area arranged with different elements.

In the case of a square standing on a corner, both pairs of sides lying symmetrical to the medial plane are especially closely joined together. We can say that both lines of a pair are always prominent at the same time in our awareness. But if I observe a square lying on its side and combine two lines that come together in a corner into one unit, I cannot say that both sides intrude simultaneously in awareness, although I have the same impression of this square as with the square standing on a corner. The fact that I become aware of two sides at the same time cannot be relevant for the impression of unity that I have of them. On the contrary, one can say that this figure divides into an upper and a lower half. Each half gives the impression that it is isolated and the whole is simply the sum of both parts. Each of the two pairs of closely associated lines therefore works as a whole.

This explanation of the term *unity* will no doubt be supplemented by further experience. Probably there is a sensory factor that is not further definable as a last step in awareness that we can mostly only clarify through example.

Whether the unity that is shown by consonant tones is identical to the unity spoken about here, or whether the two phenomena are only similar, is not very easy to decide definitely, although much speaks for the former assumption. In any case, there is a further analogy between the two phenomena, in that they are both closely related to an agreeable feeling: a square appears more agreeable than a rectangle with sides of different lengths of lines, and the same is true of all figures with equal lengths of sides. If one divides a square, on the one hand, with a vertical and horizontal middle line into four small squares, and on the other hand, into four rectangles of different sizes, the former unitary figure appears determinedly more agreeable. If we draw a background of similar black squares in regular patterns, they work more agreeably than a board with many different colored squares. These examples can be further augmented. I only want at this point, to mention that even the lines that form known agreeable symmetrical figures join together into one whole, as we saw above.

8. The discussion in the preceding paragraphs shows that I was quite justified in my critique against proof of alleged "rigorous stringency" by v. Ehrenfels (Über Gestaltqualitäten, Vierteljahrsschrift f. wiss. Philos. Vol. 14, 1890, p. 269), who claimed to establish the existence of specific contents of the mental image, as a genuine property of the "spatial figure" configurations.

Ehrenfels starts from the opinion that an area is made up of innumerable spots ("local entities") and concludes in the following way: If a spatial figure, e.g., a square area, was nothing other than the sum of "local entities," different spatial figures should be more similar, the more similar their single elements. Because the "local entities" are dependent on their position in the visual field, and would be even more similar the closer they were to one another, it cannot be understood why two squares always stay the same no matter how far apart they are in the visual field and why another spatial figure near a square would not appear much more similar to it than to a distant square. Ehrenfels concludes that the similarity of spatial figures, which join together in awareness, must be due to something other than the similarity of their elements, and he thought he could assume the existence of a new mental element that brings together the elements and which immediately introduces the impression of similarity. This new one which combines the elements, Ehrenfels calls *gestalt quality,* which he understands to be "such concrete mental contents which join complexes in awareness, which themselves consist of elements that can be separated from one another, i.e., do not require each other to be conceived."

Without a doubt, it is correct that the similarity of spatial figures does not have an effect on the similarity of the purely fictive element. The observations shown here, cited on the qualities of squares, oblongs, etc., also clearly show that it is not a new mental content that is responsible for the similarity in our awareness, but something completely different. A square and an oblong differ from one another in that in the former, all four sides are equivalent and equally closely associated with one another, whereas with an oblong, the longer sides are more strongly associated and stand out.[1] Further, a square and a rhombus both have four sides that are equally joined with one another, but they differ in that the square has right angles. The properties by which we recognize a square—at least, a square lying on its side—in different positions in the visual field are the equal association of all four sides and the right angle. The

---

[1] A second paper will show in more detail that the properties really are characteristic for the square and oblong. (Ed. note: This was published as "Beiträge zur Analyse der Gesichtswahrnehmungen." Zweite Abhandlung. "Zur Schätzung raumlicher Grössen." *Zeitschr. f. Psych.* 24, 1–3.)

equality of the association is not a new mental element, because this would only be a further member in a sum of mental images, so that five mental images would be specified instead of four. At the most, one could say that the fifth additional mental image had this special attribute: to join the others uniformly together. It is considerably easier, however, to ascribe to the four border lines the property to join themselves uniformly together, as soon as they are similar to each other.

In the demonstrated cases, the relationships are also quite similar to those in consonant tones. If I have on the one hand, two deep tones which are an octave apart, and on the other hand, two high tones also an octave apart, the similarity between both complexes is not a case of similarity of elements, or of an addition of special mental images, but a case of a strong tendency to blend, which is shown by all complexes of simultaneous tones that are an octave apart.

Thus, in addition to the contents of the mental image, we have to consider the strength of the connection of the mental contents into units, as a special phenomenal fact of our awareness.

Addendum

Ehrenfels had maintained the existence of "gestalt qualities" for many other complexes of mental contents which form unique wholes and always gave the proof analogously. As he ascribed to his proof, " a rigorous" stringency I felt myself obliged, in an earlier work dealing with some of these complexes (Zeitschr. f. Psych. 17, 128), to investigate whether the existence of the gestalt qualities had really been so definitely proven. I came to the conclusion that for the present, one should exercise some restraint.

Meinong (1899), who in an earlier work had already tried to lend further support to the Ehrenfels article, has now in a new very comprehensive paper (Zeitschr. f. Psych. 21, 183) objected to my arguments of that time. It would be too much to go into detail here on all the points of difference. I also have little hope of bringing about an understanding because our fundamental ideas are too different. However, I cannot avoid touching upon at least some points of his paper.

Against Ehrenfels' line of argument, I had maintained among other things that because the fields of sound and spatial sense had not been thoroughly investigated psychologically, the further development of the science could easily bring surprises, in that the similarity of the complexes might be explained in a way that cannot be foreseen. Meinong writes against this:

Schumann finds the facts of sound and spatial sense not thoroughly enough investigated to attract empiricism in these fields. But where could Ehrenfels have found a more thoroughly studied field? Consistently, then, Schumann insists that one should refrain from thinking about what he claims are "difficult questions" until—until when? In all good faith, such restraint must be derived from an extreme conscientiousness: but if the human research instincts had to be quelled each time, then I fear we would have a somewhat short history of the science, if we had one at all.

These comments would be quite justified if I had really insisted that one should "refrain from thinking" about the difficult questions referred to. But I did not do this at all. I only insisted that for the time being, the existence of gestalt qualities should be seen as not definitely proven. In stating the reasons for such behavior, I pointed out that in a little studied field, development in the science could bring surprises. If Ehrenfels had seen the existence of gestalt qualities as only probable, I would hardly have considered them more closely in my earlier paper. In that work, the experiment I undertook was to describe the laws of mental events in which I left out all hypothetical mental contents and concentrated first of all only on the contents that could be stated with certainty with the help of introspection. Because it had been maintained that "gestalt qualities" could also be stated with certainty I felt compelled to show that a proof of "rigorous" stringency had not yet been furnished.

Secondly, I would like to clear up another misunderstanding. Meinong writes,

If Schumann therefore means that introspection does not allow an inclusion of that that is decided in the decision, but only shows that the representation of that that is decided causes the decision, of "unknown size" (!), I must question whether the factual findings are correctly described by introspection.

The description is too little concerned with "inclusion" as well as too much concerned with causation, which in my opinion Hume has already done adequately, so that they cannot be perceived either outwardly nor inwardly.

As I read this for the first time, I was completely surprised, because up to then, I had also not once even fleetingly thought to be able to establish by introspection that the representation of that that is decided could cause the decision. Actually, I find neither in the article cited by Meinong (Zeitschr. f. Psych. 17, 118) nor in any other part of my earlier article, one comment that would allow such a view of mine to be assumed.

Shortly before the end of this study, a paper by H. Cornelius appeared (Ueber Gestaltqualitäten. Zeitschr. f. Psych. 22, 101) in which the author also defends the existence of gestalt qualities against my attack. He writes:

These similarities between complexes are, however, in no way always due to the similarities of their relevant contents. On the contrary, similarities between complexes also occur when the relevant contents are completely different. We are therefore here concerned with a new type of similarity between complexes, that is not dependent on this similarity of the contents. Depending on these similarities, new features of the complex arise, which differentiate the complexes from those that are the mere sum of their contents.

The properties of this new characteristic type of similarity that occurs only between complexes, we call "gestalt qualities of the complex."

If "gestalt qualities" are understood to be only properties which differentiate the complexes from their elements, I can see their existence as assured, because as one "property" one can also see the large unity of a complex. But Ehrenfels did not speak of the newly stated "properties," but of "concrete mental contents." Cornelius certainly thinks that here there is only a difference in terminology. He writes:

Ehrenfels describes the gestalt qualities not as properties, but as concrete mental contents that belong to the elements of the relevant complexes. Only those mental contents, he thinks, are "bound to the existence of these complexes"—which is to be understood that they are not separable from these complexes, but are something that occurs with them in the same way that the properties of simple content (pitch, intensity, etc.) are not separable but only imaginable in and with it. These properties are also often described as contents; concerning this terminology, the gestalt qualities could also be named "concrete mental contents." But this, like the other are not concrete, but abstract contents."

I cannot agree with these comments. Cornelius interprets too much from the remark that the gestalt qualities should be "bound to the existence of these complexes." From this it is by no means sure that abstract contents are meant, because even concrete contents could be "bound to the existence of the complexes." Secondly, I can recall an article by Meinong (Zeitschr. f. Psych. 2, 245), which appeared immediately after the well-known Ehrenfels article and which studied whether gestalt qualities were necessarily a "concrete mental content," or whether other possibilities existed. From this article it is clear that Meinong did not attribute abstract contents to the gestalt qualities. When he, for example, remarked (see p. 259 in the above article) that one must be prepared for the existence of a blending or similar relationship between the elements of a complex and the gestalt qualities, it is clear that he thought of a concrete content. Because Ehrenfels did not object to this and because a close scientific relationship exists between Meinong and Ehrenfels, I cannot accept that Meinong had interpreted wrongly.

Acknowledgments. The translator gratefully acknowledges the help of Dr. W. Ehrenstein and Professor L. Spillman in the preparation of this translation.

CHAPTER 3

Modifications of the Brightness Phenomenon of L. Hermann*

Walter Ehrenstein (Translated by Anne Hogg)

Hermann's Phenomenon (Hering's Contrast Grid Phenomenon)

Many readers must know from casual observation the phenomenon that readily occurs when one looks at a lattice window, especially when the bright sky is seen as a background through the window: the points at which the lattice bars intersect appear considerably brighter than the remaining parts of the bars. In the psychological literature, this phenomenon is usually referred to as Hering's contrast grid (Elsenhans-Giese, 1939) although this description is neither historically nor factually correct. According to Hering's own account the phenomenon was first described, not by himself, but by L. Hermann (1870), and as we will see, it is not a contrast effect but a brightness effect, which needs to be discussed and interpreted in these terms.

Ewald Hering described the phenomenon in the following way:

A further example of the decrease of simultaneous contrast with distance is shown in Fig. 29 [Fig. 3.1 here] to which Hermann first drew attention. The point at which two white lines intersect when seen indirectly and with normal eye movements appears as a pale gray spot. This is because this point is more completely surrounded by brighter areas than is any other part of the white stripe of comparable size (see Chapter VII). The phenomenon quickly disappears

with steady fixation, because of a local adaptation that will be described later. However, even with stabilized vision, the phenomenon can be perceived in the first few seconds after presentation, in the parts of the figure seen indirectly, and belongs in this respect to the phenomena of pure simultaneous contrast: when I laid the figure in direct sunlight and exposed it for only 1/40 sec, I could perceive the gray spots in indirect vision.

In the following study, the conditions that induce the phenomenon will be manipulated in a variety of ways in order to test whether the phenomenon can be described in terms of brightness contrast, as Hering proposed, or whether other factors requiring further study are involved.

Modifications of Hermann's Phenomenon

The experiments that I carried out, as well as, in most cases, simply the observation of the figures (Figs. 3.1–3.11) that I designed to vary factors influencing the brightness phenomenon, allow the following statements:

1. When the stripes or lines of the grating pattern do not actually cross, or radiate from one point, but stop a certain distance from the point of intersection, then the brightness of the central white area between the ends of the lines is considerably increased in comparison to the brightness of the surrounding area (Fig. 3.2). This has been demonstrated by A. Prandtl (1927) with the help of a range of grid patterns.

* Translated from Uber Abwandlundgen der L. Hermannschen Helliskeitserscheinung, by W. Ehrenstein, 1941. *Zeitschrift für Psychologie, 150,* 83–91. Copyright 1941 by Verlag von Johann Ambrosius Barth. Translated with permission.

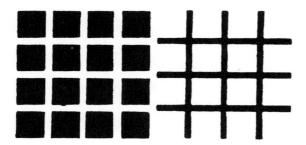

FIGURE 3.1.

2. One can still see this increased brightness of the central area when the radial lines, used as described to induce the illusion, are extremely fine and thin. The lines can be considerably thinner than those in the upper figure row in Figure 3.3 without causing the illusion to disappear. The brightness of the central field increases with increasing thickness of the rays. If the lines finally become so broad that their ends enclose the central white area (see the second bottom row of figures in Figure 3.3), the phenomenon changes. The central white area that is almost or completely enclosed loses its characteristic bright appearance, as seen in the four upper rows of figures in Figure 3.3.

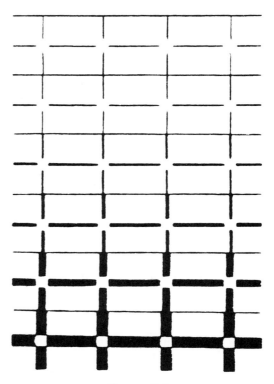

FIGURE 3.3.

3. The brightness of the central area increases up to a certain point not only with increasing thickness of the rays, but also with increasing number of these rays. This can be seen in Figure 3.4 by comparing the patterns having more rays with those having fewer. The numerous lines in the figures on the right of Figure 3.4 together cover the same size area of black as the less numerous, but there are comparatively thicker lines in the figures on the left of Figure 3.4. Nonetheless, the increase in brightness of the central area is greater in the figures on the right.

4. Figure 3.5 shows three brighter areas, next to each other, which are produced by lines having the same area but which are different in geometrical form. The lines or rays of the figure in the middle of Figure 3.5 resemble narrow rectangles, those on the left of the diagram are like thin triangles pointing outwards, and those on the right of the diagram are triangles pointing inwards. A comparison of the figures shows that the radially arranged black areas around the area to be

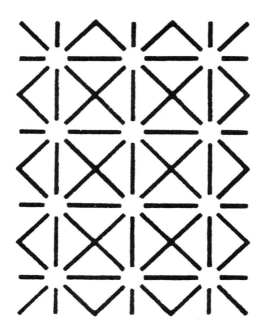

FIGURE 3.2.

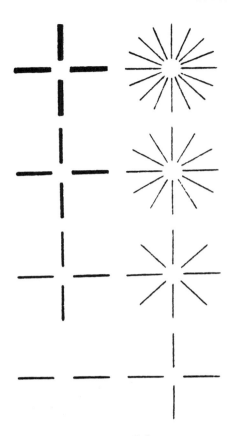

FIGURE 3.4.

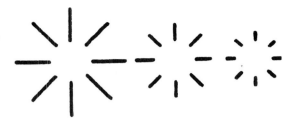

FIGURE 3.6.

As Figure 3.7 shows, the brighter area in the illusion on the left of the diagram disappears when viewed from normal reading distance, because the visual angle subtended by the brighter area is larger than that necessary to induce the illusion. The phenomenon remains with decreasing visual angle even when hair-fine lines are used, with bright areas that are proportionally spotlike and in any case extremely small.

7. The phenomenon is critically dependent on eye movements. If the figures which demonstrate the phenomenon are fixated now and then, with one eye, in the middle of the brighter area, then the illusion disappears completely. This observation, along with other points still to be discussed, shows that Hering's assumption that the brighter appearance is due to simultaneous brightness contrast cannot be correct: steady fixation facilitates brightness contrast, whereas eye movements are detrimental to its occurrence. If Hering's explanation is correct, the phenomenon would become stronger with steady fixation. Instead, we see that it disappears.

brightened have an influence on the strength of the increase of induced brightness within the enclosed central white area. Moreover, the influence of the black lines on inducing the brighter central area quickly decreases with increasing separation.

5. Figure 3.6 shows that the phenomenon is dependent on the length of the rays. The phenomenon disappears in the right of this diagram, because the lines do not have the necessary minimal length to induce the effect.

6. The phenomenon is similarly dependent on the extent (visual angle) of the brighter area.

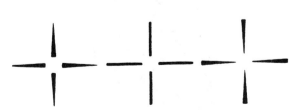

FIGURE 3.5.

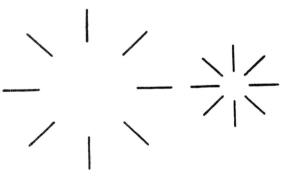

FIGURE 3.7.

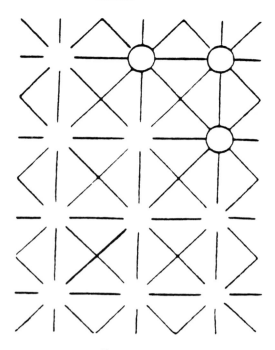

FIGURE 3.8.

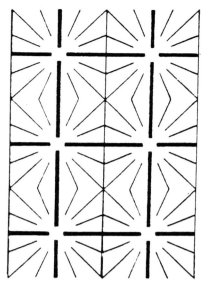

FIGURE 3.9.

8. The fact that the phenomenon can be seen even when extremely fine lines are used, as mentioned above, also speaks against Hering's explanation for the phenomenon in terms of simultaneous contrast.

9. In addition, if brightness contrast did play a role, one would expect the strength of the phenomenon to increase when the brighter area is enclosed by a black circle, as depicted in the upper right corner of Figure 3.8. Instead, the phenomenon again disappears under these conditions of increased contrast.

10. In Figure 3.9, brighter areas are induced by relatively thin lines. In the center of these brighter areas, even brighter smaller areas are induced by thicker lines. In terms of figure–ground phenomenology (Ehrenstein, 1936) this is an example of the induction of the first degree on figures of the second degree as their ground. The ground for the figure of the "second degree" is the white paper.

11. Figures 3.10 and 3.11 show that the phenomenon of brighter areas induced by radial lines also appears as an analogous phenomenon with dark areas, when one uses white lines on black paper, instead of black lines on white paper.

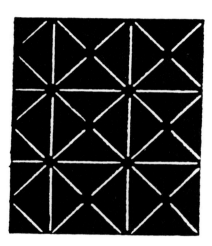

FIGURE 3.10.

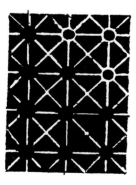

FIGURE 3.11.

Towards an Explanation of the Phenomenon

An explanation of the phenomenon could be sought in the first instance in the simple process of color mixture. Imagine that one of the figures with a brighter area induced by black rays rotates around the center of the brighter area. The black of the lines around the brighter area will be mixed with the white of the paper. Accordingly, the white paper will appear gray, whereas the white of the central area, within which no mixing with black takes place, appears brighter. Even if we do not rotate the figure, it could simply be assumed that the eye moves round in a circle so that the image on the retina would be similarly displaced. However, if the eye moves irregularly in all directions it is still the case that the central white area is crossed less often by black lines, which would cause it to appear gray, than the white area bordering on the brighter circle. It is conceivable that color mixture, produced by irregular eye movements might be considered as the cause of the phenomenon.

This possible explanation also explains why the illusion disappears when very thick lines are used, as well as when the inner central area is enclosed by a circle. In both cases, eye movements cause the central area to be traversed by a black stimulus equally as often as the surrounding white paper. If we assume that the brighter area is induced by relatively thin lines displaced horizontally on the retina, then the brighter central area will be crossed only by the upper or lower ends of the rays which are not horizontal. The larger inner part of the central area remains unaffected by such movements, with the exception of the horizontal rays towards each other. In the case of thick lines, on the other hand, which almost entirely enclose the central area, horizontal retinal movement will cause a black stimulus to cross this central area equally as often as the surrounding white paper. Similarly, this holds for the retinal movement in other directions, not only in the horizontal. If the central area is enclosed by a circle, it will be mixed with black with every direction of retinal movement. This explains the disappearance of the illusion, although contrast effects are enhanced, as was the case when thick lines were used.

The assumption that, due to eye movements, a mixing takes place between the black of the rays and the white of the background provides no difficulties in the light of an experiment by A. Prandtl (1927). Prandtl showed that we can judge the total brightness of hatched areas almost as well as the brightness of black and white sectors, which will merge to gray when rotating the discs.

One difficulty remains, however, for the above explanation: the brightness phenomenon also exists when extremely thin lines are used, which under such mixing conditions should have no significance for the graying of the surrounding field. Other explanations are therefore not to be excluded.

Acknowledgments. The translator gratefully acknowledges the help of Professor L. Spillmann, Dr. T. Troscianko, Dr. N. Wade, and Dr. W. Ehrenstein in the preparation of this translation.

CHAPTER 4

Quasi-Perceptual Margins in Homogeneously Stimulated Fields*

Gaetano Kanizsa (Translated by Walter Gerbino)

Lines and Contours

If one wants to describe the visual world as it appears at a given time, one can simply enumerate and describe the objects located in the perceptual space. This is certainly the most natural and spontaneous description that a naive observer could give. If one adopts a more critical or analytical attitude—without leaving the phenomenological domain—one could describe the very same visual world not as made of objects, but as constituted of a given number of different lines and variously colored surfaces.

When we speak about surfaces, usually we refer to bounded regions of the visual field, to chromatically homogeneous areas adjacent to other homogeneous areas of a different color. A surface is differentiated from an adjacent one to the extent to which it possesses a contour. The presence of a contour is a basic condition for the segmentation of the visual field into extended perceptual units. Therefore, the problem of the phenomenal existence of segregated surfaces, although not coinciding with the problem of the existence of its contours, is so connected with it that the former cannot be solved without also solving the latter.

In fact, some observations by Rubin (1921), Galli and Hochheimer (1934), and Werner (1935) show that the shape of a surface, although not equivalent to the shape of its contours, can be considered a function of it. Phe-

nomenally, a surface exists only in relation to its contour or edge.

As a consequence, the study of contours has an important role in the solution of some central problems of visual perception, namely, the phenomenal genesis of chromatic surfaces, the segmentation and articulation of the visual world into stable and ordered perceptual units, and the formation of solid objects.

We must distinguish contours, which correspond to borders separating two differently colored surfaces, from simple lines, which cross a homogeneously colored region. Geometrically, the latter too may be considered to be thin surfaces bounded by two parallel borders. Phenomenally, however, they exist not as surfaces but as wires, in which the border character prevails over the surface character. Something similar happens to a point that, although physically a surface, is perceived as unextended.

When it is closed, a line segments the visual field and delimits a portion of it; hence, the visual field becomes divided into an inner region and an outer region. In this case, it frequently happens that one loses the distinction between a true contour and an outline contour. A closed line is frequently perceived as the contour of the inner region, which consequently acquires not only a shape, but also a specific function (i.e., a figural character, with respect to the groundlike character of the outer region) and specific material properties (i.e., texture, brightness, and cohesiveness).

If we analyze the stimulus conditions that give rise to the phenomenal appearance of either a contour or a line, we can ascertain that

* Translated by permission from Kanizsa G: Margini. Quasi-percettivi in campi con stimolazione omogenea. *Rivista di Psicologia* 1955; 49: 7–30. © by Giunti-Barbéra, Firenze, Italy.

the presence of some discontinuity or heterogeneity is a necessary condition.

Normally, phenomenal contours or lines correspond to abrupt, steplike variations in the distribution of either intensity or spectral composition of the light stimulating the retina (Bartley, 1941; Kanizsa, 1954; Kardos, 1934; Koffka & Harrower, 1931; Liebmann, 1927; Mach, 1886; MacLeod, 1947). However, the phenomenology of vision reveals several situations that do not allow us to exhaust the problem of contour formation simply by this psychophysical statement.

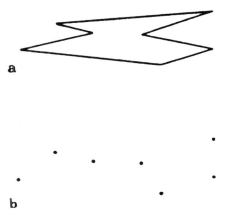

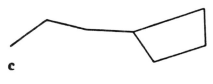

FIGURE 4.2.

Virtual Lines

First of all, it is well-known that very special kinds of lines exist—so-called "virtual lines"— that do not correspond to any stimulus discontinuity.

The dots of Figure 4.1 are spontaneously grouped into two configurations with a well-defined shape. We perceive them in Figure 4.1a as connected by an open curved line, in Figure 4.1b as connected by a closed sequence of three straight segments. These virtual lines run from each dot to the other and cross homogeneously stimulated regions. Although we cannot say that we see them in the literal sense, they are phenomenally present and far more real than merely imagined or thought connections.

This distinction is worth emphasizing. There is a substantial difference between virtual lines connecting a dot pattern and all lines thought as

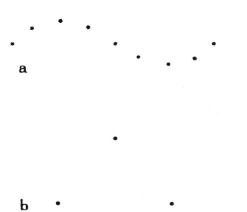

FIGURE 4.1.

geometrically possible interpolations. In order to realize this point, let us remember that we can think of many linear paths connecting dots of Figure 4.1a. They are possible only in an abstract sense, because they are far from possessing the perceived requiredness and compellingness of the curved virtual line.

The same fact is demonstrated, even more clearly, by an example by Hertz (1929). The seven stars of the Big Dipper shown in Figure 4.2b can be mentally connected in many ways, for example as in Figure 4.2a; but the familiar solution depicted in Figure 4.2c is what coercively imposed itself over centuries upon people and astronomers of different countries, as well as upon the child that looks at the sky for the very first time.

Analogously, four dots equally spaced on a hypothetical circumference are perceived as unified into a virtual square; it is possible to think of the circle circumscribing the square, but it is very hard to "see" it. If we regularly add other dots, as shown in Figure 4.3, a limit is reached where it becomes impossible to perceive a polygon, and a circular connection imposes itself. After this limit, one can imagine a

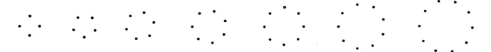

FIGURE 4.3.

polygonal straight connection, but not experience it.

If one actually draws the straight segments between the stars of the Big Dipper or between the dots located on the circumference, we merely enhance some connections that *already exist,* as Metzger (1936) properly noticed referring to these figures. I will call virtual lines only those connections that are perceptually experienced.

What factors generate these virtual lines, which may be considered as lying between really perceived and merely thought lines? They are the result of unification processes, which follow the general principles of figural grouping discovered by Wertheimer (1923) just by using dot patterns. It would be easy to show that they occur between some specific dots but not between others, because the former but not the latter instantiate those conditions of proximity, similarity, good continuation, and closure that represent the organizational factors of our visual experience.

Such an interpretation can be applied also to other instances of *phenomenal doubling,* which occurs whenever two phenomenal dimensions come to correspond to a single stimulus dimension. The most common instance of phenomenal doubling is figure/ground articulation, where the ground is psychologically present behind the figure, even in the absence of any modal property. For this reason, such a presence has been recently called *amodal* by Michotte (1954).

However, more than the general phenomenon of figure/ground articulation, some particular instances of it seem relevant to this research. Figure 4.4a (slightly modified from Koffka, 1935) can be perceived as a single rather irregular shape or, more easily, as two partially overlapping identical shapes. When the second outcome occurs, the inner black area appears to be divided by borders not corresponding to any stimulus discontinuity.

The unifying forces produced by the uniform stimulation of the black area are counterbalanced by the segregating forces generated by the tendency towards the formation of shapes that are "better"—i.e., more symmetrical and balanced—than the single homogeneous shape. The same occurs in Figure 4.4b. Unlike common figure/ground situations, here one observes something more than mere amodal continuation of the background figure; i.e., one perceives the foreground figure as having a complete contour, even where there is no stimulus discontinuity.

A similar situation is shown in Figure 4.5, one that I observed when studying the influence of marginal gradients on the mode-of-appearance of color (Kanizsa, 1954). Many subjects see a cross completing itself in front of the square. Hence, the central, physically homogeneous,

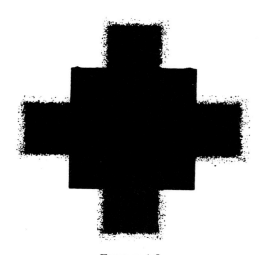

FIGURE 4.5.

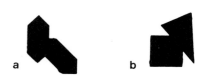

FIGURE 4.4.

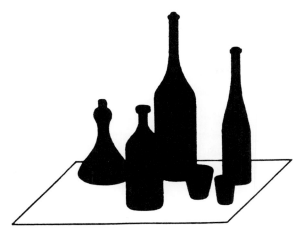

FIGURE 4.6.

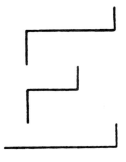

FIGURE 4.7.

region is phenomenally segmented into five zones divided by a fuzzy border.

As shown in Figure 4.6, the effect is greatly facilitated if past experience interacts with other organizing factors. Past experience is active also in Figure 4.7, in reference to which Brunswik (1935) coined the term *empirical Gestalt*.

Segmentation of homogeneous fields and the phenomenal genesis of virtual borders are strongly favored by motion, which is one of the most effective factors structuring our perceptual world (Musatti, 1937). Studying conditions for apparent rest, Metelli (1940), Praturlon (1947), and Bejor (1947) described several examples where a homogeneous field, in translatory or rotary motion, is segmented into two regions. One region is perceived as still and the other moving, and they appear divided by a border. For instance, when the whole pattern in Figure 4.8a is rotating, only the black bar forming the diameter is seen as moving, on a resting ground made of a white circle and a black ring; in this way, the central part separates itself from the peripheral one. Analogously, when the whole black region depicted in Figure 4.8b slides horizontally behind the rectangular window, one perceives as moving only a small vertical bar that disconnects itself from the resting black/white ground.

These borders described by Metelli (1940), which are purely due to the kinetic factor, are as compelling as those observed in the screen-effect (Michotte, 1950), in the tunnel-effect (Sampaio, 1943), and in the so-called Rosenbach effect (Rosenbach, 1902), recently studied by Glynn (1954).

Quasi-Perceptual Margins

These phenomena seem to demonstrate the existence of contours and lines which do not have, as normally occurs, a counterpart in a stimulus discontinuity. They arise as a consequence of translocal tensions in the visual field, and occupy, as far as their phenomenal presence is concerned, an intermediate place between

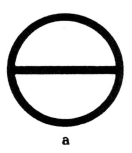

a

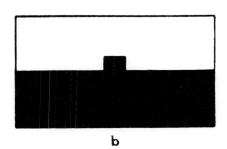

b

FIGURE 4.8.

merely imagined lines and those perceived as actually real.

What about the existence of other instances between these two extremes? How could the degree of perceptual salience of virtual lines be increased? Can one create conditions where amodal presence becomes modal presence? In other words, when stimulation is completely homogeneous, can one find margins that approximate, or even equate, the perceptual effectiveness of a true physical contour?

I will now present some stimulus configurations that seem to allow a positive answer to these questions.

More than 50 years ago Schumann (1900), in a paper on visual perception, observed: "These margins do not emerge only when two differently colored areas come into contact; under favorable conditions, they can emerge also in areas that are objectively colored in a totally homogeneous way" (p. 14). In order to support his statement, Schumann showed Figure 4.9 and remarked that, at the center, one can see a white rectangle with margins that cross homogeneously stimulated zones. He added: "Nevertheless, under favorable conditions I have been able to generate only straight and never curvilinear margins."

Curiously enough, this phenomenon captured my attention for the first time when I, unaware of Schumann's work, observed Figure 4.10, where a clear circular margin appears. Since then, I have found no particular difficulty in generating other compelling curvilinear margins.

In my opinion, the notably high degree of perceptual presence distinguishes these phenomena not only from merely thought margins but also from virtual lines. For instance, let us con-

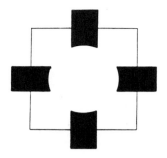

FIGURE 4.10.

sider Figure 4.11, where, according to a geometrical description, there are only three black sectors and three outline corners symmetrically located on a completely uniform white ground. However, all observers clearly see a white triangle upon an outline triangle and three black disks; furthermore, several of them claim that they could not discriminate the foreground figure from a triangular piece of paper glued on the background.

The modal character of these margins—i.e., the fact that they may be confused with the effects of stimulus discontinuities—makes them different from virtual lines, whose perceptual presence has only an amodal character.

These margins can acquire a quasi-perceptual or, for some subjects, a wholly perceptual character, supported by the fact that the central region subjectively undergoes a strong transformation in its brightness and hue. This looks like a paradoxical case of color contrast which I will discuss later on. Let us consider some other situations, that can help in identifying the causal conditions of the phenomenon. In Figure 4.12, which represents the negative version of Figure 4.11, the foreground triangle is much

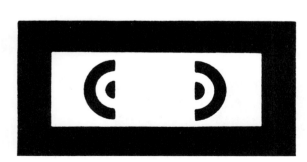

FIGURE 4.9.

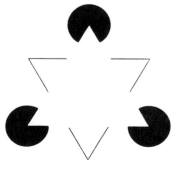

FIGURE 4.11.

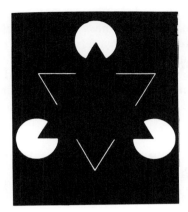

FIGURE 4.12.

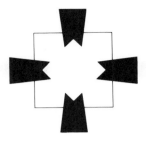

FIGURE 4.14. The color plate of this figure can be found on the color insert on page xv.

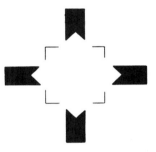

FIGURE 4.15.

blacker than the ground. Let us compare the clarity and compellingness of its margins with those of margins observed in Figures 4.4 and 4.6, and realize that segmentation and stratification of the black surface are here (Fig. 4.12) quite vivid indeed, and possess a more real character.

In Figure 4.13, the same configuration is modified in order to reduce to a minimum the number of physical borders of the foreground triangle. The effect, although diminished in its intensity, is still there.

For the sake of economy, I present only one colored plate (Fig. 4.14; see color plate of this figure on page xv), which is sufficient to show that chromatic displays are as effective as black and white displays, regarding the occurrence of quasi-perceptual margins (see Fig. 4.15).

An appropriate configuration of inducing elements allows us to multiply figural layers and to obtain several margins on different depth levels (see Fig. 4.16). Figure 4.17 illustrates that curvilinear quasi-perceptual margins are, contrary to Schumann's opinion, as easy to obtain as straight ones.

Figure 4.18 reproduces, with some modifications, a situation utilized by Matthaei (1929) to argue against a merely summative theory of brightness contrast.

In Figure 4.19, borrowed from Ehrenstein (1942), the white disks stand out, extraordinarily brighter than the ground, over the crossings

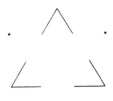

FIGURE 4.13.

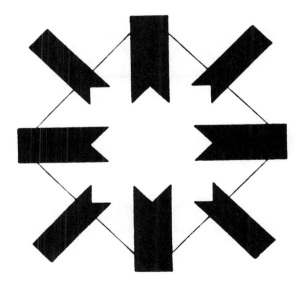

FIGURE 4.16.

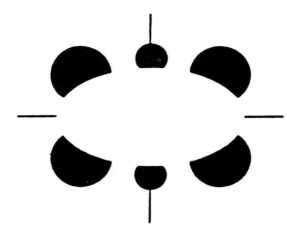

FIGURE 4.17.

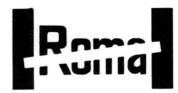

FIGURE 4.18.

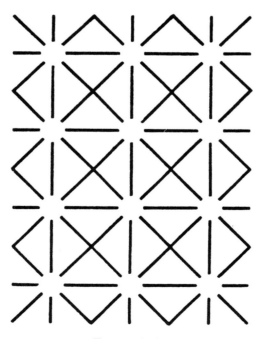

FIGURE 4.19.

of the black grating. Ehrenstein focuses his attention on the brightness effect, which would also represent to him a falsification of Hering's traditional theory of simultaneous contrast, and neglects both figural stratification and margin formation, which are particularly clear in this situation.

Quasi-Perceptual Margins: Properties and Causal Factors

The phenomenal properties common to all of the above stimulus configurations are:

a) In a particular region of the visual field, transformations of brightness and/or mode-of-appearance occur that phenomenally distinguish that region from contiguous regions, even though stimulation from all regions is the same.

b) Phenomenally, the region undergoes a displacement in the third dimension, and is seen as situated in front of or over the rest of the field.

c) The region possesses a more or less clear margin, which separates it from the contiguous areas, and also crosses regions where there is no quantitative or qualitative change in the stimulation.

d) When conditions are optimal, all above interconnected phenomenal aspects (chromatic transformation, displacement in the third dimension, presence of the margin) are compelling and acquire a modal character that distinguishes them from the perception of merely virtual lines.

If one examines these situations with the aim of singling out the factors that determine the segmentation of an objectively homogeneous field into phenomenally different regions, one may notice that a specific condition is always present. This is the existence of elements that, by themselves, are not perfectly regular, and require some completion in order to achieve regularity. By completion, the inducing elements can transform themselves into stable, ordered, symmetrical, and simpler figures.

The pattern in Figure 4.10 can be objectively described as made of *four* black shapes, almost rectangular apart from a slightly curved side, connected by *four* rectilinear corners. In exceptional cases, highly analytical subjects might describe the pattern in the above way. But the same pattern is normally seen in an entirely different way which is compelling to the majority of subjects: that is, an opaque white disk over a black cross, which in turn is covering an outline square.

With respect to the first, the second perceptual outcome possesses an obvious superiority from the point of view of its simplicity and regularity. The condition for this figural improvement is the possibility of perceiving the central white region as a disk, behind which the four black elements complete themselves in a single cross. Hence the disk, by lying in a different spatial plane, does not "belong" any more to the white ground, and looks separated from it by a sharp edge.

Analogously, in Figure 4.11 the three outline corners exhibit a strong tendency towards unifying themselves into an equilateral triangle that represents not only a unitary but also a "better" form with respect to simplicity and internal balance. Furthermore, the three circular sectors acquire stability and *Prägnanz* by completing themselves into three disks. Such a completion, in order to possess an amodal character, necessitates an occluding opaque surface that arises at the expense of the unity of the white region; hence, this region splits into different depth layers along border lines constrained by the given figural conditions.

This analysis can be easily repeated for all other configurations, and suggests the hypothesis that these margins, which arise in the absence of any stimulus discontinuity, are a direct consequence of *stratification,* which in turn is determined by the process of *amodal completion* of some pattern elements.

If this hypothesis is correct, one should be able to demonstrate that, all other conditions being equal, the phenomenon does not occur in the absence of *completion,* just because this is the primary and necessary factor.

In this regard, the two following examples seem to constitute rather convincing evidence. Let us consider the different perceptual outcomes in Figures 4.20 and 4.21. In the first, the prevalent outcome is the stratification of an opaque white rectangle over four black regular octagons. In the second, even perceptually there are only four black crosses on a white ground; in this case, the ground is homogeneous and unitary. Internal corners can be connected by virtual lines enclosing a rectangle,

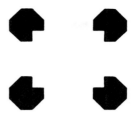

FIGURE 4.20.

but they do not achieve the quasi-perceptual character of the margins of the white rectangle visible in Figure 4.20.

Apparently this is due to the figural properties of black elements which are different in the two patterns. By themselves, crosses are good, balanced, closed shapes, without any need for completion: therefore, the internal corners belong to them and not to the ground which, uninterrupted by any border, continues under the crosses. Conversely, black elements of Figure 4.20 are open, incomplete; only when perceived as partially covered regular octagons they achieve, through this closure, a much higher degree of stability and compactness. By this organization, the internal corners do not belong to black elements, but to a white rectangle that, in order to stand in front of octagons, must detach itself from the ground and acquire its own margins.

A fully analogous argument may be developed for the comparison between Figures 4.22 and 4.23.

This hypothesis is supported also by the results of the following simple demonstration. Instead of steady drawings, one can utilize movable pieces of cardboard on a homogeneous ground, and observe that the quasi-perceptual margins can arise also when the resulting figure is not perfectly regular, provided that summa-

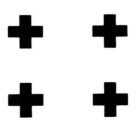

FIGURE 4.21.

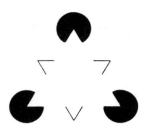

FIGURE 4.22.

tions of incomplete elements are possible. This demonstration simply requires cutting four incomplete shapes, as those of Figure 4.20, out of white cardboard, and arranging them on a perfectly flat black surface. The central black figure promptly emerges, even when the white pieces are not exactly located at the four corners of a rectangle. Furthermore, it is possible to move some or even all pieces within a rather large range without destroying the stratification effect. The black figure strains and deforms itself, showing a resistance that elicits some surprise in the observer; but it does not vanish, unless the pieces are reciprocally displaced too much.

As a general conclusion, I would stress that, in all situations here examined, some incomplete regions "improve" their form by completion. This completion is amodal and occurs behind a nontransparent figure which, as a consequence, is perceptually differentiated from the ground and located on the foreground plane, although the stimulus conditions are perfectly identical for both the figure and the ground. But a figure cannot exist without its margins: hence the necessity of the splitting of

the homogeneously stimulated field and the emergence of quasi-perceptual margins.

These results may contribute to solving some difficulties that Metelli (1940) found when trying to explain the phenomenon of apparent rest in a rotating field. He hypothesized that apparent rest could be a by-product of perceptual completion, but his hypothesis was not in agreement with the fact that completion does occur in kinetic but not in static displays.

Such a difficulty is specific to Metelli's displays, and is removed in the present stimulus configurations in which completion and stratification occur just in static conditions. As a consequence, it seems plausible to propose that both phenomena—apparent rest and quasi-perceptual margins—are due to stratification, which is the way by which forces in the perceptual field reach a better final equilibrium.

However, one can consider another possible explanation, suggested by the remarkable color transformations of the foreground surface. Although there are some differentiations of hue and particularly of mode-of-appearance, the most important change is in regard to brightness. For instance, in Figure 4.11, the foreground triangle looks brighter than the ground. The opposite happens in Figure 4.12.

One may wonder whether this difference in brightness should be considered as a *consequence* of figure formation or, on the contrary, whether it should be considered as its *causal factor*. In fact, one may contrast my previous explanation with the hypothesis that the true factor determining this kind of figural organization is not amodal completion, but an illusory brightness change due to processes of antagonistic color induction. Stratification and quasi-perceptual margins would be only an effect of color transformations, which would constitute the primary phenomenon.

This hypothesis is not supported by some facts, particularly by all cases where brightness modifications occur in a direction opposite to what one should expect on the basis of simultaneous contrast. In Schumann's pattern (Figure 4.9), the white hemi-ring, which is almost completely surrounded by black areas, should undergo a stronger antagonistic induction than the central rectangular region; nevertheless, the latter appears brighter. The same argument ap-

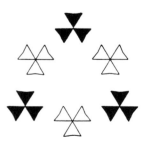

FIGURE 4.23.

plies to Figure 4.18, where the transverse bar, which is coextensive with the white ground at several places, looks brighter than the completely surrounded holes of the letters. And in Figure 4.13, according to this hypothesis, the central resulting triangle should owe its brightness increment to the action of three small black dots, which appears implausible.

Examples may be multiplied, but the previous arguments should suffice in order to reject the hypothesis that contrast is the primary factor determining the phenomenon. Figures 4.20 and 4.21 show that, all conditions for contrast being equal, the formation of a stratified figure occurs only when it is supported by organizational requirements, i.e., when it is necessary to the phenomenal totalizations of incomplete elements of the visual field. Hence, brightness transformations would be dependent upon the particular figural and spatial articulation that, under certain conditions, prevails in the perceptual field.

In my opinion, the phenomena studied in this paper have some interest for theories of chromatic and figural perception, and are worthy of further investigation.

1986 Addendum

At the time of the writing of this paper, I considered the phenomenon of illusory contours and surfaces as beautiful proof of the existence of a tendency towards Prägnanz in the segmentation of the perceptual world, which is one of the most fascinating hypotheses of Gestalt theory. The emergence of illusory contours seemed to me a consequence of such hypothesized tendency, because amodal completion of gaps or missing parts in the inducing elements allowed the formation of simpler, more regular, more prägnant units. I naively reinforced this belief by using as inducing elements only figures that could become regular through completion (truncated disks, triangles, or hexagons). Later on, empirical evidence forced me to modify my interpretation (Kanizsa 1974). In fact, one can obtain good illusory figures by using inducing elements that do not become regular forms through completion. Therefore, I have abandoned the hypothesis that a tendency towards maximal regularity is a causal factor in the genesis of illusory figures. By the way, I am now convinced that such a tendency towards regularization of the visual field does not exist in general (Kanizsa, 1975; Kanizsa and Luccio, 1986).

SECTION II
Theoretical Analyses

Theories have been developed to explain illusory contours to an unusually great degree. In
this section, the authors present discussions of
the major theoretical accounts of illusory contours.

Chapter 5, by Day, presents a new approach
to illusory contours and object perception in
general. Going beyond his earlier work and including data from a wide variety of sources,
Day proposes a treatment of illusory contours
as possessing the relevant cues for edge perception.

In Chapter 6, Rock presents a detailed analysis of illusory contours as prime examples
of hypothesis testing mechanisms in perceptions.

Written from a Gestalt framework, Minguzzi's Chapter 7 presents an extension and modification of this approach. He emphasizes the role
of amodal continuation rather than completion
of illusory contour-inducing elements.

In Chapter 8, Parks questions the relationship
between illusory contours and picture perception. Writing from a cognitive perspective, he
also discusses the role of cognitive mechanisms
in illusory contour perception.

The final chapter in this section, Chapter 9,
by Gregory, also analyzes illusory contours
from a cognitive point of view. Gregory
presents here a new characterization of illusory
contours based on rule-generating perceptual
processes, which he calls an Algovist approach.

CHAPTER 5

Cues for Edge and the Origin of Illusory Contours: An Alternative Approach

Ross H. Day

Introduction

In perception objects are characterized by numerous properties, including surfaces and edges, texture and pattern, solidity and depth, and lightness and color. They can also be characterized by opacity, translucency, or transparency. These properties are signaled by what in accord with traditional usage can be called cues. Thus object depth is signaled by retinal disparity, motion parallax, vergence and accommodation, and various "pictorial" cues such as linear perspective, overlay, and elevation in the visual field. Of greatest relevance here is the contrivance of cues by various forms of artifice to convey the *appearance* of an object property where none exists physically. For example, retinal disparity can be contrived by means of two-dimensional stereograms viewed in a stereoscope. The outcome in perception is a compelling appearance of depth when none is present in the distal stimulus array. Similarly, linear perspective and overlay can be effectively contrived by means of drawing and photography to convey the appearance of depth in pictures and photographs.

The central thesis of this chapter is that edges are also correlated with specific features of the stimulus array. These will be called *edge cues*. It is proposed that these cues can also be contrived artificially, with the result that edges can occur in perception where none exist in reality. In short, illusory contours, like illusory depth, occur when the cues which are normally correlated with real edges are contrived by artificial means. It is also proposed that other object properties including form, transparency, and

movement are associated with cues which can be produced independently of the physical properties themselves. In such circumstances these properties are perceived when they are not present in the stimulus pattern. From this standpoint illusory contours are regarded as instances of a broad class of perceptual effects which emerge when one or more of the cues that normally signal an object property are generated by artifice.

It is to be noted that this interpretation of illusory contours in terms of cues for edge is a marked departure from that proposed earlier (Day, 1986; Day & Jory, 1978) primarily in terms of the spread of induced brightness to partially delineated borders. It is therefore appropriate first to outline this earlier explanation and to describe the observations which led to its rejection and its replacement by that set out here.

Illusory Contours and the Spread of Induced Brightness and Color

Three experiments (Day, 1983; Day & Jory, 1980; Jory & Day, 1979) led to the development and consolidation of a theory of illusory contours based on differences in induced brightness between regions of uniform luminance separated by partially delineated, i.e., discontinuous, borders. These borders can be composed of the ends of lines, regularly or irregularly spaced elements, sections of real edges, or combinations of these elements. The central feature of the explanation is that the stimulus pattern induces changes in perceived brightness. These changes may take the form of enhanced brightness or darkness such as simultaneous brightness contrast and line-end contrast, or reduced brightness or darkness as with assimilation of brightness. The induced effects spread more or less evenly to incompletely delineated borders. The illusory contours form along these borders when brightness is either enhanced or reduced in the regions on either side of the border. They are particularly compelling when enhancement occurs on one side of the border and reduction on the other.

In these terms illusory contours are the outcome of step-function differences in brightness when the differences occur in consequence of brightness induction rather than in consequence of luminance changes. Since essentially similar induced effects occur for color, illusory contours due to color differences or to a combination of color and brightness differences can also

form. Simultaneous brightness and color contrast, line-end contrast (which may be a special case of the first), and brightness and color assimilation can be demonstrated independently of illusory contours and have for long been subjects of independent experimental enquiry (see Day, 1986; Day & Jory, 1978). The spreading effect has also been demonstrated independently.

This explanation was based mainly on the outcome of three separate sets of observations. The first (Jory & Day, 1979) involved eight stimulus figures similar to those of Kanizsa (1955) and Ehrenstein (1954), shown in Figure 5.1. These were constructed from Munsell papers so that for half (two of each figure) there was a difference in Munsell value between the figure and its ground and for the other half no difference. Thus for four figures there was a difference in hue and brightness between figure and ground and for the other four a difference in hue only. One group of subjects rated the

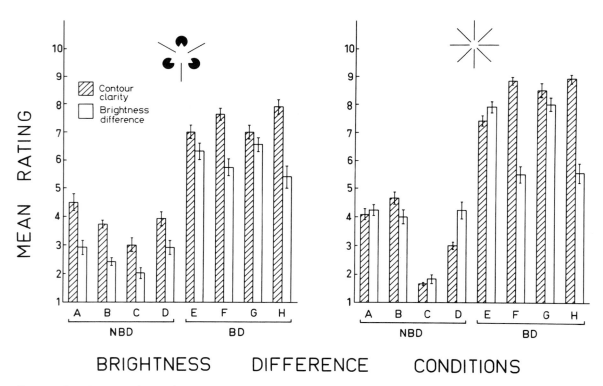

FIGURE 5.1. Mean ratings of the clarity of illusory contours and the differences in brightness on either side of them in the Kanizsa and Ehrenstein figures with a difference in Munsell value (brightness) between the figure and its background (BD) and no differences (NDB). From Jory & Day (1979), with permission.

strength of the illusory contour in the two figures and another the brightness difference induced between the region within the illusory contour and that of the same luminance surrounding it. The results, which are summarized in Figure 5.1, were clear in showing that the strength of the contours in each figure and the degree of induced brightness were in close accord. This outcome was taken to indicate that the spread of induced brightness is strongly implicated in the generation of the contours around the region in which induction occurs.

The second set of observations involved a crosslike figure originally reported by Koffka (1935) and shown in Figure 5.2. Landauer (1978) pointed out that at the center of this figure there is a diffuse, roughly circular region of enhanced brightness. This is presumably due to line-end contrast generated by the inner ends of

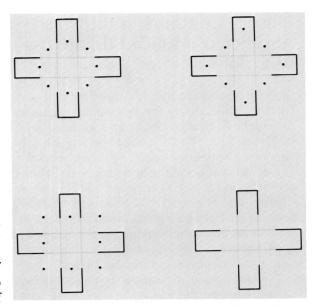

FIGURE 5.3. A version of the van Tuijl spreading effect. The light gray of the thin lines spreads to the square, diamond, and circular regions partially delineated by eight dots. From Day (1983), with permission.

the four pairs of lines making up the arms of the cross. Day and Jory (1980) showed that if the borders of a square, a diamond, or a circle are partially delineated by either four or eight dots, illusory contours coincident with these borders are clearly discernible. The contours, which can be seen in Figure 5.2, do not occur when the same shapes are partially delineated by very short lines in the absence of the crosslike figure.

Van Tuijl (1975) described a curious color effect occurring in line patterns in which sections of the lines are colored. Day (1983) showed that this so-called neon-color spreading also gives rise to illusory contours along partially delineated borders in the Koffka cross. These contours can be seen in Figure 5.3, in which the van Tuijl effect is generated by thin, light-gray lines instead of by colored lines.

Together these three observations were interpreted as indicating that the spread of induced brightness and color to incomplete borders is the primary determinant of illusory contours. More recent data showing that illusory contours occur in the absence of induced brightness or color and that they are stronger in figures with apparent depth are not consistent with this interpretation.

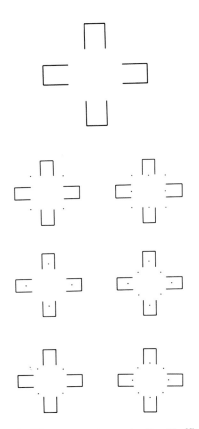

FIGURE 5.2. Illusory contours in the Koffka figure from the spread of line-end contrast and assimilation of brightness to borders partially delineated by either four or eight dots. From Day & Jory (1980), with permission.

Illusory Contours in the Absence of Induced Brightness or Color

Illusory contours are visible along the diagonal borders delineated by the right-angle corners of the regularly arranged black and white squares in Figure 5.4A. There is a compelling impression of a continuous edge coincident with the line of the corners along both diagonals. These contours were first noticed by chance when Crassini and Broese (1983) presented a similar figure as part of a paper concerned with perceptual alternation in ambiguous figures. Kennedy and Chatterway (1975) had earlier drawn attention to these contours in Figure 5.4B.

The main point of interest in these illusory contours is that there is no reason to suppose that there is an induced brightness difference between the regions on either side of the borders delineated by the right angles. This is not to claim that there are no induced brightness effects in Figures 5.4A and 5.4B. There quite probably are. Localized enhancement of brightness is likely to be generated at the corners themselves, a special instance of line-end contrast, and reduction of brightness due to assimilation is likely in the interspaces between both the black and the white squares. Both effects could be expected to spread and respectively to increase and decrease brightness in the interspaces. However, in neither case would a *difference* in brightness on either side of the diagonal line defined by the corners be expected.

A   B

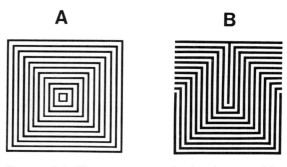

FIGURE 5.4. Illusory contours in the absence of induced brightness or color. The contours occur only on the diagonals marked by apexes of the right angles. Figure 5.4B after Kennedy & Chatterway (1975), with permission.

However, there is another possible basis for a difference in brightness. It is known that blurring of edges can result from regular astigmatism. If this is so then, as Wade and Day (1978) have pointed out, focusing on lines in one orientation would render those orthogonal to them blurred. As a result, black and white bars in one orientation in Figure 5.4 would appear grayer than those at right angle to them. Color difference between the two orientations would also be likely to occur due to chromatic aberration. In other words, differences in brightness and color between the horizontal and vertical bars in the two figures in Figure 5.4 could conceivably occur in consequence of regular astigmatism. That this is unlikely can be demonstrated by the occurrence of illusory contours of about the same strength when the figures are rotated through 45° so that the black and white lines are diagonally oriented. Blurring due to astigmatism is uncommon for oblique orientations. Yet all observers shown Figure 5.4A with the bars obliquely oriented reported illusory contours as strong as those with the bars in the vertical and horizontal axes.

In summary, the strong illusory contours in Figures 5.4A and 5.4B cannot be attributed to differences in either brightness or color due to induction or to aberrations in the optical system of the eye.

Illusory Contours and Apparent Depth

Two groups of experiments (Day & Kasperczyk, 1983a, 1983b) have shown that illusory contours are consistently stronger in figures with apparent depth due to overlay or linear perspective than in those that are without such cues. The first group of experiments were designed to test Kanizsa's (1979) claim that illusory contours form around figural regions that are apparently separated in depth from the rest of the figure due to overlay. Day and Kasperczyk (1983a) used two of Kanizsa's figures (Figs. 5.5C and 5.5F). According to Kanizsa's argument perceptual completion of the incomplete octagons and crosses in Figure 5.5C would because of overlay give rise to "layering" of the white rectangle with the consequent formation of illusory contours around it. Since in Figure

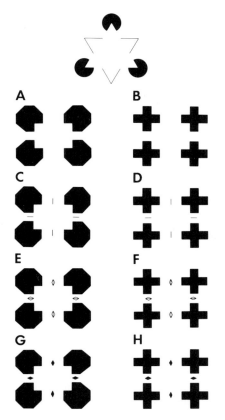

FIGURE 5.5. Illusory contours in Kanizsa's figures formed from perceptually complete (crosses and diamonds) and incomplete (incomplete octagons and short lines) corner and side elements. Figures 5.5C and 5.5F are Kanizsa's (1979) original figures. From Day & Kasperczyk (1983a), with permission.

lay is evident. In short, illusory contours were clearly present in figures without apparent separation in depth due to overlay and present but consistently stronger in those with simulated overlay.

In a later experiment Day and Kasperczyk (1983b) produced an appearance of depth in a line pattern by means of simulated overlay and linear perceptive (see Figure 5.6D). Subjects estimated the strength of illusory contour along a border that was partially delineated by the ends of the lines forming the figure. The results indicated that illusory contours along the border in the form of an "outside" corner due to simulated perspective were as strong as one along a similarly delineated edge due to overlay. An illusory contour along a border in the form of an "inside" corner due to both perspective *and* overlay was stronger than one along a border due to either of these cues alone.

Illusory Contours and Cues for Edge

It is clear from the experiments briefly reviewed in the last two sections that illusory contours occur and do so quite strongly and consistently in the absence of either brightness or color. Moreover, whereas illusory contours occur along partially delineated borders in figures without apparent depth they do so consistently more weakly than in figures with it (Day & Kasperczyk, 1983a). Contours in line patterns in which apparent depth is attributable to both overlay and perspective are stronger than in patterns in which it is due to either of these cues alone (Day & Kasperczyk, 1983b). An alternative interpretation in terms of cues for edge is therefore proposed.

Cues for Edge

Various features of the physical stimulus array are correlated with the perception of edges. For the most part these cues are in the form of sudden, i.e., step-function, changes in object properties. These properties include luminance, color, regular and irregular texture density, and depth (as with ridges and the corners of three-dimensional objects). Movement of one part of

5.5F the elements (crosses and diamonds) are complete in themselves, neither depth separation nor illusory contours would be expected. As can be seen in Figure 5.5, the completeness of the corner and side elements was systematically varied. Subjects estimated the strength of the illusory contours around the white rectangle relative to those around the Kanizsa triangle which is uppermost in Figure 5.5.

The results of this and subsequent experiments in the series showed that illusory contours consistently occur in figures like Figure 5.5F in which the elements are complete and in which therefore there should be no simulated overlay. However, the illusory contours around the white rectangles were consistently stronger in figures like Figure 5.5C in which the elements were incomplete and in which simulated over-

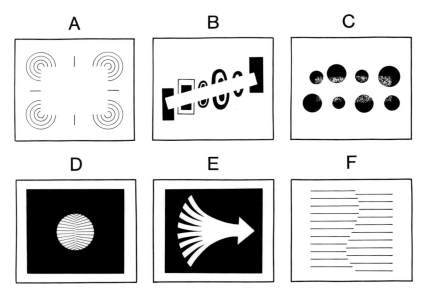

FIGURE 5.6. Illusory contours from different combinations of cues for two- and three-dimensional edges. See text. Figures A, B, C, and F are from Karizsa (1979), D from Day and Kasperczyk (1983b), and E from Kennedy (1979), with permission.

an otherwise edgeless region also gives rise to the perception of edges.

It is proposed that when one or more of these edge cues is artificially contrived in the absence of real edges, *apparent* edges, i.e., illusory contours, occur. It is now suggested that change in brightness and hue by induction is simply *one* such contrivance. Before setting out this reinterpretation it is necessary first briefly to identify some of those properties of the stimulus array that are correlated with the perception of edges in the real world.

Edges occur in surfaces and in depth. For convenience these will be referred to as two- and three-dimensional edges. In both cases the perceived edge is correlated with a step-function change in a spatially extended object property. For two-dimensional edges such changes occur in luminance, color, and texture. For three-dimensional edges the step-function changes occur in respect to the direction and relative depth of surfaces. For example, a step-function change in luminance on a surface gives rise to a dark-light edge and a change in the direction of surfaces in depth to an inside corner. Both classes of edge may involve more than one step-function change. Thus a two-dimensional edge may derive from abrupt changes in both luminance and texture density.

Likewise, a three-dimensional edge may derive from changes in the orientation of surfaces and in luminance, as when a dark wall meets a light one at a corner.

It is emphasized that whereas it is possible to name some of the more obvious stimulus correlates of two- and three-dimensional edges, a more exhaustive treatment than can be given here would be necessary to identify all of them, in particular those involving relative movement of parts of the figure.

Artificial Cues and Illusory Contours

Some cues for two- and three-dimensional edges can be generated in the absence of real physical edges. When cues are so contrived, observers experience edges that cannot be detected independently of vision. Visual edges generated in this way are called variously illusory, subjective, or anomalous contours. Artificial contrivance of edges is well illustrated in Figure 5.6A taken from Kanizsa (1979). First, there is a discontinuous edge formed by the ends of circular and straight lines and this forms a rectangle. In addition, a step-function change in brightness is produced along this discontinuous edge by means of assimilation of brightness between the circular lines and line-end contrast at the ends of the circular and straight lines. Both effects spread to the discontinuous, i.e., partially delineated, boundary (Day & Jory, 1978). Finally, overlay is simulated by means of the incomplete circles and the incomplete cross. Thus a step-function difference in brightness is added to the discontinuous edge by means of two forms of induction, and the rectangle has the appearance of overlaying complete elements. The outcome is a compelling, apparently continuous edge around the bright rectangle.

The contrivance of these and other cues to edge is illustrated in Figures 5.6B–5.6F. In Figure 5.6B (Kanizsa, 1979) simultaneous contrast is induced and spreads to the discontinuous edge of the apparently overlaying strip. In Figure 5.6C (Kanizsa, 1979) an abrupt change in texture is added to that of brightness from simultaneous brightness contrast in the apparently overlaying rectangle. The basis of the illusory contour in Figure 5.6D (Day & Kasperczyk, 1983b) is a discontinuous edge from vertically displaced line-ends together with simulated perspective producing the appearance of a ridge. In this case, as in the two figures in Figure 5.4, there is no reason to suppose that a brightness difference occurs at the discontinuous border. The contour in Figure 5.6E (Kennedy, 1979) is attributable to assimilation of brightness in the splayed elements of the tail of the figure and line-end contrast at the ends of the pointed black interspaces of the splayed elements. This figure is of special interest since there are no cues for depth. Thus the illusory contour along the pointed ends of the tail region is presumably due to the induced brightness effects spreading to the discontinuous border formed by the pointed ends of the black interspaces. Likewise, there are no cues for depth in Figure 5.6E (Kanizsa, 1979). Nor is there any reason to expect a step-function brightness difference at the discontinuous edge. The illusory contour must therefore be due to other discontinuities, presumably the ends of the lines themselves and their lateral displacement. Both of these, it is interesting to note, are spatial discontinuities.

Two rather speculative issues are worth raising. They concern cue "saliency" and the effect of multiple-edge cues in generating illusory contours. As far as is known, perceived edges

have not previously been conceived of in terms of cues for edge. It is therefore not surprising that there are no data concerning the relative saliency of the cues. Casual inspection of Figure 5.6 does suggest that the discontinuous edge from vertically displaced line-ends (Fig. 5.6F) produces an illusory contour as compelling as one from assimilation of brightness, line-end contrast, and overlay (Fig. 5.6A). The issue of edge-cue salience deserves closer attention. Second, the experiments reported by Day and Kaspercyzk (1983a, 1983b) showed that whereas illusory contours are present in two-dimensional figures they are stronger when simulated depth is added. There is also a need for a more systematic examination of the strength of illusory contours as a function of the number of two- and three-dimension edge cues.

Illusory Contours as a Member of a Class of Perceptual Effects

Illusory contours can be regarded as instances of a broad class of perceptual phenomena that occur when one or more stimulus correlates, i.e., cues, are artificially contrived. Other members of this class include illusory depth, illusory form, illusory (apparent) movement, and illusory transparency. There are no doubt many other examples. Since it is considered important to remove illusory contours from the state of splendid isolation which they have so far enjoyed and place them in the company to which they rightfully belong, some consideration of the company is relevant.

The term *cue* is most commonly associated with the perception of depth and distance and includes oculomotor, binocular, and "pictorial" correlates of absolute and relative distance (see Sekuler & Blake, 1985 for a detailed description). Any, some, or all of these correlates when synthesized in the absence of real depth will convey an impression of depth, i.e., of illusory depth. Illusory impressions in a picture or by means of stereoscopic presentation of equidistant stereograms are cases in point. The artform called *trompe l'oeil* is particularly notable in this regard.

No equivalent analysis has been made of the correlates of form. The instantaneous perception of an object or a person, including a particular person, in a cartoon suggests that outline, prominent features, and shading are involved. Johansson (1973, 1975) has shown in his well-known demonstrations that points of light attached to a person are not perceived as a recognizable form when the person is stationary. They are almost immediately recognizable as a human form when the person engages in an activity such as walking or dancing. That is to say, a recognizable human form emerges when the points of light move together in the characteristic fashion of the body parts to which they are attached. It is therefore possible to conclude that the dynamic relationships between moving parts constitute a cue to form and that when these are presented alone, i.e., in the absence of the form itself, a form is perceived. The effect lends itself to computer simulation.

In another series of well-known demonstrations Metelli (1974a, 1974b) has shown that the perception of transparency—the perception of one surface seen through another—is marked by specifiable stimulus correlates. When these are synthesized on a single surface a strong impression of one surface seen through another occurs. Kanizsa has made the point that "physical transparency is not a necessary condition for the occurrence of a strong visual impression of transparency. Indeed, it is quite simple to arrange things so that an entirely opaque surface will be experienced as obviously transparent" (Kanizsa, 1979, p. 155).

The last example is more speculative and is bound therefore to be more controversial. A compelling impression of movement occurs when two or more spatially separated elements, usually points of light, are presented sequentially. Under specified conditions of duration and interval between the presentation of each element, a single moving element is perceived. Recent evidence (Barbur, 1981) suggests that motion perceived when one element actually moves and when one is presented after another in a different position are indistinguishable. It is suggested that the occurrence of a stimulus element in two or more discriminably different spatial locations is among the stimulus correlates of movement. When this correlate is contrived by presenting two elements one after the other in different locations, movement of a single element is experienced.

The point to be made is that there is a variety of perceptual experiences of states of affairs in the real world that are signaled by specific stimulus features. When some or all of these features—stimulus correlates or cues—are synthetically produced in the absence of the states of affairs which normally give rise to them, that state of affairs—edges, depth, form, transparency, movement—is experienced. Since the experiences occur as a result of artifice in the absence of the actual situations which normally trigger them the term *illusory* can appropriately be applied. Thus illusory contours, the subject of a now considerable body of recent research, are no different *in principle* from various other illusory effects which have not so far been considered as related. The common thread is the synthesis of those proximal stimuli that normally signal object properties—edges, depth, form, transparency, movement—in the absence of the physical properties themselves.

Concluding Comments

In concluding this approach to illusory contours in terms of artificially contrived cues for edge, three issues deserve comment. These are the appearance of illusory contours, the processes associated with them, and, more broadly, the point of studying them.

The Appearance of Illusory Contours

It is relevant to note Metelli's (1982) call for careful phenomenological description of perceptual effects. He has pointed out that, leaving aside the importance of such description for contemporary Gestalt theory, particularly in regard to the isomorphic hypothesis, phenomenological observation provides the data that are the main object of perceptual research. Such observation of illusory contours reveals two features that deserve close consideration. First, contours in different patterns are often different in appearance. For example, those in Figure 5.6A around the rectangle are characterized by a difference in brightness between the bright rectangle and the less bright background. No such difference marks the nevertheless strong contours along the discontinuous, diagonal edges defined by the regularly spaced corners in Figures 5.4a and 5.4B. In Figure 5.3 the contours surround areas which have the appearance of transparency. It was observations of this kind that suggested that different stimulus features can alone or together give rise to the perception of edges.

Second, illusory contours have a somewhat "unreal" appearance and seem less stable in perception than real edges. With sustained inspection they frequently waver and disappear. This unreal character is not unlike that of other artificially contrived properties. For example, apparent depth in stereoscopic displays often appears oddly static, with human forms resembling cardboard cutouts rather than solid figures. This appearance may well be due to the absence of other cues such as motion parallax that are normally operative in real-world situations. Likewise the instability of illusory contours with prolonged inspection could be due to the absence of cues that are normally involved in viewing real edges. Such observations suggest that the greater the number of cues for edge that are contrived the more indistinguishable from real edges will the illusory ones be. It is conceivable that the type and number of cues involved are the key to the unresolved issue concerning whether real and apparent movement are distinguishable (see Sekuler & Blake, 1985).

The Question of Processes

Illusory contours have been identified with various sensory, perceptual, and cognitive processes. These include the activity of neural "edge detectors" (Smith & Over, 1975, 1976; Stadler & Dieker, 1972), neural interactions associated with simultaneous and line-end contrast (Brigner & Gallagher, 1974; Day & Jory, 1978; Frisby & Clatworthy, 1975), amodal completion of a figure overlayed by another (Kanizsa, 1975; Kanizsa & Gerbino, 1982), and higher-order cognitive processes (see Pomerantz & Kubovy, 1981). Evidence has frequently been adduced in support of one of these processes or for the rejection of another. Such evidence has occasionally taken the form of a particular figure in which it would be difficult or even impossible to attribute an illusory contour to, say, the neural interactions associated with brightness or color contrast.

An explanation of illusory contours in terms of contrived artificial cues for edge implies more than a single process. It is hardly to be expected that the processes set in train by contrived cues as diverse as step functions in brightness resulting from induction and apparent depth from simulated perspective will be the same. Nor does it seem likely that the processes invoked by, for example, simulated motion parallax and overlay would be the same. For the time being it can be assumed that the processes associated with illusory contours are as diverse as the artificial cues that alone or together generate them. It is also reasonable to suppose that, depending on the cues that are contrived, the processes that they initiate may operate at the sensory-neural, perceptual, or cognitive levels.

Why Study Illusory Contours?

A perceptual effect that is not fully understood and for which there is no agreed explanation is presumably worth investigating. However, there is another and perhaps less trite reason for studying illusory contours and this applies to other members of the class. If, as suggested, illusory contours are visible when one or a few cues for edge are contrived in the absence of a physical edge, a means is thereby provided for systematically exploring the range of edge cues and assessing their relative salience. That is to say, stimulus features believed to be implicated in the veridical perception of edges and contours in two- and three-dimensional arrays can be manufactured, so to speak, and the strength of the resultant experience of edge assessed by means of magnitude estimation or some such technique.

This procedure can, of course, be followed for the systematic exploration and assessment of stimulus features suspected of involvement in the perception of other object properties such as depth, form, and transparency. After all, the early and recent history of enquiry into the role of retinal disparity in depth perception (Wheatstone, 1838; Julesz, 1971) is one of contriving retinally disparate images in two-dimensional arrays and observing the consequent experiences of apparent depth where none exists physically. The technique of contrived cues is a powerful one for establishing what features in a stimulus array are primarily responsible for the perception of those qualities of the environment which we so readily perceive. The study of illusory contours is in this tradition.

CHAPTER 6

A Problem-Solving Approach to Illusory Contours

Irvin Rock

In the illustration shown in Figure 6.1, one can see a white diamond on top of black rectangles (or, alternatively, on top of a black cross). While not all illusory contour effects are identical, the best known and most studied is of this kind, devised by Kanizsa (1955a; 1974). This is the kind of effect I will discuss here. There are three aspects of the illusory contour (IC) phenomenon that require explanation: (1) A contour is perceived where none is present in the display or in its retinal representation, (2) the region bounded by the illusory contours appears to differ in lightness (typically whiter) than the background of the remainder of the display of the same physical luminance, and (3) the fragments that constitute the display tend to appear as amodal representations of larger, more complete entities.

The Sensory Theory: Contrast

One explanation of IC is that the fragments (typically black) generate a contrast effect so that the region they surround appears lighter than the remainder of the display. More accurately stated, the claim is that a lightness enhancement effect occurs for the regions adjacent to the black fragments based on the elimination of or release from inhibition. This effect presumably spreads to the entire region surrounded by the black fragments. If a region appears lighter than its surroundings, then, ipso facto, it will have a perceptible boundary or outer contour. (As we see later, it is possible to reverse this argument and maintain that it is the IC that is fundamental and brings about the

lightness effect.) I would like first to give my reasons for finding a contrast theory of IC wanting and then to devote the remainder of the paper to outlining a problem-solving type of theory that sees top-down cognitive intervention in the ongoing processing as a necessary part of the sequence of events.

There are a number of assumptions that must be made concerning how and why the contrast is only perceptible in the specified region.[1] Apart from the question of whether these assumptions are justified, however, there are the following difficulties. The IC effect is not ineluctable, although this point is not obvious for two reasons. First, we who study the effect are not naive, and, second, we tend to use figures that are particularly "good" in generating the effect. Patterns of the kind shown in Figure 6.1 will not typically lead to the IC percept in naive subjects. Figure 6.2 illustrates the same point (see Rock & Anson, 1979). Prior to the moment when the IC *is* perceived, there is no lightness effect, and that can hardly be because of failure of attention or failure to fixate the appropriate region. This single fact then seems to me to be of critical importance. If and when observers do succeed in perceiving the central region as a

---

[1] Among these are (a) that contrast is below threshold in most of the area around each black fragment but summates in the areas that tend to be "surrounded," such as in the gaps facing inward in Figure 6.1. (b) Since, however, contrast is not readily detectable when only *one* fragment is viewed, perhaps even with such hypothetical summation, contrast is still below threshold in the "gaps." (c) This below-threshold contrast spreads to the entire white region between all of the black fragments.

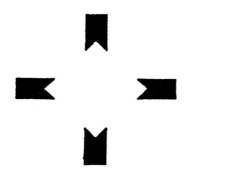

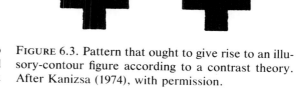

FIGURE 6.1. Figure perceived as four black photo mounts by naive observers or as a white diamond covering either four black rectangles or one black cross. After Kanizsa (1974), with permission.

FIGURE 6.3. Pattern that ought to give rise to an illusory-contour figure according to a contrast theory. After Kanizsa (1974), with permission.

diamond or triangle, then and then only does the extra whiteness emerge.

Which brings me to a second, completely neglected, fact. In all figures of this kind, the perception of the IC entails *figure–ground reversal*. At the outset, the central region of Figure 6.1 is ground. Only the black fragments are figural and this is why they can be perceived and recognized as photo mounts. Their innermost contours are organized as belonging to them and, thus, give them shape. When the reversal occurs those contours belong to and give shape to the white diamond, which becomes figure. The black fragments no longer look like irregular shapes but like the visible portions of rectangles or of a large cross. Thus, we see that the illusory figure is perceived if and only if figure–ground reversal occurs. Such reversal, I would argue, is not a bottom-up process. In our laboratory we have found that reversal often does

not occur when subjects are not informed that they are viewing figures that can be reversed, such as Rubin's well-known vase and faces figure or reversible perspective figures similar to the Necker cube (Girgus, Rock, & Egatz, 1977). Knowing about reversibility is a critical factor, which means that to the extent that this is demonstrable, by definition, top-down processing occurs.

A further difficulty for a contrast theory is that illusory-figure percepts do not occur with some patterns at all even for informed subjects, although they ought to occur if contrast is the underlying cause. Figure 6.3 is an example. The reversal is unlikely to occur here because a white rectangular figure in the center would usurp the inner borders of the black crosses. These contours would then belong to the rectangle, and that means that the crosses would be occluded by the rectangle, would be ground with respect to the rectangle. They would, therefore, not be crosses at all. They would be incomplete figures, the shape of which could be the one shown in Figure 6.4.

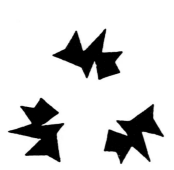

FIGURE 6.2. A pattern that typically does not spontaneously yield an illusory-contour effect when viewed by naive observers, but yields a curved triangle percept when the illusory figure is achieved.

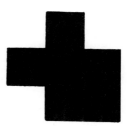

FIGURE 6.4. How each corner fragment (or cross pattern) of Figure 6.3 might appear if it is perceived as occluded by a central white rectangle.

So we see that to achieve the illusory-contour figure in this example entails giving up the initial perception of four corner crosses. One might speculate that the perceptual system is loath to surrender that percept because it is "good" in the Gestalt sense of the term, or alternatively because it is familiar and already complete.

A Problem-Solving Theory

In what follows, I will outline a problem-solving theory of illusory contour.[2]

The Formation of the "Hypothesis"

For some finite period of time the pattern (such as that in Figure 6.1) is perceived, literally, as several circumscribed figures (the fragments) on a homogeneous background. Each fragment is a closed region surrounded on all sides by a uniform region of a differing luminance. Such surroundedness is a known principle of figure-ground organization. The processing will stop here if the pattern of lines and other fragments is not too "good," and if no set or expectation is created to guide the system to try to perceive anything else. Nothing else but these figural fragments will be perceived even with prolonged inspection. This much then might be the result of bottom-up processing. I will refer to it as the *stage of the literal solution.*

If, however, as is generally the case in the IC patterns, the fragments resemble familiar figures with a region missing, then it is plausible to suppose that a hypothesis will be generated that an object is occluding the missing region. If only one such fragment is given, such a hypothesis will die on the vine, as it were. It receives no support. Familiarity is not the only possible basis of an impression of incompletion. An otherwise symmetrical object with a region missing that eliminates the symmetry might also trigger the hypothesis. Often familiarity and symmetry reinforce one another because the incomplete fragment is both familiar and potentially symmetrical (an incomplete circle, square, or the like).

FIGURE 6.5. A pattern in which the corner fragments do not suggest incompletion nonetheless typically yields an impression of a central white triangle, presumably because of alignment of the edges of the corner gaps across fragments. From Rock & Anson (1979), with permission.

Incompletion is not the only possible cue to the hypothesis of an occluding object. The alignment of the edges of the gap in the fragments *across* fragments can serve as a cue. In an experiment in our laboratory we constructed fragments that did not suggest incompletion of the fragments themselves (Rock & Anson, 1979) as shown in Figure 6.5. Nonetheless, if certain edges were aligned, i.e., collinear, a figure with ICs was perceived in the central region. To be sure, each fragment then appeared as if a gap in one region was occluded by an opaque white figure, but that impression was part of the phenomenal *outcome*. The gap could not have functioned as a cue in the sense of appearing as an incomplete part of the fragment prior to the emergence of the hypothesis. When the critical edges were arranged so as *not* to be aligned across fragments (as in Fig. 6.2), then very few subjects perceived an illusory figure. For in this case there is neither the cue of incompletion nor of alignment. In the experiment, needless to say, subjects were naive about the possibility of perceiving illusory figures. I hasten to add that the reader who is not naive will experience no great difficulty in achieving the illusory figure here. This suggests that still another cue to the hypothesis is set, expectation, or knowledge.

The more contour alignment in the stimulus pattern, the more likely it is that it will be noticed and the sooner it will be noticed. That is why patterns such as those of Kanizsa will

---

[2] For a more complete discussion of this kind of theory, see Rock (1983). Many points I bring out in this chapter are identical to those made by others, such as Kanizsa (1955, 1974), Gregory (1972), and Pritchard and Warm (1983), both with regard to limitations of a sensory or contrast theory and to features of a more cognitively based approach.

seem to lead immediately to the figure-ground reversal that brings about the IC percept. This is what I meant when I referred to "good" IC patterns. While the IC figure is experienced as immediate, I would maintain that it is preceded, however fleetingly, by an earlier stage of processing, the literal perceptual solution.

Maintaining the Hypothesized "Solution"

The observer constructs the perceptual solution that has been cued, if and only if it has been cued, by incorporating the visible fragments into it in a fitting way. The solution must account for the proximal stimulus or rather for the components that are part of the literal solution. The constructed solution is that of a white object covering the black fragments (or line fragments).

The shape of the constructed figure must account for the orientation of the edges of the fragments. From the standpoint of a problem-solving approach, if a figure is constructed to fit the requirements of an object occluding the three corner fragments, then in the case of the pattern in Figure 6.2, its edges must be curvilinear. This is a good example of the principle that *the solution must conform to the proximal stimulus*. Because the illusory figure is covering the fragments, their precise phenomenal shape depends upon a number of factors which I will not be able to discuss further in this paper.

Above all, if the solution is to be viable, there must be adequate stimulus support for it. What this means is simply this: Wherever the solution—considered as a description of a particular object or arrangement of objects—would entail the presence of a certain stimulus feature, then it must be present for that perceptual solu-

tion to survive. If not present, its absence must be accounted for. For example, if the solution is an outline figure, then a pattern with only some of the outline in it will not support that solution as in Gregory's well-known figure (Fig. 6.6a). But a pattern in which the missing segments of outline are replaced by an occluding figure does support that solution (Fig. 6.6b).

Internal consistency is critical. If the solution is that a white opaque figure is present on a white background, then its physical borders will only be visible where it happens to occlude a region (fragment) of a differing lightness. It would be inconsistent, then, if certain other parts of the borders of the hypothesized figure were included in the stimulus pattern. Why are they visible and not the remainder of the figure, the homunculus would have to ask. This analysis may explain why a pattern such as the one shown in Figure 6.7 is not a good one for producing illusory-contour figures. It undoubtedly generates the hypothesis of an inner triangle. But it fails to support it because of the internal inconsistencies that arise. Compare this with Figure 6.8, which works quite well, but when some contours are added as in the previous fig-

_____

[3] The fact that patterns containing only lines of the kind shown in Figure 6.8 produce striking IC and lightness effects is of special interest because there are no solid black regions to generate lightness enhancement. Although one might consider this fact to be formidable evidence against the contrast theory, advocates of the theory have presented arguments and evidence that strong contrast effects occur at the ends of lines (Brigner & Gallagher, 1974; Day & Jory, 1978; Frisby & Clatworthy, 1975; Jory & Day, 1979; Kennedy, 1979). For further discussion of this issue, see Frisby and Clatworthy (1975) and Rock (1986).

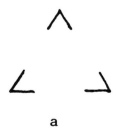

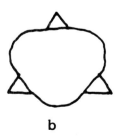

a   b

FIGURE 6.6. a. A pattern that does not support the perception of a triangle although it undoubtedly cues that perception. From Gregory (1972). 6.6b. This pattern does support the perception of a triangle although it contains only the same fragments of such a triangle as are present in 6.6a.

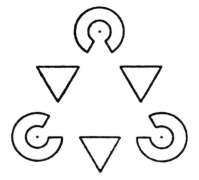

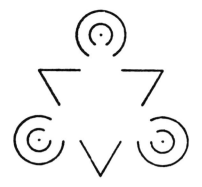

FIGURE 6.7. Despite the addition of extra lines along the perimeter of a central triangular region, no illusory white triangle is perceived. From Kanizsa (1974), with permission.

FIGURE 6.8. In comparison to Figure 6.7, this figure yields a vivid impression of a central white figure although, except for the end points of lines, none of the contours of such a figure are physically present. From Kanizsa (1974), with permission.

ure, the effect disappears.[3] This occurs despite the fact that the added contours are along the locus of points that would constitute the IC. Although the presence of these contours puts less of a burden on constructive processes, the illusion is not likely to occur. If I am right about this example, we can see that subtleties of consistency play an important role in the construction of the percept.

A blatant contradiction is, of course, an internal inconsistency par excellence. It would be inconsistent if one were able to see through the central region hypothesized to be a solid *opaque* figure. We investigated the effect of a striped pattern seen within the central region of an illusory-contour pattern (Rock & Anson,

1979). When depth cues such as retinal disparity or motion parallax led to an unequivocal impression that the stripes were behind the fragments, the observers were unable to perceive an illusory figure, as is illustrated in Figure 6.9b. When, however, the stripes were seen as in front of the fragments, the illusory figure was perceived (Fig. 6.9c). Thus, the detrimental effect of the stripes in Figure 6.9b was not of some inhibitory kind based simply on the mere presence of such contours in the vicinity of the region expected to be seen as a figure with illusory contours. A similar effect based on depth contradiction was demonstrated in a well-known experiment by Gregory and Harris (1974).

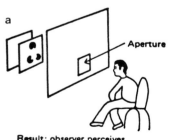

Result: observer perceives
white triangle

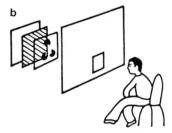

Result: observer perceives
three circular segments
in front of stripes

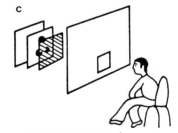

Result: observer perceives
white triangle behind
stripes

FIGURE 6.9. a. An illusory white triangle is seen occluding black circles at its corners. b. The illusory triangle is not seen, presumably because it would be incompatible with depth information that the critical region is not opaque. c. An illusory triangle is perceived despite the presence of stripes in the central region. However, here the stripes are seen as in front of the triangle. From Rock and Anson (1979), with permission.

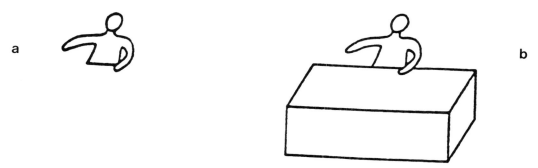

FIGURE 6.10. Although the same part of a person is represented in a and b, in a the person is seen as truncated, whereas in b the person is seen as amodally completed. From Kanizsa & Gerbino (1982), with permission.

Completion

A neglected aspect of the IC phenomenon is that the stimulus fragments are perceptually completed. The amodal completion that occurs with these figures is of the kind occurring in interposition patterns in depth perception. We now know that such completion is based on perceptual processing and is not merely an act of interpretation. Otherwise the two people in Figure 6.10 would not look so very different to us. Gerbino and Salmaso (1985) have shown that reaction time to identify amodally represented figures is about as rapid as time to identify the figure when it is entirely represented and much more rapid than time to identify a truncated version of the figure that is a proximal stimulus copy of the incomplete pattern (Fig. 6.11).

The important point is that the stimulus for the interposition-completion effect is not present in IC patterns, so even if one were to invoke a bottom-up theory to explain this kind of effect in the more typical example in line figures or in daily life occurrences, it would be difficult to do so for IC patterns. That is because the central contour between two enclosed regions giving rise to T junctions at its end points does not exist in these patterns. Stated otherwise, there is no interposition pattern (a point to bear in mind when one invokes depth cuing as the explanation of IC). Thus, it would seem plausible to conclude that the completion effect is a fundamental part of the solution, a top-down hypothesis imposed on the stimulus and not a perception we should expect to occur without such cognitive intervention.

Preference

There is a further question to be addressed. Assume it is correct to speak of two possible solutions to the problem posed by the IC stimulus pattern, a literal solution of a group of fragment figures and the illusory figure solution. Why is

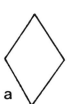
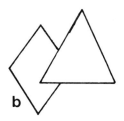
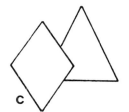
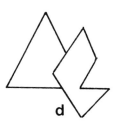

FIGURE 6.11. The reaction time to identify the presence of the target figure a in b, where it is only amodally represented is almost as rapid as in c, where it is entirely represented, whereas in d, the reaction time to identify the presence of a diamond is significantly increased although the truncated representation is physically and categorically identical to that in b. After Gerbino & Salmaso (1985), with permission.

the latter preferred? My answer is that the literal solution is not satisfactory. The other solution accounts for the incompletion and/or contour alignment, whereas the literal solution does not. These features remain as pure coincidence within the context of the literal solution. When, however, the IC solution entails unexplained coincidence, as in the case where the corner fragments are crosses (Fig. 6.3), then the literal solution is preferred.

The Lightness Effect

How is the lightness effect to be explained? One possibility is that the perceptual system *invents* a lightness difference in order to rationalize the IC solution. There are many examples of rationalization in perception. The common denominator for its occurrence would seem to be the presence of an inconsistency. Rather than relinquish a particular solution that is favored, the perceptual system achieves an interpretation of the contradiction that is consistent with that solution. An example in IC perception is shown in Figure 6.12. Some of the lines if seen *behind* the central region would contradict the interpretation of that region as an opaque object. Hence, they are perceived as weaving in and out, in front of that opaque object where necessary and behind it where necessary. In the case of the lightness effect, such a process would have the effect of accounting for the perception of the contour on the basis of a lightness difference between the illusory figure and its background. An interesting fact supports this interpretation.

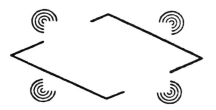

FIGURE 6.12. Perceptual rationalization. Rather than preventing the illusory-contour perception, the oblique lines are perceived as parts of an elongated diamond that go above or below the illusory white rectangle. From Kanizsa (1974), with permission.

If the illusory pattern in Figure 6.13 is outlined as shown, the lightness effect is very much diminished if not entirely eliminated (Coren & Theodor, 1975; Kennedy, 1979; Parks, 1979; Parks, Rock, & Anson, 1983). The contour eliminates the need for an invented lightness difference since its presence explains why the figure's borders are visible. Were the lightness effect the direct result of contrast, it is hard to see why it would be all but eliminated by the addition of the outline.

An alternative is that the lightness effect is the result of contrast, but of a special kind. It is one that depends upon the construction of the illusory contour figure, so it is a very different theory than one in which the illusory figure results from contrast. It has been known for over a half century that the effectiveness of contrast is very much a function of figure-ground organization. I am referring to the effect discovery by Benary (1924) in which a region

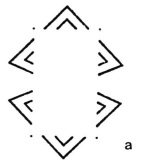
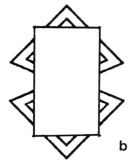

FIGURE 6.13. Little if any extra-whiteness effect occurs in b, where the rectangle's contours are physically present, in comparison to a, where they are not. This suggests that the Benary contrast effect requires solid black regions and does not occur with contour lines. After Kanizsa (1974), with permission.

that appears to belong to a background region contrasts more with it than one of equal luminance that appears only to be adjacent to it. This effect itself can be regarded as one that challenges a purely bottom-up account of contrast.[4]

The Benary effect can be invoked to explain the lightness effect in IC figures *but only after the appropriate figure-ground organization has occurred.* If no such reorganization has occurred, one only perceives black figural fragments on a white ground. Whereas, if reorganization has occurred, then the illusory figure is perceived to lie *on* the black corner fragments. The illusory figure would then be expected to contrast more with the black fragments than would the white regions surrounding the fragments on all other sides. That a white region will appear to be whiter than it would otherwise appear to be as a result of just such a perceptual organization is clearly shown in Figure 6.14. It is quite reasonable, then, to suppose that such an effect will occur when this organization happens with an IC display. But, to repeat, it can only be expected to occur after the illusory-figure percept is achieved.

At the moment, then, there are two possible explanations of the extra whiteness effect that are compatible with a problem-solving approach. One is that it is of the nature of a cognitive invention. The other is that it results from that kind of contrast that depends upon figure-ground perceptual organization, which in this case means perceptual reorganization. In both cases, the effect is secondary to the prior emergence of the illusory-contour organization, rather than being the primary effect. Certain facts argue against the generality of the Benary explanation, for example, that little if any contrast occurs for patterns consisting only of line components, as shown in Figure 6.13b. Yet the rectangle figure here is perceived as on or belonging to the background elements just as much as is the illusory rectangle in Figure 6.13a.

There is, however, one remaining problem for the cognitive-invention theory. The illusory

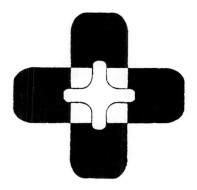

FIGURE 6.14. The white region that is perceived to be on or to belong to the background (the curved cross) appears whiter than the enclosed white region that does not (the square). After Kanizsa (1975), with permission.

figure could just as well be lighter or darker than the surrounding region. Either direction of a lightness "invention" would solve the problem of rationalizing the perceptibility of the illusory figure borders. Why then is the choice one in which this figure appears whiter than the white background? Perhaps contrast only plays a role in resolving this ambiguity. It sets the direction or "sign" of the effect. With black fragments, solid or line, the perceptual system "decides" that the lightness of the illusory figure that differentiates it from the overall background is opposite in color to that of the covered fragments, namely, white.

Final Remarks

That a perception can occur either spontaneously or only after it has been suggested or otherwise facilitated is a fact that has generally been ignored by investigators. Although spontaneous perception may or may not indicate bottom-up processing, the other, facilitated, kind would surely seem to indicate top-down processing.

Such examples are instructive because they stop the action, as it were, in the normal rapid processing that leads to the final, preferred, world-mode perception. They thus serve to bring out the two stages or phases of perceptual problem solving. We see that some cue is needed to lead to the appropriate solution. In these cases, that cue is either absent from the

---

[4] See also the research of Coren (1969), Gilchrist (1977), Kanizsa (1975), and Wolff (1935) concerning the effects of perceptual organization on lightness perception.

stimulus (or from the literal solution to which it gives rise), not noticed, or the cue is camouflaged. It is therefore worth emphasizing that despite this, the final percept, once it occurs, can be perfectly adequate. A pattern such as the one in Figure 6.1 or 6.2 may not spontaneously yield the effect until one is told where to look and what to look for, but once this is known, the effect can be every bit as adequate as when the effect spontaneously arises based on strong cues.

If these various examples illustrate adequate perception despite poor cuing, then there are also examples of the opposite, inadequate perception despite good cuing. Figures 6.3, 6.6a, and 6.7 are examples of this kind. The key factor is the quality of stimulus support. It must be adequate if the cued perception is to be adequate. Needless to say, conditions can be such that neither the cue nor the stimulus support is adequate, or they can be such that both are adequate. An element in a pattern can have the dual role of serving as a cue (or as part of a cue) and as stimulus support. The line segments between the corner fragments orthogonal to the illusory contours in many of Kanizsa's figures serve in both of these capacities: Their inner ends are aligned with the edges of the corner fragments so that they are part of the alignment cue and thus improve it. But they also support the solution because of their location in the long stretch of space between fragments, appearing as longer lines, parts of which are occluded. Such local support is needed to yield the IC throughout the empty space between corner fragments. So we see that there is another meaning to "good patterns" besides the one concerning cuing discussed earlier.

Some further comment about the role of past experience in perceptual problem solving is warranted. The solving of a problem should not be identified with prior experience, as the Gestaltists were at pains to point out, although such experience, if relevant, will often be utilized in the process (Duncker, 1945; Wertheimer, 1945). Understanding of the problem, reformulating the problem, searching for an appropriate object or method of solution are not processes that are reducible to past experi-

ence. In perception, in the case of the IC effect, we have seen that the cue of incompletion quite probably is generally based on experience, because it is through such experience that we know what configurations are incomplete departures from the norm. But the cue of alignment is not necessarily based on past experience. The hypothesis of the presence of an occluding opaque object need not necessarily derive from any experience with object occlusion in daily life. Phylogenetic "experience" is an alternative possibility. It is unlikely that the lightness effect, whether it be a cognitive intervention or a kind of contrast based on figure-ground organization, derives in any way from prior experience. Finally, the viability of a cued solution that depends on stimulus support and internal consistency and the preference for that solution over the initial, literal solution are characteristics of the perceptual process rather than contents in the mind that are acquired by previous perceptual experience.

In short, "cognitive intervention" is not to be regarded as equivalent to "the effect of acquired knowledge" on perception. Moreover, where past experience does enter in, it should not be regarded as knowledge in the ordinary sense of the word. Perception is generally immune to any effect based on having information about what is or is not actually present in the environment. For example, illusions do not cease on learning that what is perceived is illusory. Perception is usually autonomous with respect to conscious thought and knowledge. Thus, it is likely that when past experience does affect perception, it does so in the form of specific memories of prior perception or in the form of unconscious rules acquired in the past.

Acknowledgments. Portions of this chapter are based on work that appeared in Cognitive intervention in perceptual processing, by I. Rock. *In* T. J. Knapp & L. C. Robertson (Eds.), *Approaches to cognition: Contrasts and controversies.* (1986) Hillsdale, NJ: Lawrence Erlbaum Associates. Permission for use of these portions is gratefully acknowledged.

CHAPTER 7

Anomalous Figures and the Tendency to Continuation

Gian Franco Minguzzi*

Amodal Completion and Amodal Continuation

Throughout the paper, I will call the phenomena studied in this volume *anomalous figures,* in order to stress that perception of a figure occurs in conditions different from the normal ones.

Two of the many hypotheses used to explain anomalous figures have frequently been considered to be in opposition. One hypothesis posits amodal completion of inducing figures to have a primary causal role; first formulated by Kanizsa (1954, 1955a), it has been supported by others, though differing in their general theoretical positions (Gregory, 1972; Parks, 1979; Pastore, 1971; Rock & Anson, 1979). The other hypothesis posits the local effects of brightness contrast to constitute either the only or the primary factor (Brigner & Gallagher, 1974; Frisby & Clatworthy, 1975; Spillman, Fuld, & Gerrits, 1976). I would like to make some remarks in support of the first hypothesis, emphasizing that in my view it is more suitable to speak of a tendency to *continuation* rather than a tendency to figural *completion.*

This reformulation seems necessary for two reasons. First, the word *completion* implies the concepts *incompleteness* and *gap.* In the classical Kanizsa triangle, and in many other displays, the incompleteness of the inducing figures is obvious: the pies are disks lacking a sector, and they do not change even when they are isolated. However, this does not always happen with other inducing elements—for example, lines. Thus, Ehrenstein's illusion is composed of bars which, if isolated, do not lack anything.

Second, the outcome of amodal presence behind the anomalous surface is not always a completion. The irregular fragments employed by Rock & Anson (1979) and those of Day & Kasperczyk (1983a) remain jagged. Sometimes the outcome is not even the unification or grouping as in Kennedy's configuration (1978b), where the bars remain perceptually isolated (Fig. 7.1). But what happens in every case is the continuation of the inducing figure beyond its physical edge, i.e., behind the anomalous figure. This continuation sometimes completes the inducing figure or unifies it with another, and sometimes it is only a figural spread, obviously amodal. I will come back to this point later. Now, however, I would like to consider in more detail arguments against the role of brightness contrast in the emergence of anomalous figures.

The Role of Brightness Contrast

First of all, I would emphasize that Kanizsa and other authors who argue for the fundamental importance of completion (or, in my view, continuation) do not deny the existence of brightness contrast effects. Instead, they believe that these effects are secondary and, according to Parks (1982b), they serve the "need of perceptual expression" of an occluding surface under which the inducing figures may continue. Many facts support the view stated and developed by Kanizsa and others (for review of the literature see Parks, 1984). It is generally known that the

---

* We were saddened to learn of the death in March 1987 of Gian Franco Minguzzi. He was a man of exceptional kindness and wisdom and he will be missed very much.

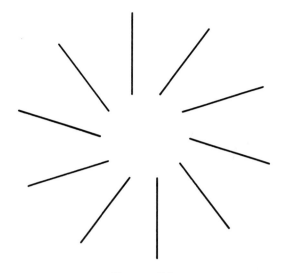

FIGURE 7.1.

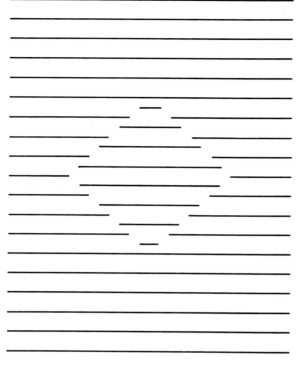

FIGURE 7.2.

anomalous brightness disappears when a complete or partial physically defined border is added (Coren & Theodor, 1975; Kanizsa, 1974; Parks, 1979). Since this circumscribed area is isolated by physically defined borders, its differentiation from the background is no longer necessary to express the character of an occluding surface. In these cases not only does the anomalous brightness disappear, but so does the anomalous figure. In other cases the anomalous figure is maintained. This happens when it is "evident" in some way that the region which may be thought of as performing the function of covering the underlying continuation of inducing figure has the quality of a solid surface, as in Figure 7.2 from Bachmann (1978) and my own Figure 7.3.

Moreover, Kanizsa (1974) has already pointed out the independence of anomalous brightness and anomalous contours in the case of Figure 7.4, later republished by others (Kennedy, 1975; Day & Kasperczyk, 1983b).

This interpretation of the brightness effect seems also to be supported by studies of the anomalous Necker cube (Bradley, Dumais, & Petry, 1976), where the change in perceived brightness depends on the general organization.

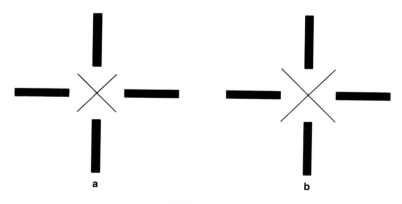

FIGURE 7.3.

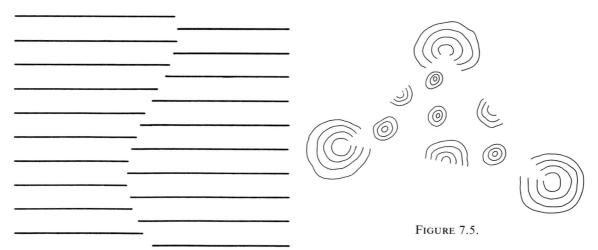

FIGURE 7.4.

FIGURE 7.5.

Thus, if the cube is perceived behind the plane of the paper, it appears brighter than when perceived in front of the plane. We have a similar result in Figure 7.5, where the central region may be perceived as a surface behind or in front of the plane of the paper. In the latter case it is perceived as being darker, in the former a little brighter, but not as much as is usual in anomalous figures.

As a final example, in Figure 7.6, an anomalous bright triangle can be seen (often described as a convex surface with semitransparent

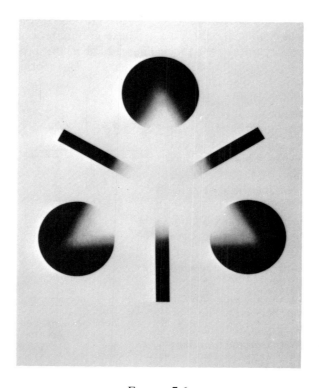

FIGURE 7.6.

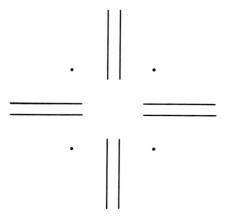

FIGURE 7.7.

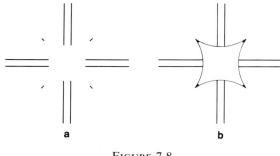

FIGURE 7.8.

boundaries). However, an explanation of this triangle in terms of local brightness contrast effects is at best difficult, due to the absence of a sharply defined contour.

The Role of Points and Ends of Lines as Inducing Elements

Other results of my investigations concerning the form modification of anomalous figures provide an additional argument against ascribing a primary role to brightness contrast effects. Points placed in the immediate vicinity of a critical region produce meaningful distortions in the shape of the anomalous figure, though brightness contrast effects are not involved. In Figure 7.7 observers see a quadrilateral form with curved contours, the points fixing or anchoring the perceived angles. This effect has also been noted by Sambin (1974a) and Day & Kasperczyk (1983a), but has had little systematic investigation.

A new, interesting, and theoretically significant phenomenon emerges when the points are replaced by bars (Fig. 7.8a). Some observers still perceive the same kind of anomalous figures as obtained from Figure 7.7, whereas others perceive a quadrilateral with curved sides which incorporate the bars (see Fig. 7.8b for representation of the percept). It may be observed that a bar does not continue amodally under the figure but becomes part of it.

I plan in the future to study the limits and the parameters of the phenomenon of perceptual

incorporation quantitatively. In the meantime, I can report some informal observations. If pairs of parallel bars are used as secondary inducers, the shape of the anomalous figure is that of an irregular octagon and the bars appear to continue for a short length under the anomalous surface (Fig. 7.9a). If the bars form an angle, the perception varies according to the size of the angle. When the angle is very acute (Fig. 7.9b), the effect is similar to that obtained with parallel bars. When the angle is increased, the bars complete the anomalous figure, and they continue the anomalous contours (Fig. 7.9c). The phenomenon of perceptual incorporation of secondary inducers is more pronounced if the bars are curved (Fig. 7.9d).

These preliminary observations indicate that lines added in the proximity of an anomalous figure may: (1) perform the function of an induc-

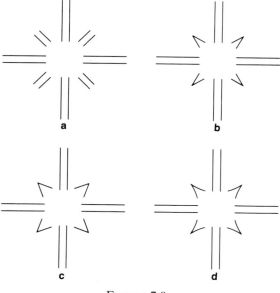

FIGURE 7.9.

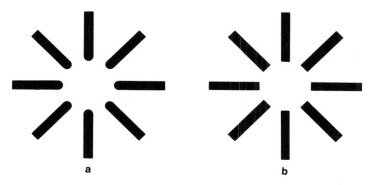

FIGURE 7.10.

ing figure and amodally continue for a short length under the anomalous surface, or (2) complete the anomalous figure and modally continue the anomalous contours. Both phenomena may be interpreted as a consequence of a tendency of lines to continue beyond their physical end.

Hence the tendency to continuation seems to act in more than one way. It is perhaps a hazardous generalization to say that just as an event developing over time tends to continue phenomenally beyond its stop—an effect of phenomenal permanence studied by the Louvain school (Michotte, 1962)—so also a figure tends to continue beyond its edges. Anomalous patterns, more so than the cases of amodal completion behind physically present figures, are particularly suitable for the discovery of conditions underlying this tendency.

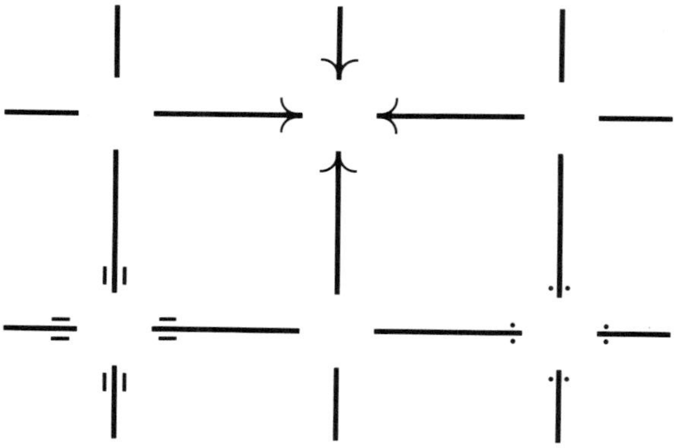

Thus, convex borders of bars apparently inhibit continuation and influence the presence of the anomalous figure, as demonstrated by the comparison between Figure 7.10a and Figure 7.10b. The role of borders recalls Rubin's old studies on the influence of the shape of borders on figure–ground organization (Rubin, 1921). Even more impressive is the fact that minimal details, added close to the end of an inducing line without modifying other local conditions, anchor it and stop its amodal continuation (Fig. 7.11).

In summary, in this paper I have tried to show that the primary factor in the emergence of anomalous figures is the tendency to continuation. This tendency is hypothesized to be a general principle of perceptual organization, and to account for the effectiveness of lines in inducing anomalous figures.

FIGURE 7.11.

Acknowledgments. This work has been supported by a National Research Council (CNR) grant no. 81,00049.04. The author wishes to thank Nicholas Pastore for his help in preparing the manuscript.

CHAPTER 8

Illusory Figures and Pictorial Objects

Theodore E. Parks

Of all the things that can be said about illusory figures—and are said so well elsewhere in this volume—I will content myself with bolstering one familiar conclusion and cautioning against a second conclusion that might seem to follow from the first. On the positive side of this dual purpose, I would argue that illusory contours are cognitive creations and that, as such, they present an important example of the ability of the visual system to supplement (and not merely resonate to) the information gathered by the eyes. Now in our perception of pictures—particularly of effective but minimal outline sketches—it seems obvious that some such supplementation must also occur. That is, to the extent that such sketches arouse in us something more than merely an awareness of markings and paper, that extra something has been added by the brain. But herein lies the potential for error: despite that similarity, I would further argue that neither illusory figures nor the stimuli that evoke them can be accurately characterized as pictorial.

First, however, it behooves any author to look to his defenses when working around (if not stumbling into) such philosophically thorny entanglements as the epistemology of picture-perception. I claim no expertise in the epistemology of representative art. Nor, for that matter, am I fully conversant with the epistemological problems inherent in the sort of cognitive theory of perception which will be put forward here. As to the former, however, it seems to me that the present point can be made quite independently of a thorough-going account of how representation is possible or, indeed, what representation is. As to the latter, I

can only say that I find the specific arguments I have read against the logical acceptability of such a theory (e.g., Katz and Frost, 1979) to be unconvincing, at least as long as the posited processes are understood to be heritable outcomes of natural selection (e.g., Jerison, 1973, 1976). Now to the present arguments.

Illusory Figures Are Cognitive Creations

First of all, the mere fact that the triangle seen in Kanizsa's classic pattern is obviously a creation—it isn't there—is not sufficient to show that it is a cognitive creation. This is so because that triangle could be the product of relatively less interesting processes, processes which sometimes and under some circumstances lead the visual system to error. Clearly, not all such errors should be glorified by the name "cognitive creations," as that phrase is intended here. Indeed, most such errors are not at all what those who argue for supplementation have in mind. For example, it is well known that visual neurons are interconnected in quite complex networks and, so, can affect one another in terms of the neural message that each passes forward. One result of these interactions is illusory alterations in the apparent lightness of various parts of various displays which are produced at a very early stage within the visual system. Such is the commonly accepted explanation for such familiar effects as so-called Mach Bands and the Hermann Grid illusion.

But what if such is not the case for illusory-figure lightness? What if the illusory alteration

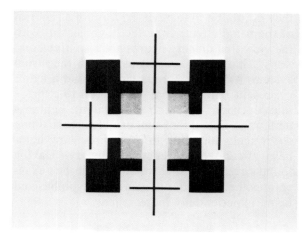

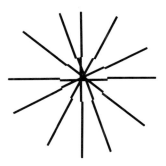

FIGURE 8.2. A circle is usually seen here, but it is often difficult to decide how that area differs from the surrounding area, if at all. From Letter to the editor, by T. E. Parks, 1980. *Perception, 9,* p. 723. Copyright 1980 by Pion Limited. Reprinted by permission of Pion Limited.

FIGURE 8.1. A pattern which produces an impression of altered texture (filminess) rather than or in addition to altered lightness. From Subjective figures: An infrequent, but certainly not unprecedented, effect, by T. E. Parks, 1981. *Perception, 10,* p. 589. Copyright 1981 by Pion Limited. Reprinted by permission of Pion Limited.

in lightness seen in illusory-figure patterns is created by the visual system as a *late* step (rather than a very early one) in processing? And, specifically, what if that processing can be characterized, as Irvin Rock suggests in his contribution, as a problem-solving search for an answer to the question, "What is it that is there?"

Consider, for example, certain facts about illusory figures and how they are experienced:

1. *Patterns that produce illusory figures do not always produce an illusory-lightness effect.* For example, the illusory figure may appear as an area of altered "texture" instead of, or in addition to, altered lightness. This may happen in patterns very like Kanizsa's (Parks, 1981), but such texture effects are especially common if the inducing elements suggest the presence of a translucent occluding figure (Kanizsa, 1974; Parks, 1981; see Fig. 8.1).

In addition, there are cases in which it is very hard to decide exactly how the illusory figure differs qualitatively from the surrounding paper, if at all. This seems to be especially true for some patterns in which several elements are included within the area of the illusory figure (Parks, 1980b; see Fig. 8.2). Such effects may not be as compelling as some others, but that

they occur at all argues that an illusory-lightness effect is not a necessary component of all illusory figures.

2. Even when an illusory figure does appear as an alteration in apparent lightness, *the direction of that lightness alteration can be influenced by a variety of factors.* For one thing, unspecified factors can sometimes produce an illusory figure which appears to some observers to be darker than the surround even in patterns that usually produce the lighter-than-surround effect (Parks, 1982a; Richardson, 1979). Furthermore, when a pattern that generally produces a light illusory figure is presented on a background which is not homogeneous, but instead is darker at its center than at its edges, many observers experience an illusory figure whose edges are darker (rather than lighter) than the paper just to the outside (Parks, 1982b; see Fig. 8.3). Thus, real lightness differences can contribute to the appearance of an illusory figure and can even reverse the effect that is usually seen.

3. Even when the usual lightness effect occurs, *there is more involved in the contribution of its various sources than their mere occurrence within the illusory area.* That is, the usual lighter-than-surround appearance of an illusory figure is probably an exaggeration of (rather than merely an incorporation of) very weak illusory-lightness effects. For example, we know that when any white area which is adjacent to black elements comes to be seen as figure against them as background, there will be a ten-

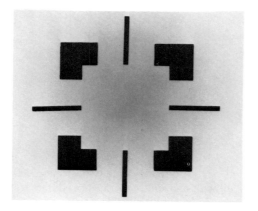

FIGURE 8.3. Black elements such as those in this pattern generally produce a lighter-than-surround illusory figure. Against a background such as this, however, a darker-than-surround square is often seen. From Illusory contours: On the efficacy of their need for expression, by T. E. Parks, 1982. *Perception and Psychophysics, 32,* p. 286. Copyright 1982 by the Psychonomic Society. Reprinted by permission of the Psychonomic Society.

dency for that white area to appear very slightly (almost unnoticeably) lighter than it did before it became figure to that ground (e.g., Coren, 1969). In the case of illusory figures, that part of the homogeneous field which becomes such a figure is so lightened, but again the point here is that the lightening effect is much stronger than usual (Parks, Rock, & Anson, 1983). In fact, the same could be said regarding another potential source of illusory-figure lightening: the possibility that illusory "buttons" of lightness occur just beyond the ends of line segments or next to abrupt changes in contour (Frisby & Clatworthy, 1975; Kennedy & Lee, 1976). If such "line-end contrast" occurs in Kanizsa's pattern, it too is weak, so weak that virtually no one will notice a lightness effect in Kanizsa's pattern prior to the emergence of a completely realized illusory figure (e.g., Bradley & Mates, 1985). Apparently, then, if such lightness buttons are a source of illusory-figure lightness, they too are exaggerated when the illusory figure emerges.

This suggestion that the lightness effect that is usually seen within an illusory figure is an exaggeration of weaker effects, together with the previous observations that illusory figures need not involve illusory lightness at all or, if

they do, that it may be in the form of a reversal of the usual effect, is perfectly consistent with the view that illusory figures are cognitive creations. That is to say, it is as though the visual system, having gathered evidence that a figure is present, may (or may not) go on to express that decision by altering apparent lightness within the area of that supposed figure. In doing so, it seeks direction in other prevailing lightness effects, both real and illusory. Having found direction in such conditions, it then exaggerates them in order to make the hypothesized figure experientially more salient.

Illusory Figures Are Not "Pictured"

If then, as Richard Gregory put it long ago, an illusory figure is a "cognitive fiction" (Gregory, 1972), are the patterns that induce them pictures and are the fictions, themselves, pictorial? For example, can we say with any satisfaction—indeed, without the risk of being seriously misleading—that Kanizsa's pattern is "a *picture* of a triangle"? If not, in what way is it different from any picture of anything?

First of all, it must be understood that any picture is, to be more precise, a picture "of an X-shaped thing." Thus, "a picture of a horse" is, in and of itself, a picture of a horse-shaped thing since it cannot be distinguished, in and of itself, from a picture of a statue of a horse or any other horse-shaped thing. Moreover, any common picture of any object is, itself, produced by *producing a thing of that shape:* a picture of a horse-shaped thing is produced by producing a horse-shaped arrangement of carbon streaks, ink stains, or whatever (putting aside, of course, matters of scale and of the third dimension). But—and this may be crucial—that is precisely what Kanizsa did not do: he did *not produce a physical triangle* within his pattern. Is that pattern, nevertheless, a picture? Is the very point of Kanizsa's demonstration that he has freed the artist from the harsh rule that to picture some shape you must produce something of that shape? The matter hinges, I would suggest, on how we *respond* to it.

John Kennedy made the interesting point that our experience of both ordinary sketches and of illusory-figure patterns is "bicameral" (Ken-

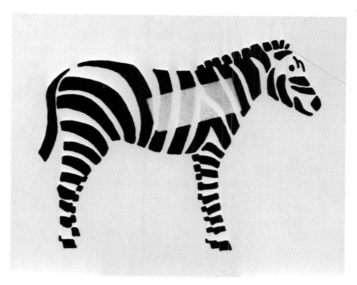

FIGURE 8.4. A "piece of tape on a picture of a zebra" (?) From Humor, by T. E. Parks, 1982. *Perception, 11,* p. 240. Copyright 1982 by Pion Limited. Reprinted by permission of Pion Limited.

nedy, 1976a; Ware and Kennedy, 1978 see Kennedy, this volume, for a fuller discussion). That is to say, in both cases we have two contradictory experiences. For example, in the case of sketches we are (a) perceptually aware of the fact that something is depicted, but we simultaneously perceive that (b) what we have before us is, in fact, only some marks on a surface. Now, as Kennedy further argues in this volume, we also have a duality in our experience of illusory figure patterns: typically we perceive (a) the illusion, itself, and (b) the fact that all that is really there is the set of dark inducing elements. Clearly the second halves (the physically accurate halves) of these two bicameralities are identical: in looking at sketches or looking at Kanizsa's pattern, we can be aware of physical truth. But what of the first halves? If we can be fooled by a picture in exactly the same manner in which we are fooled by Kanizsa's pattern, the latter could, indeed, aptly be called a picture.

My contention, to the contrary, is that there is a fundamental and critical difference between the nonveridical experience of ordinary sketches and the nonveridical half of our experience of good illusory-figure patterns. Specifically, our "error" in looking at pictures consists of a recognition of what is depicted by, *but not actually present in,* the physical stimulus. By contrast, in the case of illusory figures our "error" consists of our impression of an *actual presence* in the physical stimulus itself. For example, the erroneous experience produced by Kanizsa's pattern is the impression that a triangular area has been physically altered by bleaching or by a coat of paint or by an added piece of paper or whatever. Thus, in our experience of illusory-figure patterns, but not in our experience of sketches, both sides of the bicamerality have to do with impressions about what the producer physically did with his materials. In the case of pictures, the nonveridical side has to do, instead, with merely what the producer intended to remind us of.

Perhaps the point will be clarified by the example seen in Figure 8.4 (Parks, 1982c). I submit that one's experience (that is, one's nonveridical experience) of this figure is captured more accurately by the sentence "A piece of tape on a picture of a zebra," than by "A picture of a piece of tape on a zebra." And, for that matter, what of the zebra itself? Are the white parts of its edges only "pictured"?

In Conclusion

To return to a question raised earlier, it follows (rather ironically) that one could say that Kanizsa showed us how to "draw a picture of a triangle," but *only* if one quickly adds that he did so in a way that does not completely violate the principle that to draw a triangle you must produce one. True enough, he did not physically include a triangle in his pattern, but the point is that to some extent his pattern tricks the visual system into responding as though he did. His triangle is not a response to depiction, but more like the raw material of depiction.

CHAPTER 9

Illusory Contours and Occluding Surfaces

Richard L. Gregory

The question we are addressing here might be put: "Is the notion that illusory contours are *cognitive fictions* true, or merely science fiction?" The answer turns on what is "cognitive"—which leads to how we should think of perception generally, and to experiments of many kinds.

Approaches to Views of Perception and Illusions

On some accounts of paradigms of perception, illusions present no special problems; on others it is hardly credible that perception can play us false. There is, indeed, a great divide between theories of perception, such that phenomena and experiments are interpreted very differently according to which side one stands on. The great divide is between *passive* and *active* accounts. The most distinguished recent exponent of a passive view (which has generally been held in some form by philosophers) is the late James J. Gibson, especially in his well-known books *The Perception of the Visual World* (1950) and *The Senses Considered as Perceptual Systems* (1966). The most authoritative voice, and very much the originator, of an active account is the great nineteenth-century polymath scientist Herman von Helmholtz, especially in his *Physiological Optics* (1867) and his essays, "The Relation of Optics to Painting" (1871) and "The Facts of Perception" (1878). These accounts are extremely different: Gibson holds that all the information needed for perception is in the external world (in the "ambient array of light") simply to be "picked up"

by the observer, who has little to do but select what is needed. The Helmholtzian view is that perceptions are rich creations, based on limited sensory data, which as they are essentially inadequate have to be interpreted, or "read," from various assumptions—which may or may not be appropriate. This "active" (because active perceptual processes are invoked) account is essentially *cognitive*, for it stresses the importance of *knowledge* of objects and how they interact causally (among themselves and with the observer) in various situations.

Any illusion looks very different from a "passive" or an "active" theoretical account of perception. Illusions are, indeed, largely played down or even denied by the passivists—as they think of perceptions as directly related to the object world. Very differently, activists—who see perceptions as created from inadequate data—seize upon phenomena of illusions as suggestive failures of perceptual processes and procedures to make sense of the world in some circumstances—even to producing perceptual fictions. It is this latter, cognitive active view of perception and illusions, that I have argued in *Eye and Brain* (1966), *The Intelligent Eye* (1970), and *Mind in Science* (1981), where perceptions are regarded as predictive hypotheses—much like hypotheses of science. On this active view, perceptions are far richer than the available sensory data, and since they are not restrained by stimuli or data, are liable to dramatic illusions of various kinds, these phenomena being extremely useful for discovering the procedures by which perceptual hypotheses (perceptions) are created. In particular, the active processes generating perceptual hypotheses (which on this view are perceptions) may go overboard to produce fictions such as visible but nonexistent surfaces and contours.

An analogous case of fiction-production, on this view, is drawing a line on a graph. For, a line drawn to fit experimental data is always a fiction since it fills gaps between data points; and the best fitting line may not touch even one of the data points. Graph lines may, also, extend beyond the range of the data, and may represent more-or-less expected or ideal curves—and so are, appropriately or not, "cognitive." It is important to note that although these fictional graph lines can be misleading they are very often highly useful, as they marshal complicated and often disparate data into simple consistent forms which can be compared with other data. It may also be noted that, in the practice of displaying data in science, the procedures of curve fitting are automatic and are readily carried out by computer programs following quite simple algorithms, which may be applied in a wide variety of situations, though perhaps not always appropriately.

The notion that perception works by following simple rules, or algorithms, is important in current Artificial Intelligence (AI) visual research. It provides a potential bridge across the Great Divide, between what I have called the passivisits (stressing bottom-up from stimuli) and the activists (stressing top-down from knowledge) accounts of perception. To these we may now add the *algovists*. Since useful algorithms must be general, they cannot be based on specific object knowledge—so they cannot be richly cognitive. Also, since they work from, and provide, rather simple generalizations of object shapes, they cannot be strictly stimulus-driven. So, as they cannot be markedly top-down or bottom-up, the algovists lie in the Great Divide between the activists and the passivists. Having set this up, only experiments can classify phenomena in these terms. Whether the terms are useful depends on whether they suggest or help to clarify experiments.

Illusory Contours and Ghostly Surfaces

Returning to illusory contours: if we accept, at least for the moment, that normal visual contours are generated from somewhat scattered retinal signals, by procedures somewhat similar to line-fitting for graphs, we might well expect such procedures to produce illusions in odd situations. Then (just as artifacts of graphs) they might be powerfully misleading—even to creating ghosts. It is a curious and generally ignored fact of these and *all* illusions that we see the "ghosts"–or distortions or whatever—*perceptually* while, at the same time, we know *conceptually* that they are illusions. This separation of perception and conception, as revealed in illusions, is a highly disturbing fact—that we can experience illusion while knowing it is illusion—which is not sufficiently considered by philosophers concerned with epistemology. Yet we experience this separation of perception and explicit knowledge (which may be a problem for cognitive theories of perception) every time we study illusory contours: for we see them yet know they are not "really" there. Why should perception and conception be so separate? An explanation will be suggested at the end of this chapter.

Figures such as Schumann's early example (Fig. 9.1) or the very well-known Kanizsa triangle (Fig. 9.2) elicit illusory contours bounding an illusory surface, which may be slightly lighter or slightly darker than the background. There are, however, illusory contour figures (such as Fig. 9.3) which do not produce surfaces—but only contours. Here we are concerned with illusory surfaces having bounding contours or edges, rather than with cases of isolated illusory contours, which though of undoubted interest have not been studied so fully. Strictly speaking, phenomena associated with the edges of illusory surfaces (such as their binocular fusion, which will be discussed below) should be checked, to make sure that they hold

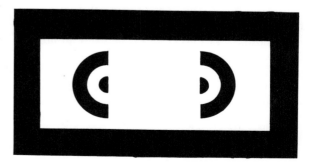

FIGURE 9.1. Schumann's figure. This is the first known cognitive contour figure (1900).

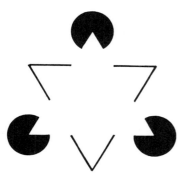

FIGURE 9.2. Kanizsa's triangle. This is the most famous example of an illusory surface bounded by illusory contours. It is suggested that the illusory surface is a postulated occluding surface to account for the gaps, perceptually.

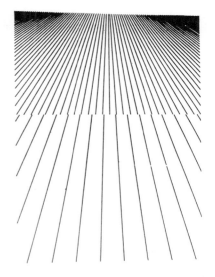

FIGURE 9.4. An isolated contour produced by a sudden change of slope, as indicated by perspective (though this also has displacement).

also for isolated contours (such as those of Fig. 9.3) to be sure they are closely related phenomena, having much the same neural basis. This should be done; but meanwhile it may be assumed that they have similar neural and phenomenal characteristics, even though what generates them is somewhat different. Preliminary (unpublished) experiments suggest that they do have very similar properties.

Invoking Surfaces

Illusory surfaces are given by "gappy" figures, such as Figures 9.1 and 9.2. Isolated illusory contours can be produced by evidence of a discontinuity, especially in depth (Fig. 9.3) or perspective evidence of a corner or change of slope (Fig. 9.4). Discontinuity of depth in random dot Julesz (1971) steroe pairs, in which planes or

dots lying at various depths are clearly seen, give smooth edges even when the dots are few and widely spaced.

It was suggested in 1972 (Gregory, 1972), that the illusory surfaces of the Kanizsa triangle and many other examples may be perceptually postulated surfaces, accounting for unlikely gaps as due to eclipsing or occlusion by some nearer opaque object or surface. This notion depends very much on an "active" view of perception, such that perceptions are *hypotheses,* based on, but frequently going beyond, available sensory data—sometimes to generate fictions such as these. Thus, in the 1972 paper:

The cognitive paradigm of perception regards perceptions as hypotheses selected by sensory data, but going beyond available data, to give "object hypotheses" (Gregory, 1970). This paradigm would be satisfied by supposing that the illusory object is "postulated" as a perceptual hypothesis to account for the blank sectors and the breaks in the triangle.

This continues:

As these features are removed from the figure, the hypothesis becomes weaker, until the postulated masking object is no longer seen.

In the same year Coren (1972) also suggested that these phenomena are related to depth perception. Coren supposed that the figures provide evidence of depth, presumably by what are usually called depth-cues. I did not suppose

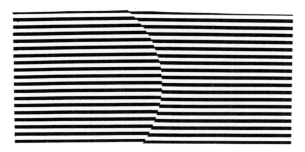

FIGURE 9.3. An isolated illusory contour. This is given by a displaced grating. Possibly this is a "depth cue," normally indicating a discontinuity of surfaces.

that the depth seen in illusory contours was cue-driven, but rather that the illusory surfaces and contours are postulated, to account for these gaps when they are surprising, as due to some occluding object or surface getting in the way. This often happens in normal perception as nearer objects often partly hide further objects, though they are still recognized and assumed to be complete. Such assumptions of completeness, though parts are missing, is clearly important for object perception in typical scenes. The illusion-generating figures are strikingly "gappy." Inspection of many figures suggests that illusory surfaces only appear when (a) the gaps are *unlikely;* (b) they form a *likely* object shape. This is also a prediction of this theoretical account. Inspection of a wide variety of examples seems to confirm it without exception.

An implication is that the visual system computes probabilities of whether gaps are likely to occur by chance, or are so unlikely that they are probably due to eclipsing by some nearer object or opaque surface. This probability balancing must be in terms of what are likely object shapes. Whether this is based on *particular* knowledge of objects, or on *generally* likely object shapes is surely the key question for deciding whether illusory surfaces should be thought of in inference from top-down specific knowledge activist terms, or by the more general algovist rules for what are likely to be objects. Here I reject an extreme Gibsonian "visual cues" account—for it is extremely hard to think of surprising gaps as simple cues giving depth directly, without some inference or rule-following. This, indeed, is exactly Gibson's own view (Gibson, 1950) when he considers occlusion and figure–ground phenomena. In his earlier writings, he concedes (in spite of his extreme passivist view of perception) that occlusion is not a simple depth-cue. Gibson (1950, p. 142):

The phenomenon of the superposition of objects is actually not a clue to the depth of objects but a perception which requires explanation. A man knows that a near object can partially obscure a far object but his retina does not, and the retinal explanation should be sought first. . . . There is no texture, double imagery (stereopsis), or relative motion in these drawings. They suggest the principle that the more complete, continuous, or regular outline tends to be

the one which looks near. Is completeness, then, a sign or clue for distance?

Gibson goes on to give remarkably nonpassivistic suggestions to account for selection of object over ground: that a nearer object tends to have the more *regular, complete* and *closed* contours (Fig. 9.5). These, he thinks, are best described not as "stimuli for perceptions of space" but as special, "probable signs, secondary to the others, or as having doubtful status." This seems an eminently reasonable account, though it is hardly in the Gibsonian passivistic tradition, as he evidently realizes.

We may accept that most figure–ground effects can be handled with the minimal cognition of algovism; but consider cases such as Rubin's vase-face figure. Here one might think the balanced probabilities of the vase and the face is the crucial point. But perceptual effects from specific knowledge of vases and faces would clearly be top-down, and would fit the activist paradigm. Evidently there is a gold mine here for experiments to investigate the claims of passivism, algovism, and activism.

An algovistic account demands that illusory contours should always be simple smooth curves—and should only be induced by or follow smooth closed curves. John Kennedy (1979) shows illusory surfaces produced by pointers arranged to converge on a circular area. This suggests experiments with adjustable

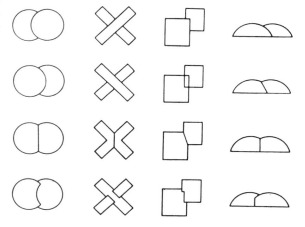

FIGURE 9.5. Occluding surfaces. These, surely, show something of the rules by which the perceptual system decides what is hiding and what is hidden, in an overlap situation (from J. J. Gibson, 1950, with permission).

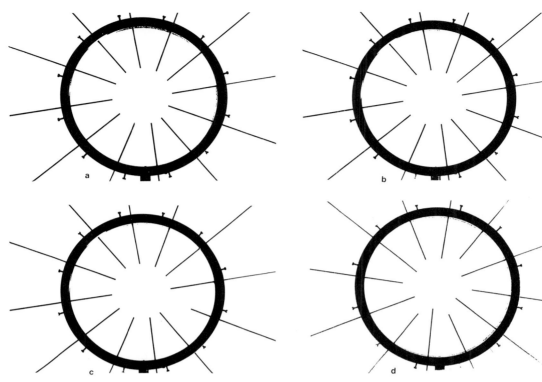

FIGURE 9.6. Spokes that speak of meaning. a. The converging wires forming a circle are seen as touching an illusory surface with a faint but distinct illusory contour. b and c. The contour will follow a displaced wire—up to a certain point—then "reject" the abberant wire. d. When the wires are random-ized, the contour and ghostly surface vanish. This suggests that it must represent a likely (smooth-edged) object. The extent to which this is given by an algorithm (like graph fitting) rather than by knowledge of specific objects is an important question as to how images convey meaning.

wires mounted in rings (Fig. 9.6) to find out how irregular or random an outline can be to support an illusory surface, as in Figure 9.6a,b,c,d. It may be seen that when the ends of the wires form a simple smooth shape (a circle) there is a strong illusory disc; but when the wires are individually pushed in and out to give a more and more jagged edge, the illusion is diminished, and with sufficient randomization it disappears. Also, a single wire pushed inside or outside the circle is "ignored," though several wires forming a gradual distortion of the circle drag the contour with them—to form a distorted figure with all the wires "touching" its illusory contour. It is surely interesting (though it is not possible to show it in a nonstereoscopic picture) that when the wires are arranged to form a smooth curve in *depth,* a corresponding three-dimensional illusory surface is produced—touching all the wires—provided they form a smooth curve in the third dimension. As for the two-dimensional wires, a wire too discrepant in *depth* is rejected. This observation might be significant, for the disparity at the retinas (or rather the difference in position of the wires at the two retinas) is very small. So this is not merely a matter of stimulus separations at the eye. Presumably the (algovistic) rules apply to perceptual space, in three dimensions, rather than simply to the retinal projection. This strongly suggests a postretinal origin for the phenomenon. But the situation is not entirely clear, as closely spaced wires give stronger contours. However, this could be because closely spaced wires provide more perceptual data for a contour or surface. It is likely that these contours are algovistic, while the surfaces are invoked by cognitive occlusion. Further evidence bearing on these issues will be given below: with evidence that the phenomena originate early in the visual system, though not at the retina.

Evidence from Physiology

This kind of algovistic rule-following, and activistic cognitive inference from particular kinds of known objects, is to be contrasted with contours signaled far more directly by Hubel and Wiesel type feature detectors (Hubel and Wiesel (1962, and many later papers), though this kind of account has been suggested for illusory contours. One reason why they seem very different is that the illusory contours are seldom if ever in line with, but rather *cross* the lines actually present in the stimulus pattern. This is clear in Figures 9.6a and b (which also shows the curious brightness contrast effect) and in many other examples. Electrophysiological evidence against such a feature detector account is the finding by von der Heydt, Perterhans, and Baumgartner (1984) that cells of the first stages of visual processing (area 17 of the Rhesus monkey visual cortex) do not respond to stimuli giving us illusory contours, though related activity is found further up, in area 18. We (Sillito, Gregory, & Heard, 1982) found no responses to illusory edges in area 17 in the cat, recording from cells that respond to weak actual contours; but unfortunately this study could not be completed and no cells were recorded from further along in the visual system (Fig. 9.7). This kind of negative evidence is somewhat unsatisfactory—and electrophysiologists do not like publishing records of no signals!

Evidence from Psychophysics

A somewhat unexpected finding which was reported in my 1972 paper (though it was reported earlier, by Lawson and Gulick (1967) and by Pastore (1971, Fig. 14.13, p. 296) is that the phenomena can occur through *binocular fusion* of parts of the figures—though neither eye, alone, has sufficient features to produce the illusory contours. This powerful technique for showing that a visual phenomenon is "central," and not retinal in its origin or cause, goes back to Witasek (1899). In his use of it, Pastore was discussing Gestalt-type isomorphic brain field explanations, which place the origin centrally and not retinally, which is compatible with Pas-

tore's findings that the illusory surface of the Kanizsa triangle is seen by binocular fusion from parts of the figure which are unsufficient for either eye alone. There are, however, devastating reasons for rejecting the Gestalt notion of physiological isomorphism: especially that it does not at all agree with the now known physiology of the early processes of vision.

It is interesting that *luminance*—rather than *color*—contrast is important for illusory contours, and for much of form, stereo, and motion perception. Thus stereo depth (Julesz, 1971), given by pairs of identical—except for displaced regions—random dot patterns, presented one to each eye, fails to produce apparent depth, or the bounding illusory contours of the displaced region of dots, when the dots and their background have color but no luminance contrast. Just such smooth continuous bounding contours are seen, also, when Julesz pairs are presented without stereo depth—viewed with one or with both eyes—but alternated to give *apparent motion* of the displaced regions of dots. It is suggestive that for this motion, and its associated illusory bounding contour, as for the stereo depth, there must be luminance and not merely color contrast in the display. Indeed, absence of brightness contrast, with only color contrast (isoluminance) greatly reduces Kanizsa-type illusory contours (Gregory, 1977), destroys random dot stereo depth (Lu & Fender, 1972), and destroys apparent motion from alternated dot displays (Ramachandran & Gregory, 1978). There is also general loss of form perception at isoluminance (Gregory, 1977, 1985). This shows that luminance contrast is crucial for much visual processing, and that color has a secondary role, which is not entirely surprising as color vision occurs late in the mammalian sequence (virtually only found in primates), and color can often allow recognition without precise form perception. This may indeed be its biological function. However this may be, the finding that some, but not other, visual phenomena are lost or modified with color-only contrast surely makes isoluminance a valuable diagnostic tool for classifying illusions. It has been found (Gregory, 1977) that distortion illusions believed to be essentially cognitive are not affected, while others believed to occur at early stages of visual processing, and not cognitive, such as the "cafe wall" illu-

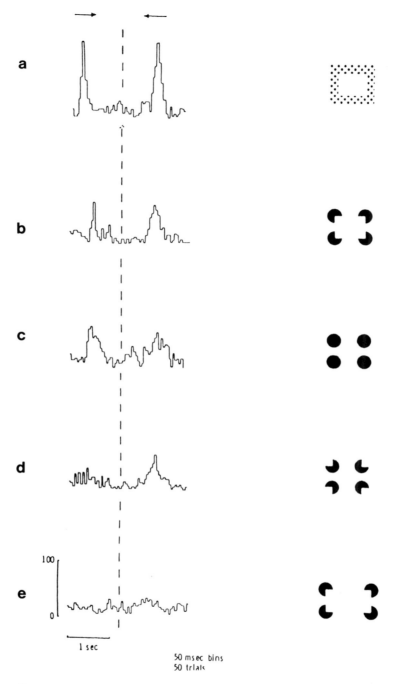

FIGURE 9.7. These figures were used to test, electrophysiologically, where associated neural activity is to be found in the cat. The stimuli were kept essentially the same—with no added or removed real contours—but the illusory contours disappeared for us by rotating the discs. Cells in area 17, which were found to respond to (weak) real contours did not respond to these illusory contours (Sillito, Gregory, & Heard, 1984). Electrophysiologists are, however, unhappy reporting *no* activity! It is a bit like publishing a picture of a black cat in a dark room.

sion (Gregory & Heard 1979), are lost at iso-luminance. The Kanizsa-type illusory surface figures are somewhat anomalous, as they are very largely though perhaps not completely lost with color but no luminance contrast.

The finding that these phenomena are ob-served through binocular fusion makes it virtu-ally impossible to suppose that the phenomena are retinal, or very early on in the visual sys-tem. This is compatible with the cognitive per-ceptual-postulate notion put forward in my 1972 paper. But the result of a later finding of ours (Gregory & Harris, 1974) is, at least at first sight, surprising on such a cognitive account. This experiment, which is easy to carry out as a demonstration given a stereoscope of some kind, starts from the fact that illusory contours can have a wide range of curves (Kanizsa, 1955a, though not extreme curvatures or dis-continuities). It also derives from the finding (which runs counter to a Gestalt ''good figure'' account of illusory contours) that *concave* curves can be produced (Gregory, 1972). John Harris and I (Harris & Gregory, 1973), using a specially designed stereoscope which allowed depth measurements to be made, presented pairs of figures giving slightly differently curved illusory contours to each eye. We found that not only would they fuse—just as true contours of the same curvatures would fuse—but also they were seen as single contours lying in *stere-oscopic depth*, as for true lines of the same cur-vatures presented binocularly in the stereo-scope (Fig. 9.8). It follows that each eye system

must be capable of generating its own illusory contours. For contours must be available for (or produced by) each eye system in order to fuse into stereoscopic depth. It follows from the first experiment that the origin of illusory contours must be postretinal, and from the second exper-iment that they can (though not necessarily in all cases) be produced by processes at or be-yond the combining of the signals from the eyes, giving stereoscopic vision. This means that illusory contours can be produced by pro-cesses not right at the start, but probably quite early on in the visual system. But if they occur in the early stages of processing, how can they be *cognitive* phenomena? How can it be reason-able to suppose that they (or at least some of them) are *postulates* based on the *improbability of gaps?* For it seems implausible to suppose that probabilities depending on knowledge of objects can be assessed early in the visual sys-tem.

The Role of Cognition

It is important to note that these phenomena are not produced by surprising absence of particu-lar objects, or features of objects, however fa-miliar—such as missing noses of faces. A face with a missing nose does not evoke a fictional nose. The ghostly shapes that are produced are reasonably shaped *kinds* of objects, rather than particular objects, or parts of objects. So al-though the probability assessment may be thought of as cognitive (as it is based on what is likely to be an object) it is a minimal kind of cognitive decision-taking compared with what must be required for full object recognition. All that is needed, on this account, is assessment—which might be provided by quite simple rule following—of whether there is an object of some likely shape getting in the way. As we do not have to suppose that illusory surfaces are postulated for specific objects, their neural ori-gin could be early in the system—preparietal—and possibly within each eye system, prior to binocular stereo fusion, in the striate cortex. It is interesting, if this is indeed correct, that pro-cessing equivalent to David Marr's (Marr, 1982) ''2 1/2-D sketch'' can take place so early in the visual system.

Is there positive evidence that illusory sur-faces are postulated to account for otherwise

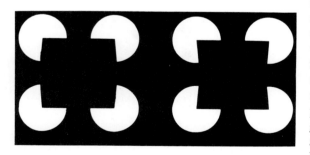

FIGURE 9.8. This stereo-pair evokes a three-dimen-sional illusory contour and surface (on the side com-ing out) by stereopsis. (The inward-going side tends to give double vision, or lack of fusion). The outgo-ing contour shows that each eye system is capable of generating its own illusory contours for fusion into depth (Harris & Gregory, 1973).

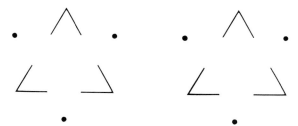

FIGURE 9.9. A stereo-pair used to force the illusory triangle back—when it disappears—or forward—when it is clearly seen in front of the gaps. The experiment used a range of disparities (Gregory & Harris, 1974).

surprising gaps? An obvious prediction is that they must (as they generally appear to do) lie perceptually in front of these gaps. A test of the notion is to see whether there is an asymmetry between near and far—as a surface cannot produce gaps by occlusion unless it is in front of the gaps, and so nearer to the observer than the gaps. So we (Gregory & Harris, 1974) presented a simplified Kanizsa triangle figure (a broken-line triangle, with three dots in place of Kanizsa's sector discs) (Fig. 9.9), in a stereoscope. For convenience this was a stereoscopic shadow projector, using collimated light (Gregory, 1969). We found that when the three dots were forced, by stereopsis, in front of the broken-line triangle, the illusory surface disappeared or was very weak. After some minutes of observation, however, it would generally reappear; but in a curious form, for its central region would pop up in front of the gaps of the broken-line triangle—bending so its corners went down to touch the dots behind the gaps. The conclusion was that the critical region of the surface must indeed lie in front of the gaps, for the gaps to be due to occlusion. When the stereoscopic disparity was reversed, the surface was clearly seen lying well in front of the gaps. This asymmetry is predicted from this account of a postulated surface. But it seems bizarre on any other account so far suggested.

Conclusion

We noted at the beginning of this chapter that we can simultaneously perceive an illusion and know that it is an illusion. This is so for these illusory figures and all other kinds of illusion, such as distortions and visual paradoxes. The key to why *perception* and *conception* are essentially separate is, surely, that they serve different purposes. Perception serves to ensure survival into the next few seconds; while conceptual understanding works over a far longer time-scale. Thus we perceive—and this is essential for survival—surrounding objects in a fraction of a second, and perception develops very fast in babies; but it takes years to generalize experiences and organize the kinds of ideas we can express in words. So perceptual intelligence is fast but "shallow," while conceptual intelligence is slow but "deep." Considering this in computational terms: it would be strictly impossible to access all our knowledge in the short time allowed for recognizing surrounding objects and seeing their significance. So (assuming as we do, that perception and thinking are given by neural computing) it must be impossible to check what we see by all we know, or bring to bear all that we know for seeing. So the intelligence of perception is necessarily a limited intelligence, with a small knowledge-base compared with the relatively vast knowledge of all our learning and understanding. Perception and conception are, and have to be, essentially separate and they cannot at all completely check each other. Thus, whenever we study illusory contours and surfaces we *see* what we *know* to be illusory.

SECTION III
Physiologically Based Analyses and Models

All the chapters in this section emphasize the role of peripheral mechanisms. In addition, several present models of illusory-contour formation, which emphasize the role of these mechanisms.

In Chapter 10, Ramachandran describes the relationship between illusory contours and motion and stereo capture. He presents a physiologically based description of illusory contours and other perceptual phenomena.

Shapley and Gordon, Chapter 11, present results of work done using a new type of illusory contour. This work is used to emphasize the role of cortical cells and nonlinear mechanisms in illusory-contour perception.

In Chapter 12, Grossberg and Mingolla present a model of illusory contours and object perception in general. While emphasizing the

role of peripheral mechanisms it also provides for input from higher-order processes.

In Chapter 13, Ginsburg discusses the role of low spatial frequency luminance changes in illusory contour detection. Presenting new supporting data, he points out that higher-order mechanisms cannot be considered until lower-order effects have been controlled for.

Sambin's Chapter 14 is a dynamic model of illusory-contour perception from a uniquely Gestalt framework. Sambin discusses the generation of anomalous figures, amodal completion, and perceptual reversibility.

Chapter 15, the final chapter in this section, by Klymenko and Weisstein is written from a direct realist (Gibsonian) perspective. It contains an analysis and model of motion-induced illusory dihedral edges.

CHAPTER 10

Visual Perception of Surfaces: A Biological Theory

V. S. Ramachandran

I doubt if we can ever guess what Natural Selection has achieved, without some help from the way function has been embodied in actual structures. The reason is simple. Natural Selection is more ingenious than we are.

—F. H. C. Crick, 1985

Introduction

There is a wealth of anatomical and psychological evidence which suggests that when you look at an object in the visual field, its various attributes such as color, motion, depth, and "form" are extracted by separate channels in the visual system. If so, how are these different attributes put back together again to create a unified picture of the object? And, in the case of a rapidly moving object, how is such perfect synchrony maintained between different features on its surface if it is indeed true that they are being extracted separately? In this essay, I shall suggest that this synchrony arises from a mechanism that I call *capture*. The visual system seems to extract certain conspicuous image features (such as occlusion boundaries), and the signal derived from these is then blindly attributed to features throughout the surface of the object. This implies that visual perception (especially in the periphery) is highly sketchy and impressionistic and that much of the richness and clarity that we experience is really an illusion.

My purpose in the chapter shall be to briefly describe some new illusions we have observed in our laboratory and to discuss their functional significance. I shall also try to provide some

conceptual links between these psychophysical findings and the recent anatomical discoveries of Hubel and Livingstone (1985).

Phylogenetic Considerations: Four Types of Contours

Since the brain is an organ that has been shaped by natural selection, a convenient starting point for the study of visual perception would be to carefully examine the different types of contours and edges that the visual system had to deal with as it evolved. Even a casual glance around you will reveal that there are at least four basic types of contours in the visual image:

Type 1 contours are continuous contours that form the boundaries of an object occluding another object or an object occluding its background. Such contours coincide with *abrupt* depth discontinuities and are always associated with depth cues such as stereopsis and motion parallax. From the standpoint of image segmentation these are the most important contours in the visual image.

Type 2 contours or discontinuous contours define texture elements, e.g., the flecks of light and shade on a carpet, the fur on a cat, or the grain of wood on a table top. Such contours are not associated with steep change in depth and they are often characterized by the presence of terminators.

Type 3 contours result from differential illumination of surfaces that meet at a corner. The corner can be convex or concave (e.g., the far corner of a room), and in the case of a convex corner there is always an associated attached shadow. The two surfaces defining the corner diverge from each other gradually; unlike Type 1 contours there is no step change in depth coinciding with the contour.

Type 4 contours form the borders of cast (or detached) shadows. Unlike Type 1 and Type 3 contours, there is no associated change of surface depth.

How does the brain distinguish between these different types of contours? Visual textures (Type 2 edges) generally continue across Type 3 and Type 4 contours but not across Type 1 contours. Similarly, color borders often coincide with occlusion (Type 1) borders but not with the other three types. That the eye must be sensitive to these regularities is evident from the sense of shock that one experiences when they are deliberately violated as, for example, in the paintings of the Belgian surrealist René Magritte. Furthermore, many similar tricks are also employed by animals which conceal themselves using camouflage. For instance, certain species of moths and flounders employ continuity of surface *texture* to conceal the Type 1 contours that would otherwise delineate them against the background. Also, many animals have evolved elaborate splotches on their coats in order to break their outlines, i.e., to eliminate Type 1 contours.

Many of the Gestalt laws of perceptual organization also begin to make sense when viewed in this context. Grouping texture elements on the basis of similarity, for example, would be especially valuable in a situation where an occluding object and its background have identical surface reflectances but dissimilar textures. Since most surface features on any single object tend to be similar it makes sense to group them together to delineate the object's outline. The law of "good continuity," on the other hand, might help preserve the continuity of Type 1 contours that are partially occluded by other objects such as tree trunks.

Since Type 1 contours always coincide with depth discontinuities, it follows that to perceive them accurately one needs to not only extract and locate edges (as emphasized by physiologists) but also to determine which side of the edge is figure and which side is ground. The Gestalt psychologists recognized this obvious fact and pointed out that the central problem in perception is the delineation of figure and ground, i.e., *surfaces* are just as important as contours.

Given the existence of these four types of contours, one wonders whether they are handled by separate physiological mechanisms in the brain. I would like to suggest that Type 1 and Type 2 contours are processed mainly by two separate anatomical pathways (the magnocellular and parvocellular systems). The magnocellular system is first used to extract and match Type 1 contours in order to construct 3-D surfaces. Type 2 contours, on the other hand, are extracted by the parvocellular system and the texture is then simply used to "paint" or fill in the 3-D surfaces—a process that we call *stereocapture* and *motion capture*. Because texture elements are highly redundant we hypothesize that the brain resorts to this "trick" to avoid the burden of having to match all the individual elements. And lastly, our evidence also suggests that color is independently processed by a separate anatomical pathway and is similarly used to "paint" the scene.

Illusory Contours

Figure 10.1 shows a striking example of image segmentation: a square defined by "illusory contours" (Coren, 1972; Gregory, 1972;

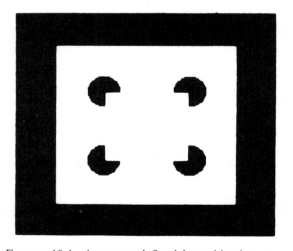

FIGURE 10.1. A square defined by subjective contours. Observers usually perceive an opaque white square whose corners partially occlude the four black discs. Faint "subjective" lines are seen to delineate the square, even though no physical lines exist.

Kanizsa, 1976; Rock, 1983; Schumann, 1904). These contours were produced by appropriately aligning black discs from which right-angle sectors were removed. One has the enigmatic impression of a contour connecting these aligned edges even though no contour exists physically—hence the name *illusory contours*. Whether these contours are physical, physiological, or truly illusory is a much debated semantic issue that need not concern us here. Whatever their epistemological implications, illusory contours are a striking illustration of the principle that a great deal of tacit knowledge of the world is built into early visual processing. Collinear edges evoke a sensation of occlusion because through millions of years of trial and error the visual system has learned that such edges are *usually* produced by occluding objects.

Since illusory contours are usually associated with occlusion, it follows, by definition, that they are also Type 1 contours. Why do illusory contours exist and how do they influence subsequent visual processing? In a world that is so rich in real contours it is hard to see what evolutionary advantage would accrue from the ability to construct illusory edges. But consider an arboreal primate trying to detect a leopard seen against a background of dense foliage. To this creature, segmenting the scene using illusory contours may be of vital importance as an anti-camouflage device. Many animals have developed elaborate splotchy markings in order to break their outlines (i.e., to eliminate Type 1 edges), and the ability to perceive illusory contours may have evolved specifically to defeat this strategy. In fact, we have argued elsewhere (Ramachandran, 1985a, 1986a) that many of the early processes of vision (including structure-from-motion, stereopsis, texture discrimination, etc.) evolved primarily as tricks to defeat camouflage rather than for seeing depth or motion per se.

It is a well-known fact that the visual system often uses many different strategies for a single purpose. For example, depth perception can be achieved through occlusion, light and shade, stereo (Julesz, 1971), and motion parallax (Rogers & Graham, 1979), and the organism can make *independent* use of each of these cues. At any given instant the visual system may try to engage all these processes simultaneously in or-der to ensure that at least one of them proves reliable. Further, the cues may also interact and complement each other in interesting ways, and in this paper we shall explore several examples of such interactions.

Physiological Considerations

The question of how different attributes of objects (such as form, color, motion, and depth) are analyzed has recently received considerable attention from physiologists. When tangential sections of area 18 in the Rhesus Macaque are stained for the enzyme cytochrome oxidase, one observes distinct dark stripes corresponding to enzyme-rich regions. There are two kinds of stripes, broad and narrow, which alternate with unstained "interstripe" regions (DeYoe & VanEssen, 1985; Hubel & Livingstone, 1985; Shipp & Zeki, 1985). Single unit recordings have revealed that cells in the narrow stripes have a double-opponent organization suitable for detecting color contrast. Cells in the broad stripes are tuned to binocular disparity, and those in the interstripes are sensitive primarily to length (form). Cells sensitive to direction of movement, on the other hand, tend to dominate the magnocellular pathway which relays through layer 4B in area 17 and terminates eventually in the broad bands in 18 as well as in area MT. In MT, the cells are tuned to both binocular disparity and motion but are insensitive to color-contrast (Van Essen, 1985).

Figure 10.2 summarizes the "flow diagram" we have just described. There is a clear anatomical separation of pathways which respond to color contrast from those which respond to movement, form, and stereoscopic depth. The separation of movement from stereo is not as clear-cut and, in fact, area MT contains cells which are tuned to both disparity and direction of movement.

Given this separation of color contrast-detecting cells from those sensitive to disparity and motion, it would be surprising if there were no psychophysical correlates of this in human vision, and in the last section of this chapter, we shall consider three obvious examples (Experiments 10, 11, and 12). Of more direct relevance to the theme of this book, however, is an observation made by von der Heydt, Peterhans, and Baumgartner (1984), who found that certain

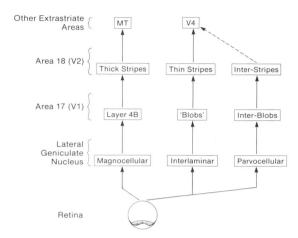

FIGURE 10.2. The flow of information in the visual pathways of primates (adapted from Van Essen, 1985). The parvocellular output actually relays through layer 4C, which is not shown in the diagram.

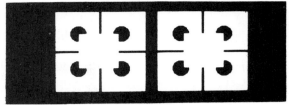

FIGURE 10.3. A stereogram produced by using two subjective squares similar to Figure 10.1. Small horizontal disparities are introduced between the vertical edges of the cut sectors. When the patterns of the two eyes are fused, a subjective square stands out in stereoscopic depth. All stereograms described in this chapter are printed in reverse to enable easy fusion; the pattern of the right eye is printed on the left and that of the left eye is printed on the right. To experience the illusions described, the reader should cross his eyes while fusing the stereograms. If the reader prefers to diverge his eyes, he should xerox and interchange the positions of the pictures.

cells in area 18 (but not 17) respond to illusory contours. Whether these cells occur in the narrow stripes, broad stripes, or interstripes is still an open question, but our observations on the loss of illusory surfaces at isoluminance (see the last section of this chapter) suggest that they would probably *not* be found in the narrow stripes.

This chapter is divided into three sections. In the first section we describe the manner in which illusory contours interact with stereoscopic disparity cues; the second section focuses on interactions with motion, and in the last section we explore interactions with color.

Section 1: Stereopsis

Experiment 1. Stereopsis from Illusory Contours

We created a stereogram using two illusory squares similar to Figure 10.1 by introducing small horizontal disparities between the vertical edges of the cut sectors (Blomfield, 1973; Gregory & Harris, 1974). The discs themselves were at zero disparity in relation to the surrounding frame. When the two patterns (Fig. 10.3) are fused by crossing one's eyes, the four black discs are seen in the same depth plane as the frame, but the white illusory square stands out quite clearly in front of the background, an

observation that suggests a high degree of interaction between illusory contours and stereoscopic depth perception.

Experiment 2. Capture of Stereopsis by Illusory Contours

Figure 10.4 depicts the "wallpaper effect." A pattern of repeating stripes is inherently ambiguous when viewed binocularly for it can convey any one of a number of different depth planes

FIGURE 10.4. A well-known stereoscopic illusion called the wallpaper effect. If the reader brings the pattern very close to his nose and changes his angle of vergence while viewing this display, he will perceive corresponding changes in the plane of perceived stereoscopic depth.

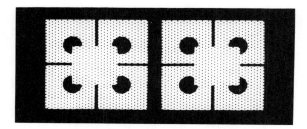

FIGURE 10.5. This figure is produced by superimposing a template of Figure 10.3 on a repeating wallpaper pattern. Eyes should be "crossed" to fuse this stereogram. The interdot separation between the elements constituting the wallpaper is 5 min of arc. A subjective square stands out in front of the background and carries the wallpaper with it, even though the elements on the wallpaper are at zero disparity. This is an example of stereocapture (see text).

(Helmholtz, 1909/1925). At any given instant, however, the entire pattern is seen to occupy only one single plane; the exact plane seen seems to depend mainly on the angle of convergence.

Patrick Cavanagh and I superimposed a template of the stereogram depicted in Figure 10.3 on several kinds of wallpaper to generate "wallpaper stereograms" (Figs. 10.5 and 10.6). In Figure 10.5 we simply used repeating vertical rows of dots (see figure legends for additional details). When the patterns of the two eyes were fused, the square defined by the subjective contours could be seen standing out clearly in front of the background. Interestingly, the corresponding dot rows on the wallpaper were also carried forward with the plane—an effect we call *stereoscopic capture* (Ramachandran, 1986a; Ramachandran & Cavanagh, 1985a). Since the disparity of the squares was several multiples of the periodicity of the dot rows, this finding implies that the subjective surface in depth created by the subjective contours was somehow pulling the dots with it even though the dots themselves were at zero disparity in relation to the background. Eight naive subjects who viewed these patterns reported this effect spontaneously. Interestingly, stereocapture can be obtained only with two-dimensional textures. If all the dots in Figure 10.5 are removed except for a single horizontal row in the middle the effect disappears completely and the dots remain flush with the background.

Experiment 3. Capture of Vertical Stripes

In Figure 10.6a we used continuous vertical lines instead of rows of dots in the background. Subjects reported that the illusion was just as

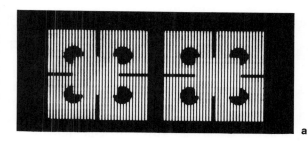

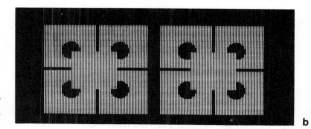

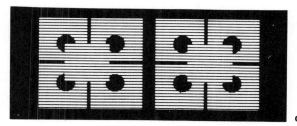

FIGURE 10.6a. A template of Figure 10.3 is superimposed on a pattern of repeating vertical stripes. (The spatial frequency of the stripes is 9 cycles/degree.) A subjective square stands out clearly from the background, carrying the lines with it. Also, the capture effect is strong enough to overcome the physical continuity of the lines and causes apparent breaks to appear on the lines. The effect is especially compelling if the disparity between the cut sectors is arranged to be an exact multiple of the grating periodicity. b. Similar to 10.6a except that the disparity has been reduced to 10 min of arc to enable easier fusion. The spatial frequency of the grating is 18 cycles/degree. c. Capture is considerably weaker if horizontal lines are used. The lines adjoining the sectors themselves are pushed forward but not the lines in between (they remain flush with the background and it is impossible to see subjective breaks).

compelling here as in Figure 10.5. Interestingly, the capture effect was strong enough to overcome the physical continuity of the vertical lines, and caused apparent breaks to appear on the lines at the upper and lower borders of the illusory square even though all the lines were at zero disparity. The effect can be enhanced by using more closely spaced lines (Fig. 10.6b).

Experiment 4. Anisotropy of Stereocapture

One explanation for the stereocapture illusion would be that the unambiguous signals derived from the cut sectors are blindly attributed to finer image features in the vicinity. This explanation is readily disproved by using horizontal lines in the background instead of vertical lines. When we superimposed Figure 10.3 on horizontal lines (Fig. 10.6c) we found that only the horizontal lines actually joining the sectors themselves were pulled forward. All the other lines on the square remained flush with the background, and it was very difficult to break the continuity of these lines in order to partition them into two surfaces. Although horizontal lines are perceptually just as salient as vertical lines, the brain is reluctant to attribute depth signals to them.

Experiment 5. The Influence of Occlusion Cues in the Perception of Stereopsis

The stereograms described so far convey *crossed* disparities, i.e., the impression of a square standing out in front of the paper (Figs. 10.3–10.6). When the disparities were reversed a new percept emerged (see Fig. 10.7). Subjects reported that instead of an illusory square they now saw four "portholes" cut out of an opaque sheet of wallpaper. The black discs which were originally opaque now acquired the subjective quality of being hollow. Through these holes they could now see the four corners of a smaller square piece of wallpaper, as shown schematically in Figure 10.8. This percept was seen only on stereoscopic fusion, which makes it different from the monocular organizational effects reported by Bradley and Petry (1977; also see Bradley, chap. 22, this volume). The effect took

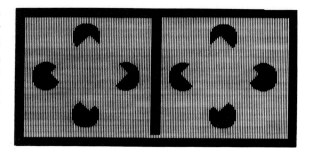

FIGURE 10.7. The "porthole" illusion produced by using uncrossed disparities. Subjects reported seeing four portholes cut out of an opaque sheet of wallpaper. Through these portholes, they could see the four corners of a smaller square piece of wallpaper which pulled the corresponding lines with them (see Fig. 10.8).

a long time to "crystallize" but once it was seen it became quite stable, and was perceptually very compelling (Ramachandran, 1986a). The illusory contours were now associated with "completion" of the holes (discs) rather than the square, and thus the corners which were seen through the holes pulled the corresponding lines of wallpaper with them. This unusual percept of seeing four deeper corners is of considerable theoretical interest for in this case, the illusory contours must be constructed *after* stereoscopic fusion. Further, once they have been constructed, these stereoscopic illusory contours must in their turn influence the subsequent processing of finer image features. This suggests that factors such as occlusion can directly influence the stereoscopic matching pro-

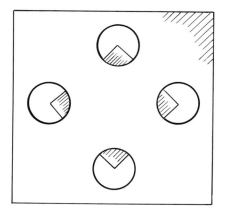

FIGURE 10.8. Schematic view of the percept obtained from Figure 10.7.

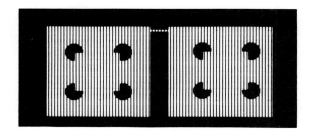

FIGURE 10.9. Disparity is introduced between the discs themselves (including cut sectors). Illusory contours are visible in the monocular image, but are actually reduced during stereoscopic viewing. Stereocapture is impossible to obtain. Hence, spread of disparity signals from the sectors alone is not sufficient to explain capture; construction of an illusory 3-D surface may be a prerequisite.

cess, and it is noteworthy that such a striking change in processing disparity signals can be induced by simply interchanging the pictures of the two eyes.

Experiment 6. Is the Presence of an Illusory Surface Required for Producing Stereocapture?

Unambiguous disparity signals can "propagate" and influence the matching of ambiguous elements in the vicinity (Julesz & Chang, 1976; Mitchison & McKee, 1985). Is stereocapture caused by a similar propagation of disparity signals from the cut sectors? To find out we tried using a "control" stereogram (Fig. 10.9) in which disparity is introduced between the discs themselves (including the cut sectors) and not just between the cut sectors alone. Stereoscopic capture could not be perceived in this stereogram even though the disparities conveyed by the cut sectors (and monocular illusory contours) are identical to those used in our previous experiments. This result suggests that the construction of an illusory stereoscopic *surface* is an important prerequisite for producing stereocapture; the mere propagation of disparity signals will not suffice.

Experiment 7. Phase Sensitivity of Stereocapture

We found that stereoscopic capture was also very sensitive to the spatial phase relationship between the wallpaper and the sectored discs;

the subjective square's disparity had to be an exact multiple of the periodicity of the lines. Thus, when the discs themselves were flush with the background, the subjective square occupied exactly the same plane as the enclosed wallpaper that was captured, and this seemed to amplify the illusion. This observation implies that the signal derived from the disparate subjective contours is not merely *attributed* to the elements of wallpaper; there must be some degree of mutual synergy between the two. In this respect stereocapture may turn out to be different from motion capture (Ramachandran & Cavanagh, 1985b; Ramachandran & Inada, 1985).

When a phase shift was deliberately introduced so that the disparity of the cut sectors was (say) 2.5 or 3.5 times the periodicity of the lines, the effect became somewhat unstable and the lines had a strong tendency to collapse into the background. In addition, some observers spontaneously reported a "transparency effect;" the illusory square acquired the appearance of a transparent sheet of glass lying on a sheet of wallpaper (Ramachandran, 1986a).

Experiment 8. The Perception of Complex 3-D Surfaces

By appropriately aligning the cut sectors it is possible to generate some rather complex stereoscopic figures such as overlapping rectangles (Fig. 10.10), bent surfaces (Fig. 10.11), or even intersecting tilted planes (Fig. 10.12). When we superimposed the overlapping rectangles on vertical stripes, capture could be perceived quite clearly (Fig. 10.13). Interestingly, the lines within the overlapping region were always captured by the *nearer* of the two rectangles, an

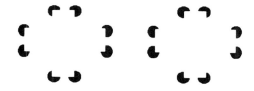

FIGURE 10.10. By appropriate alignment of the cut sectors on the discs, it is possible to generate some rather complex illusory 3-D surfaces such as two overlapping bars. The vertical bar appears nearer than the horizontal one.

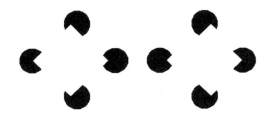

FIGURE 10.11. A stereogram depicting a diamond-shaped surface that is bent in the middle.

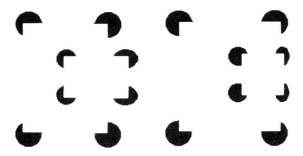

FIGURE 10.12. A stereogram depicting two tilted intersecting planes.

observation that is consistent with the occlusion principle discussed earlier (Experiment 5). Again, a simple spread of disparity signals cannot explain this effect since the region of overlap is equidistant from the cut sectors which define the vertical and horizontal rectangles.

The Role of Eye Movements

To rule out the possibility that vergence eye movements are involved in producing these ef-

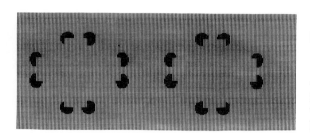

FIGURE 10.13. A template of Figure 10.10 is superimposed on vertical stripes. The lines at the intersection are always captured by the *nearer* of the two bars—in this case the vertical bar. This observation suggests that factors such as occlusion must influence stereocapture. The effect is especially vivid on eccentric fixation and tends to fade slightly on direct scrutiny.

fects we presented the stereograms (Fig. 10.5 and Fig. 10.6) in a tachistoscope to three subjects. Crossed and uncrossed disparities were flashed in random sequence while they fixated a spot presented on the background just below the subjective square. When asked to report whether the elements within the square appeared in front of or behind the plane of fixation they responded correctly on 51 out of 60 trials (3 subjects × 20 trials each). Similar results were obtained with Figure 10.6b (54 out of 60 responses were correct), suggesting that eye movements are not responsible for the effect.

Section 2: Motion

Our experiments on stereocapture were originally inspired by a very similar set of effects that we have observed in apparent motion ("motion capture"). Two uncorrelated random-dot patterns were visually superimposed and presented in rapid alternation to generate dynamic incoherent noise. When a low spatial frequency sine wave grating was superimposed on the noise patterns and made to jump left and right in synchrony with the alternating dot patterns, all the dots appeared to adhere to the grating and to move with it as a single rigid sheet (Ramachandran & Cavanagh, 1985b; Ramachandran & Inada, 1985). The motion of certain salient image features (such as the grating) masks the incoherent motion signals derived from the spots, and tends to dominate perception by a sort of "winner-take-all" process.

Experiment 9. Motion Capture with Illusory Contours

An interesting version of motion capture can be produced by a somewhat different procedure which involves the use of illusory contours. We began with illusory squares presented in an appropriately timed sequence to generate apparent motion of an illusory surface (Fig. 10.14; note that the discs themselves do not move). In this apparent motion sequence most subjects perceive an opaque oscillating square that occludes and disoccludes the discs in the background; they never report seeing pacmen opening and closing their mouths or two illusory

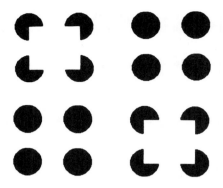

FIGURE 10.14. Apparent motion of an illusory square (Ramachandran, 1985b). The two frames of the movie are shown one below the other for clarity, but in the original experiment they were optically superimposed so that the discs were in perfect registration. One has the vivid impression of an opaque illusory surface that jumps left and right while covering (and uncovering) the black discs in the background. Note that all eight discs are present in each frame so that the discs themselves do not move.

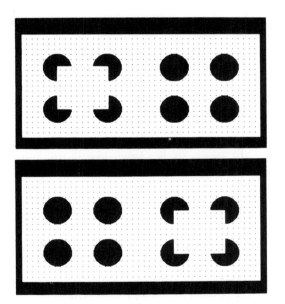

FIGURE 10.15. A template of the movie described above (Fig. 10.14) is superimposed on rows of dots. The dots are present in both frames and are exactly superimposed on each other so that they can generate no movement signals of their own. However, when the illusory square jumps, all the dots corresponding to its surface appear to jump with it as a single solid sheet—an example of a class of illusions that we call *motion capture* (Ramachandran, 1985b; Ramachandran & Inada, 1985). The motion of the illusory surface spontaneously generalizes to the dots contained within its boundaries.

squares flashing on and off. When a template of this movie was then projected on a regular grid of dots (or stripes), the dots appeared to move with the illusory surface even though they were physically stationary (Fig. 10.15). Since there is no evidence that the dots have not moved, the brain assumes, by default, that they have jumped with the illusory square (Ramachandran, 1985b, 1986a).

Two other aspects of motion capture are also worth noting:

1. When the pacmen in both frames of Figure 10.15 were made to face *outward* rather than inward, the capture effect disappeared and the pacmen were seen to simply open and close their mouths. This suggests that in Figure 10.15 capture was being produced by motion of the illusory surface rather than by the motion of the cut sectors themselves.

2. Capture was also seen when Figure 10.14 was superimposed on stripes instead of dots. Interestingly, the effect was just as vivid with horizontal stripes as it was with vertical stripes; the striking anisotropy which we observed in stereopsis was not observed in motion capture (Ramachandran, 1985b, 1986a).

Section 3: Color

Given the high degree of anatomical separation between color- and motion-sensitive cells in the visual pathways, would it be possible to discover psychophysical correlates in human vision? This question was raised by Ramachandran and Gregory (1978), who used random-dot kinematograms as a probe to study human motion perception at equiluminance. We began with two random-dot patterns which were identical except for a central square patch of dots that was displaced by two pixels in B in relation to A. When the patterns were optically superimposed (so that the background dots were in exact registration) and presented in rapid alternation, one could see a sharply defined central square oscillating left and right. Next, we replaced all the black–white elements in this kinematogram with red–green elements at equiluminance and found that the oscillating square disappeared completely. However, if two isolated spots were used instead of a kinematogram, apparent motion could still be seen to some extent even at equiluminance (Rama-chandran & Gregory, 1978). We concluded from these findings that color provides only a weak input to the motion system and that the segregation process in the kinematogram was especially dependent on brightness contrast, a conclusion that has been confirmed by Cavanagh, Boeglin, and Favreau (1985).

An elegant experiment by Cavanagh, Tyler, and Favreau (1985) also demonstrates the separation of color and motion in early vision. These authors used gratings instead of random-dot kinematograms and real movement instead of apparent movement. A red–green sine wave grating could be seen moving quite clearly so long as some brightness contrast was present but when it was made equiluminous it appeared *stationary,* even though it was observed to change location from moment to moment! The loss of motion could be observed only with low-frequency gratings and not with high-frequency ones.

More recently we have shown that the perceptual salience of texture-boundaries is also reduced at equiluminance. Textures composed of upright Ts can be readily discriminated from those composed of tilted Ts (Fig. 10.16, right) but not from ones composed of Ls (Fig. 10.16, left). Thus, oriented elements can provide tokens for texture segregation but T junctions cannot (Beck, 1966). When we repeated Beck's experiment at equiluminance (using red figures on a green background) the salience of the tex-ture-border on the right became reduced considerably and became similar to the border on the left. Since acuity for the letters would have been affected equally in both left and right panels, this dramatic reduction of texture-segregation cannot be attributed to a simple loss of resolution. Instead, the results suggest that the segregation process is at least partially color-blind.

Experiment 10. Capture of Color Borders with Moving Illusory Contours and Random-Dot Patterns

It is a well known fact that in color television the high spatial resolution of the luminance signals prevents one from noticing the very smeared low-pass images conveyed by the color channels. Also, at isoluminance, colors will tend to "bleed" across the border unless there is an associated luminance edge or a gap separating the two colors (Boynton, Hayhoe, & MacLeod, 1977). Gregory (1977) suggests that there may even be special mechanisms available in the visual system to prevent misregistration of color and luminance edges—a process that he calls *border-locking.* Grossberg and Mingolla (1985) have recently proposed an elegant theoretical model to account for some of these effects.

The separation of color, motion, and form channels observed by neuroanatomists raises three interesting questions. First, if a color boundary is deliberately blurred and superimposed over a sharp luminance edge, would the blur cease to be visible? Second, how much misregistration between the two kinds of edges will the visual system tolerate? (A high degree of tolerance is evident in the paintings of the French impressionist Raoul Dufy, who deliberately misaligned color and luminance edges in order to create pleasing visual effects.) And third, would moving luminance edges tend to capture color borders in the vicinity?

Here, we are concerned with question three, which we tried to answer using illusory contours instead of real contours. Our strategy was to create a deliberate misregistration between targets conveyed through luminance and color channels. The stimulus was a red triangle on a green background generated on an Amiga microcomputer (the triangle subtended 2°). A

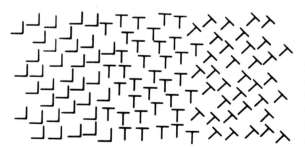

FIGURE 10.16. Tilted Ts are segmented from upright Ts, whereas Ls are not (Beck, 1966). When we repeated this experiment at equiluminance (red letters on green background), the segmentation of upright from tilted Ts was reduced considerably. Since loss of resolution would have affected Ts and Ls equally, this result implies that the texture segregation process is at least partially color-blind.

sheet of velum was then pasted over the CRT screen in order to blur the edges of the triangle. A transparent overlay of a slightly larger Kanizsa triangle (subtending 2.5° to 3.5°) was then superimposed over the velum so that borders of the illusory figure fell well outside the blurred borders of the red triangle.

Four observations were made:

1. There was a slight perceptual sharpening of the border of the red triangle.

2. When we jiggled the Kanizsa figure either vertically or horizontally, the red triangle appeared to move with it quite vividly even though it was physically stationary. The effect was especially striking on eccentric fixation; when we fixated 3° away from the center, the effect could be seen even without the velum and even for excursions of up to 0.5°.

3. When a small luminance contrast difference (20%–30%) was introduced across the color border the capture effect was reduced considerably and the red triangle usually appeared stationary.

4. Capture could also be produced if a sparse pattern of small black dots was used instead of illusory triangle. When the dots were moved, the red triangle was observed to move in the same direction.

To study the effect more carefully we used four naive subjects who were unaware of the purpose of the experiment. Both the red triangle and the Kanizsa triangle were generated on a CRT and the subjects were asked to fixate 3° away from the center of the display. The Kanizsa triangle was then made to oscillate horizontally by 0.5°. On some trials we added a 30° contrast difference across the edge of the triangle and these trials were randomly interleaved with the isoluminance trials. On each trial the subjects' task was to report whether he/she saw the red triangle moving or whether it appeared stationary. Using this procedure, we found that movement was reported on 37 out of 40 isoluminance trials and only 5 out of 40 trials when luminance contrast was present.

Interestingly, the effect was seen only if the sectored (pacmen) discs were conveyed through luminance contrast. If the discs themselves were also made red, the capture effect was abolished. Thus, moving luminance borders can capture stationary color borders, but moving color borders are ineffective in produc-

ing capture (perhaps because they generate only weak motion signals). These results suggest that motion signals are first extracted by the broad bands and perhaps applied spontaneously to color contours that happen to excite the adjacent narrow stripes.

Experiment 11. Disappearance of Apparent Motion of Illusory Surfaces at Equiluminance

We began with a stimulus similar to the one shown in Figure 10.14, except that instead of black figures on a white background we used red figures on a green background. The stimulus was generated on an RGB monitor using an Amiga microcomputer. Stimulus dimensions and SOA were identical to those used in Experiment 9. To achieve equiluminance we viewed the display through a color-flow filter mounted in front of a slowly rotating polarizer.

When a brightness difference was deliberately introduced between red and green, subjects always saw a square moving left and right to occlude (and disocclude) black discs in the background. At equiluminance, however, the moving square vanished completely and one now saw the pacmen either blinking on and off or simply opening and closing their mouths. The transition between the two states was quite striking and reported spontaneously by five naive subjects.

Experiment 12. Reduction of Stereocapture at Equiluminance

We repeated the experiment described above with stereograms (Fig. 10.6a), instead of using an apparent motion display. Again, when brightness contrast was present, stereocapture was seen quite clearly, as in previous experiments, but at equiluminance the subjective stereoscopic surface (and lines) collapsed into the background. The cut edges of the pacmen alone were seen to tilt forward from the plane of the paper, but there was no associated 3-D surface or stereocapture. These results are consistent with the findings of Lu and Fender (1972) and also with informal observations made recently by Hubel and Livingstone (1986).

Discussion

This chapter is concerned mainly with interactions between motion, depth, color, and texture. I have considered three examples: (1) Motion signals derived from certain salient image features are attributed to finer texture elements in the vicinity. (2) A similar effect occurs in stereopsis, except that there are probably two stages involved—an early stage that is similar to motion capture and a later stage in which signals derived from large-scale features interact actively with those derived from fine features. (3) Motion signals derived from luminance channels are spontaneously applied to adjacent color borders.

Unlike the "illusory conjunctions" observed by Treisman (1983), these effects occur only over a limited spatial range and are probably caused by somewhat different mechanisms. The brain tends to economize on information processing by exploiting certain regularities. Since in the real world most surface features on an object (e.g., color, texture, etc.) tend to adhere to each other, the visual system employs the simple trick of using only a handful of salient features to process motion and stereopsis. This seems especially true when rapid action is required, as when dodging a moving predator or when deciding the approximate depth of a surface that one is going to jump on. More "fine-grained" analysis of stereo and motion (Barlow, 1981) probably requires additional mechanisms, which have not been considered in this discussion.

Notice that I have left the phrase *salient features* undefined here, and one has to be careful to avoid the circularity of saying that they are features that generate capture. It remains to be seen whether feature salience in the sense of "pop out" in a search task (Treisman, 1983) also predicts motion capture.

It is important to note that low spatial frequencies are not the only features that can generate motion capture. Even illusory contours (Experiment 9) and cyclopean edges (see below) can be effective in some situations. Also, as noted under Experiment 10, a red triangle can be pulled along by a random-dot pattern, even though the triangle is perceptually more "salient." The only general rule that can be derived from these examples is that unambiguous

motion signals eliminate ambiguous ones and tend to dominate our perceptual experience. Salient features such as low spatial frequencies are simply *one* potential source of such unambiguous motion signals.

Differences Between Stereopsis and Apparent Motion

There is an obvious operational analogy between stereopsis and apparent motion (Table 10.1). In both cases, the visual system has to match two slightly dissimilar images that are separated either in space (stereopsis) or time (motion). Consistent with this analogy, we have observed certain similarities between stereocapture and motion capture. For example, our results suggest that the so-called *correspondence problem* in both stereopsis and motion is solved not by cooperative (Marr, 1982) or itera-

TABLE 10.1. Differences between motion capture and stereocapture that reflect differences in natural constraints.

Differences	
Motion	Stereopsis
Can occur unpredictably in any direction	Eyes are separated horizontally, hence disparities are always horizontal
Can occur over any distance	Eyes are a fixed distance apart, hence disparities are small and constant
Hence wider constraints	Hence narrower constraints
Hence tolerant of changes in detailed texture between successive views of the moving object	Hence not as tolerant of differences between the two eyes' images. Has time to make more sophisticated use of the constraints
Motion capture	Stereocapture
Horizontal lines are captured	Horizontal lines are not captured
Not phase-sensitive	Phase-sensitive
Works well even for uncorrelated textures	Works poorly for uncorrelated textures (Ramachandran, 1986a)
Salient features are matched first and the unambiguous signals are then simply *attributed* to the finer image features	Signal derived from salient features *interacts actively* with those arising from finer image features

tive (Ullman, 1979) algorithms alone, but by using certain salient image features that can be matched unambiguously. However, the manner in which this unambiguous signal is used appears to be somewhat different for the two processes. In motion, the unambiguous signal masks incoherent signals derived from finer image features, and the brain parsimoniously assumes that the latter have also moved with the salient features. (Or, to put it differently, the unambiguous signal is blindly *attributed* to all features in the image.) In stereopsis, on the other hand, the signal derived from salient features must actively facilitate and interact with signals derived from finer image features. This distinction[1] between stereocapture and motion capture is supported by two pieces of evidence:

1. Apparent motion of an illusory square will capture horizontal gratings almost as effectively as vertical gratings, and the spatial phase relationships do not have to be accurately maintained across successive positions. This suggests that the signal derived from the illusory surface is simply attributed to the enclosed texture elements. These findings stand in sharp contrast to stereocapture which, as we noted earlier, is anisotropic and phase-sensitive, observations that imply synergy rather than mere attribution.

2. Even textures that are completely uncorrelated in successive frames can be captured very readily, especially if sine-wave gratings are used (Ramachandran & Cavanagh, 1985b; Ramachandran & Inada, 1985). On the other hand, if the pictures of the two eyes are uncorrelated, stereocapture is reduced (Ramachandran, 1986a). The visual system is reluctant to "attribute" the signal derived from the illusory square to the rivalrous texture elements. Unlike wallpaper patterns, uncorrelated textures generate very few disparity signals and hence there is very little scope for synergistic interaction.

---

[1] It may turn out that the difference is quantitative rather than qualitative; motion capture may also be anisotropic and phase-sensitive, but to a much smaller extent than stereocapture (Ramachandran & Cavanagh, 1985b). If so, one would have to argue that the different weighting functions of the two phenomena reflect differences in natural constraints. A comparative study of capture may, therefore, provide useful insights into how the brain utilizes these constraints.

Why is there such a striking difference between the two processes? The logic of the scheme becomes clear if one considers the constraints underlying stereo and motion and the perceptual problems that the two systems were confronted with as they evolved (Table 10.1). Consider successive views of a leopard jumping from branch to branch on the treetops while pursuing one of our arboreal ancestors. For long jumps of the leopard, the excursion of the dots is beyond the displacement limit of coherent motion (Braddick, 1974) and the question arises: how does the visual system know which spot goes with which? Our results suggest the following strategy: (1) the motion of certain salient features (e.g., the leopard's outline) masks or inhibits the incoherent signals from the spots, and (2) the signal from the salient features is then spontaneously attributed to the spots as well. This strategy allows the visual system to preserve continuity of object identity while at the same time eliminating spurious motion signals through masking. The only disadvantage is that you could no longer see small local excursions of the spots themselves. For example, any slight ripple of the muscles on the leopard's flanks (or a change in its facial expression) would no longer be detected, but this is a small price to pay if you are trying to run away from him!

Motion capture "works" only because the brain can take advantage of certain statistical properties such as the fact that moving bodies normally carry their surface textures with them (e.g., spots do not usually fly off leopards). However, contrary to the views of AI researchers, we would argue that the visual system does not make *elaborate or sophisticated use of these properties*. Instead, the system appears to use a simple set of special purpose tricks (e.g., capture) to solve the problem (Ramachandran, 1985a, 1986b). By using appropriately weighted mutual inhibition between motion signals derived from different channels, the visual system solves correspondence and achives continuity of object identity without benefit from either computation or cognition.

From these considerations it follows that the motion system must, of necessity, have developed a high tolerance for changes in detailed texture (Table 10.1). The stereo system, on the other hand, operates under much narrower constraints. First, since the distance between the eyes is constant (and small), the range of binocular retinal disparities encountered is much smaller than the range of transformations encountered during motion of a textured object. Second, since the eyes are separated horizontally, retinal disparities are always horizontal whereas successive motion transformation can occur along any axis. These narrower constraints may have allowed the stereo system to evolve degrees of refinement which would not be feasible in the motion domain. Since the leopard is not moving and the two eyes are a fixed distance apart, the system can afford the luxury of carefully computing detailed depth relationships.

We have recently observed that the phase sensitivity and anisotropy of stereocapture are reduced considerably if the stereograms are flashed briefly (150 msec) and followed by a mask. Subjects tend to report that even the horizontal lines (Fig. 10.6c) are pulled forward unless they are allowed a leisurely inspection of the lines. Furthermore, even textures that are uncorrelated between the eyes are captured if a stereogram is flashed briefly, whereas on prolonged scrutiny the depth perceived in the texture elements becomes less compelling. These findings suggest that stereoscopic capture may, in fact, occur in two stages. In the first stage, which is similar to motion capture, the signals derived from coarse features are blindly attributed to finer elements in the vicinity, and this may be helpful in rapidly assigning depth values to surfaces at the expense of finer stereo discrimination. In the second stage, when scrutiny comes into play, there may be a more active synergistic interaction between signals derived from coarse and fine features. For example, wallpaper composed of vertical stripes (but not horizontal stripes) would excite multiple depth planes simultaneously, whereas the illusory contours would excite only a single plane. The latter signal may, therefore, be used to select or highlight the appropriate plane of wallpaper.

Possible Physiological Correlates

The investigations of Hubel and Livingstone (1985) and DeYoe and Van Essen (1985) suggest an anatomical explanation for the capture effects we have described here.

We have seen that the magnocellular pathway projects via layer 4B to the broad bands in area 18. Cells in these bands have large receptive fields and are sensitive primarily to stereo depth (Hubel & Livingstone, 1985) and, perhaps, to direction of movement. When a textured object is displaced suddenly in the visual field, the edges, low spatial frequencies and other as yet undefined features would tend to generate motion signals in the broad bands. These signals are perhaps spontaneously attributed to texture elements in the vicinity that simultaneously excite the adjacent interstripes. (The latter are known to have small, end-stopped receptive fields.) Using this strategy, the brain avoids the burden of keeping track of all the individual texture elements. Thus, both the old "cognitive" problem of preserving continuity of object identity during movement, as well as the more modern "correspondence problem" of computational vision, are solved by using a simple trick—a trick that incorporates the tacit assumption that in the real world textures tend to adhere to objects.

Capture of color borders is probably caused by a similar process. Since both color borders and texture borders are usually associated with Type 1 edges, the brain avoids redundancy by using the luminance edge alone to compute depth and motion and then "painting" the scene in an impressionistic way (using color and texture). Recent views on the evolution of primate vision lend some plausibility to this suggestion. Our ancestors were nocturnal insectivorous primates with very well-developed magnocellular systems, and they may have relied entirely on the broad band system for stereo and motion. Cells within this system have large receptive fields that respond well to even very low contrast (Shapley & Perry, 1986), so that spatial resolution was sacrificed for sensitivity. Later, when these ancestral primates become diurnal and frugivorous, they could afford the luxury of adding on the parvocellular system and associated color pathways and this allowed high-contrast, fine-grained texture and color to be perceived.

Cells in area 17 respond to small retinal disparities (Barlow et al., 1968) and those in area 18 respond to large disparities (Hubel & Wiesel, 1970; Ramachandran, Clarke, & Whitteridge, 1977) as well as illusory contours (Van der

Heydt et al., 1984). If we make the further assumption that cells in the broad bands of area 18 might respond to the *disparity* of illusory contours, it is not inconceivable that stereocapture results directly from synergistic interactions between cells in these two visual areas. For instance, the repeating texture of the wallpaper might excite cells corresponding to several depth planes in area 17 (or interstripes of area 18), whereas the disparity of illusory contours would excite only a single plane in the broad stripes area 18. The latter signal might then be fed back to select or "highlight" the appropriate plane—a conjecture that is consistent with the observed anisotropy of stereocapture.

The anatomical scheme suggested here may also account for the distinction between "long-range" and "short-range" motion and between "qualitative" and "patent" stereopsis that is often made by psychologists (Braddick, 1974; Ogle, 1952; Mitchell, 1969). Perhaps long-range motion and qualitative stereopsis are processed by the magnocellular pathways, and the function of "capture" may then be to simply assign the appropriate signal to underlying texture elements. The neural basis of fine-grained motion and stereopsis has yet to be discovered, but it could be based on either: (1) parvocellular pathways (e.g., the interblobs of area 17 and interstripes of area 18), or (2) a more detailed computation within layer 4B (Poggio & Poggio, 1984) and the broad stripes (Hubel & Livingstone, 1985). It should be possible to distinguish between these two models by studying the contrast-sensitivity of fine-grained motion and stereopsis (Hubel & Livingstone, 1986). Unlike the parvocellular system, the magnocellular system is sensitive to contrast levels well below 10% (Shapley & Perry, 1986); so if fine-grained stereo and motion discrimination are based on the parvocellular output alone, then they should break down at low contrast levels.

There is one observation that does not quite fit the anatomical scheme proposed here. It is found that some degree of motion capture can be produced even with cyclopean contours. A Julesz stereogram depicting a vertical cyclopean bar was displayed in Frame 1. Frame 2 portrayed an identical bar displaced to the right and this resulted in vivid apparent motion of the bar. The effect could be seen even if the elements composing the first stereogram (Frame 1) were uncorrelated with those of the second (Frame 2). Furthermore, the dots on the surface of the cyclopean bar also appeared to move with it even though they were uncorrelated in successive frames. On monocular inspection, capture disappeared and was replaced by the appearance of dynamic incoherent noise. This suggests that apparent motion can be seen between cyclopean edges and, further, that the dots that define the stereogram can be captured by the cyclopean edges. If the magnocellular pathways are picking up the motion of low spatial frequencies, how does one explain the apparent motion of cyclopean edges? Since the broad stripes and their recipient zones (MT) are sensitive to both stereopsis and motion, it is not inconceivable that these effects are mediated at some later stage within the same pathway. For instance, either the broad stripes or MT might pick up motion of cyclopean edges, and the signal might then be attributed to texture elements that excite the adjacent interstripes. The general rule might be that Type 1 edges are extracted by the magnocellular system, and that they can veto incoherent signals produced by Type 2 edges. (Cyclopean edges are, by definition, Type 1 edges.)

If the broad-band system is involved primarily in extracting stereopsis and motion from luminance borders, it must follow that these two visual processes should fail at isoluminance (i.e., it should not be possible to obtain depth or motion at equiluminance). Unfortunately, there are serious technical difficulties associated with using chromatic borders at equiluminance. First, as pointed by Hubel and Livingstone (1986), there is probably some variation of the equiluminance point with eccentricity and most investigators have not bothered to correct for this in their experiments. Second, the point of equiluminance may be different for different spatial frequencies and/or different cell types, in which case it may be impossible, in practice, to create a display that is equiluminous for all cells. Yet, in spite of these obstacles, it is possible to make some tentative generalizations. For instance, it is generally agreed that there is a considerable reduction of perceived motion at equiluminance (Ramachandran & Gregory, 1978; Cavanagh, Tyler, & Favreau, 1984; Cavanagh, Boeglin, & Favreau, 1985). Also, stereopsis is reduced (Lu & Fender, 1972), al-

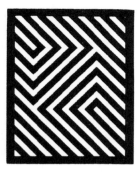

FIGURE 10.17. An ambiguous figure that can be seen either as a single occluding square or as several concentric rectangles. If the black–white edges are replaced by red–green edges at equiluminance, the square can no longer be seen. This finding suggests that the neural mechanism that mediates depth perception is at least partially color-blind.

though in a forced-choice experiment subjects can, in fact, still make some crude discriminations (de Weert, 1979). Thus, although motion and depth are not completely lost at equiluminance, it is comforting to note that at least some of the observations made so far are consistent with the known physiology.

There is some evidence that other kinds of depth perception are also reduced at equiluminance (Hubel and Livingstone, 1986). For instance, we find that the kinetic depth effect (Ramachandran & Anstis, 1986) deteriorates considerably at equiluminance, as does the sense of undulating depth that one observes in "op art" paints such as those of Bridget Riley or Victor Vasarely. Surprisingly, even depth from occlusion (Fig. 10.17) is reduced. More recently, we observed that if the blue-white edges that define the "illusory" letters on the cover of this book are replaced with red-green edges at equiluminance, then the sense of solidity disappears completely. The letters become illegible and look like Chinese characters even though there is no comparable reduction in acu-

ity. (Interestingly, reversing the *sign* of luminance contrast does not eliminate depth.) Taken collectively, these results suggest that depth information from many different sources (stereopsis, occlusion, motion parallax, shadows, etc.) may eventually converge on some higher visual area (MT?) that is color-blind.

Capture is also reduced at equiluminance. In one of our stereograms, when we replaced the black-white borders with red-green borders at equiluminance, there was a striking reduction in stereocapture. Similarly, when the movie depicted in Figure 10.14 was replaced with an isoluminant version, one could no longer see a square oscillating left and right. Instead, there was an abrupt transition to seeing the discs (pacmen) either opening and closing their mouths or simply blinking on and off. Taken together, these results suggest that motion and stereopsis associated with illusory surfaces require brightness contrast; color contrast will not suffice. Perhaps this dramatic reduction of motion, depth, and associated illusory surfaces at equiluminance is a direct perceptual consequence of the anatomical segregation observed by physiologists. The close coupling we observed between illusory contours, stereo, and motion and the fact that color contrast cannot support any of these percepts suggest that cells that respond to illusory contours are most likely to be found in the broad stripes rather than narrow stripes or interstripe regions of area 18.

Acknowledgments. I thank P. Cavanagh, F. H. C. Crick, D. Hubel, M. Livingstone, J. Allman, and C. W. Tyler for stimulating discussions, and E. Ebbesen for facilities. Experiments 2 to 4 were done in collaboration with P. Cavanagh of the Universite de Montreal and have been previously published (Ramachandran & Cavanagh, 1985b).

CHAPTER 11

The Existence of Interpolated Illusory Contours Depends on Contrast and Spatial Separation

Robert Shapley and James Gordon

Subjective, or perceptual, or interpolated contours—whatever we call them, the experience of seeing the borders in demonstrations like Kanizsa's triangle (Kanizsa, 1955) is fascinating and puzzling. Upon close inspection the apparent border may disappear, yet the initial involuntary perception of a completed contour is compelling. Explanations for the perception of such interpolated contours have ranged from cognitive processes (Gregory, 1972; Prazdny, 1983) to spatial filters (Ginsburg, 1975) to simultaneous contrast (Frisby, 1980). We have approached this problem from a somewhat different direction, based on our prior experience in studying visual neurophysiology. We have investigated the dependence of the existence of interpolated contours on the spatial separation of the inducing elements, and upon their contrast, and have found a strong dependence on these parameters. Furthermore, we have found that apparent contours may be interpolated between regions of opposite contrast (Shapley & Gordon, 1985). This latter result is of major importance, in our view, because we think it implies that form perception is performed parallel to and independently of brightness perception, and that form perception depends on a specific kind of neural, nonlinear, spatial filter. These conclusions will be discussed fully after presentation of the patterns we have used and the experimental results obtained with them.

Experimental Methods

Visual patterns were produced on the screen of a Tektronix 608 monitor (P4 white phosphor) with an electronic visual stimulator (Milkman,

Schick, Rossetto, Ratliff, Shapley, & Victor, 1980) under the control of a PDP 11/23 microcomputer. The instrument produced a 10 cm × 10 cm raster display: 256 lines/frame, 256 picture elements (pixels)/line, 270 frames/sec. It also produced four spatial luminance profiles which could be mapped into each of the 65,536 (256 × 256) pixels. The mapping was controlled by the entries in a 65,536 × 2 bit memory, the values of which set the state of a fast electronic switch at a rate of 20 MHz. The contrast on the screen was controlled by depth-of-modulation values sent to the instrument by the computer. This was done for each spatial profile independently. Thus, for example, the spatial contrast of spatial pattern number 1 could be zero, while the spatial contrast of an inducing pattern, say spatial profile number 2, could be set to 0.5. The spatial profile was multiplied by the depth-of-modulation number with a multiplying D/A converter.

Interpolated Contours and Signs of Local Contrast

We have studied the mechanisms of interpolated contours by investigating contour interpolation when local contrast changes sign along the border. We can define the local contrast across the border of an object to be:

$$(L_{obj} - L_{bg})/(L_{mean})$$

where L_{obj} is the local luminance of the object, L_{bg} the luminance of the local background, and L_{mean} the average of the two luminances. The local contrast around the border of an object can be positive or negative. It is positive if the

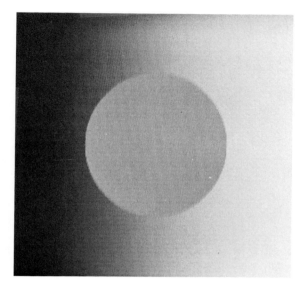

FIGURE 11.1. Circular figure at the borders of which the contrast changes sign. The background luminance is a one-dimensional linear gradient. The luminance of the central circle is constant across its extent and equal to the mean luminance of the gradient. The absence of a luminance difference across a vertical line down the middle of the picture makes the unbroken appearance of the circle's contour an example of an interpolated contour. Note that the sign of the local contrast changes from plus to minus from left to right across the picture. This is a reproduction of a photograph taken with Ilford FP4 film from the face of a Tektronix Model 608 CRT monitor. The pattern was created with the electronic instrument described in Milkman et al. (1980).

luminance of the object is greater than the luminance of the local background, and negative if the luminance of the background exceeds that of the object. The study of contour interpolation between a segment of border that has positive local contrast and a segment with negative local contrast is of theoretical interest. The existence of contour interpolation in this case rules out some models.

Figure 11.1 is a picture that contains a circular object of constant luminance on a background which is a continuous gradient of luminance. The background luminance profile can be described formally by the equation:

$$L_B(x) = L_0(1 + mx)$$

where x is horizontal position in the picture referenced to the middle of the picture, at which place $x=0$, and m is the slope of the gradient.

The mean luminance of the gradient is L_0 and that is also the luminance of the circle. Thus the circle's luminance is equal to the luminance of the background along a vertical line located at the middle of the picture. The local contrast at the border of the object is positive to the left of such a midvertical line and negative to the right. Of greatest relevance to the investigation of interpolated or subjective contours, the local contrast along the border is close to zero near where the circle's border crosses the midvertical line. At normal viewing distances of this figure at this level of average contrast, the border does not disappear where the contrast goes to zero, but rather is interpolated from a segment of border with negative contrast to a region of positive contrast. A similar circular figure bounded by border segments with opposite contrast is shown in Figure 11.2. However, in this picture the border contrast never goes to zero but jumps abruptly from positive to negative. It is apparent that the circular shape is the same in the two pictures. Although not shown, the identifiable form of a circular object with one sign of contrast around its border, for example a dark disk on a bright background, is the same as these two circles with changing con-

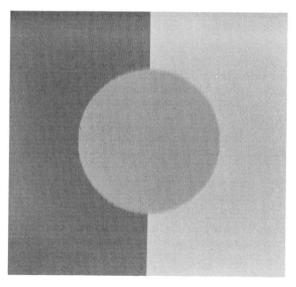

FIGURE 11.2. Circular figure on a bipartite field background. Like Figure 11.1, this is a circle of luminance equal to the mean of the luminance of its background. In this case, the background is a square wave of luminance. Again, the contrast changes in sign from the left side of the picture, where it is positive, to the right, where it is negative.

trast around the borders. Thus, the shape or form of such objects is not contingent on the sign of the contrast, while the apparent brightness is very much dependent on the sign of the contrast (Heinemann, 1955; Shapley and Enroth-Cugell, 1984). The existence of interpolated contours in Figure 11.1 suggested to us a way to characterize the spatial integration properties of the visual mechanisms that must be activated for forms to be recognized, as described below.

Spatial Integration of Contour Detectors

In our initial experiments reported earlier (Shapley & Gordon, 1985) we estimated the spatial integration of the border-sensing mechanisms by varying the viewing distance of a picture of fixed average contrast like that shown in Figure 11.1. The rationale for this procedure is that as the viewing distance becomes smaller, the absolute visual angle subtended by the low contrast gap down the center of the circle will become larger. The larger gap will eventually become so large that it is longer than the longest contour-detecting mechanism in the brain, and the perceptual interpolation across the large gap should break down. It is a significant fact that contour interpolation does break down under these conditions, for the picture in Figure 11.1 as for Kanizsa's triangle. By measuring the distance at which contour interpolation in this pattern does fail, one can calculate the length of the contour-sensing mechanisms. With this approach, we arrived at a value of the length of the contour detectors of about 1.75°. This estimate depended on assumptions about the contrast thresholds for the inducing borders, and also the assumption that change in screen size (in visual angle) and viewing distance would have little effect on spatial integration estimates. To obtain a more accurate estimate of the spatial integration length of the contour mechanism, we have designed a better experiment.

In the experiment on spatial separation reported below, the following procedure was used. The subject controlled the depth of modulation, or contrast, of an inducing pattern. Contrast of the inducing pattern is defined conventionally as $(L_{max} - L_{min})/(L_{max} + L_{min})$, where L_{max}

is the maximum luminance in the inducing pattern, and L_{min} is the minimum. The PDP 11/23 initially set the contrast to be 0.1. The luminances and therefore the contrasts were calibrated at the beginning of the experiment by means of a Photo Research 1980b photometer. During the experimental runs, the subject adjusted the contrast of the inducing pattern by pressing keys on a keypad connected to the computer, which then varied the depth-of-modulation numbers it sent to the electronic visual display. When a threshold for just seeing an interpolated contour was reached, the subject pressed a terminator key on the keypad, and the value of the contrast was recorded. Three settings were obtained for each condition and then the values were averaged. Mean luminance on the screen was 100 cd/m², and the screen was viewed binocularly at a distance of 114 cm so tht 1 cm on the screen was equivalent to 0.5° visual angle. The subjects were instructed to fixate the border, so we believe that the spatial summation results describe foveal vision only.

The estimation of spatial integration was performed using the patterns depicted in Figure 11.3. These are based on Figures 11.1 and 11.2, but have the added feature that the luminance of the variable width strip down the middle of the picture is kept constant at L_0, the mean luminance of the background and also the luminance of the circle. For contour interpolation to work, some neural mechanism(s) in the brain must bridge this gap by responding to the border of the circle at the ends of the gap. As we increase the width of the gap, contour interpolation becomes more difficult to experience and eventually fails. In this experiment, the viewing distance was kept fixed at 114 cm, so that 1 cm on the screen subtended 0.5° visual angle. Gap width could be varied in approximately 1 min arc steps. By measuring the width of the gap in degrees of visual angle above which contour interpolation fails to occur, we have determined an upper bound to the length summation of contour sensors in the human visual system.

The spatial integration experiment was conducted as described above, by adjustment of contrast from below until the interpolated contour was just visible at each gap width. Results for two subjects, the authors, are graphed in Figure 11.4. Confirmatory results were obtained with two other subjects, who were naive about the purpose of the experiment. The more

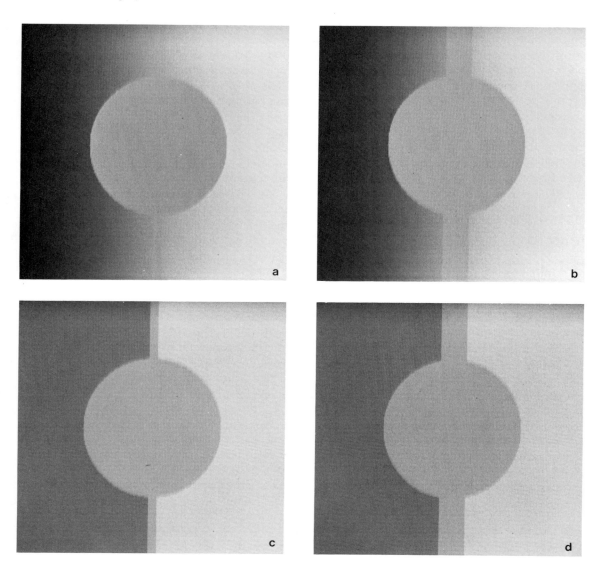

FIGURE 11.3. Circles on backgrounds with added gaps in the contour. Rectangular strips of luminance equal to that of the circles' luminance were painted on the screen. a and c: The gap was 0.16° of visual angle at our viewing distance of 114 cm. b and d: The gap was 0.46° of visual angle. The contrast of these demonstration pictures was 0.8 on the screen when the photographs were taken. In each pair, one of the backgrounds was a uniform linear gradient of luminance like Figure 11.1; the other member of each pair had a background which was a bipartite field as in Figure 11.2.

complete results of subjects R and J are reported here. The results obtained with increasing gaps in a gradient background (as in Fig. 11.1) are graphed as filled symbols, and are denoted "ramp" in the key. The results obtained with a gap placed over a bipartite background (like that in Fig. 11.2) are graphed as empty symbols and are denoted "sqwave" in the key. Although there are intersubject differences in the degree to which the nature of the background influences the contrast required to obtain satisfactory contour interpolation, we feel these intersubject differences are less important than the remarkable agreement for all four subjects in the following result: contours could never be interpolated across a gap that was wider than 0.5° of visual angle. This is our present estimate of the upper bound for the

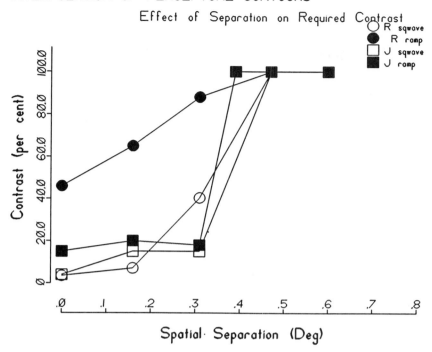

FIGURE 11.4. Dependence of contrast threshold for perceiving interpolated borders as a function of spatial separation of inducing borders. Experimental procedure described in text. The points plotted as having a contrast threshold of 100% included those cases when the subject saw no interpolated contour at any contrast; these are spatial separations at which the contour interpolation phenomenon fails.

length summation of contour interpolation in the human fovea.

The discrepancy between the present measurement of 0.5° and the previous estimate of 1.75° may be due to a number of factors. The most important factor is probably position in the visual field. In the earlier experiments, subjects were not instructed to fixate the region of border interpolation, but in the present experiments, they did fixate. It is likely that spatial integration extends over larger areas when the interpolated borders are located in the peripheral visual field away from the fovea. The measurement of 0.5° for length summation should, therefore, be interpreted as the value of length summation for the fovea. It is worth noting that border interpolation seems to depend on position in the visual field for other patterns (e.g., Kanizsa's triangle). Central fixation of the region of the interpolated border usually makes the apparent contour disappear. Fixation away from the region of border interpolation, so that the region of the illusory contour is placed into the periphery of the visual field, restores the illusion. We have argued previously that this phenomenon indicates the finite length of contour integration, and the smaller length of integration in the fovea than in the periphery (Shapley & Gordon, 1985). The finitude of border interpolation and its variation with retinal position suggests a neural as opposed to a cognitive explanation for interpolated contours.

The Nonlinear Border Detector

One consequence of the rather small estimate of length summation is that neural, mechanistic explanations are reinforced and cognitive explanations are weakened. The reason is that there is no convincing reason why a cognitive, problem-solving mechanism would have any length limit at all in this experiment. At the contrasts at which contour interpolation is success-

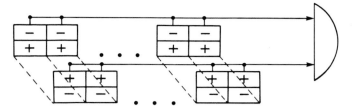

FIGURE 11.5. Diagram of a nonlinear border-detecting mechanism. It is supposed that signals from local contrast-sensing neurons of one polarity, indicated by the + and − receptive fields, are summed in a nonlinear manner with signals from local contrast-sensing neurons of the opposite sign, indicated by the − and + receptive fields. The fields of the border detectors are supposed to be elongated compared with the shape of the local contrast-sensing neurons, because of nonlinear summation along the length of the border detector's field. The results of experiments shown in Figure 11.4 give a maximum length of this detector's length summation of 0.5° visual angle. The nonlinearity of summation, indicated by the circular sector symbol in the diagram, may be an absolute value or any other even-order nonlinearity.

ful with small gaps, what the subjects experience with the large gaps is simple failure of the border to appear complete. This is just the sort of result one would expect from a hard-wired contour detector mechanism. We have previously proposed a nonlinear border detector to be the front-end for the perception of form, on the basis of our previous experiments (Shapley & Gordon, 1985). The present results, presented here for the first time, reinforce this proposed mechanism. A diagram of such a nonlinear border detector is shown in Figure 11.5.

If one assumes the existence of a nonlinear border detector, like that shown in Figure 11.5, then one would predict that there should be interpolated contours in figures analogous to Kanizsa's triangle but with alternating positive and negative contrast at the inducing corners. We created such figures in 1982, and presented them at the annual meeting of the Association for Research in Vision and Ophthalmology in Sarasota in 1983 (Shapley & Gordon, 1983). We were surprised to see a similar picture appear in the paper by Prazdny (1983)! As far as we can tell, this is a case of independent discovery. Our figure can be seen in Figure 11.6. The alternating, pacman-like, inducing bodies alternate black to white, and the interpolated contours lie on a gray ground. Such pictures make plain that the interpolated contour phenomenon is not inextricably linked with the brightness induction which is also seen in Kanizsa's figures (Kanizsa, 1955) and other variants. Thus, both Prazdny and we concluded that linear spatial filter explanations like Ginsburg's (1975) and si-

multaneous contrast explanations like Frisby's (1980) were incorrect. Both these theories would require linkage between the interpolated border and the observed brightness difference. Basically that is because both theories presume that the operative mechanisms respect the *sign* of the inducing borders. But Figures 11.1, 11.2, and 11.6 refute this theoretical position and that is why they are so important. Brightness and

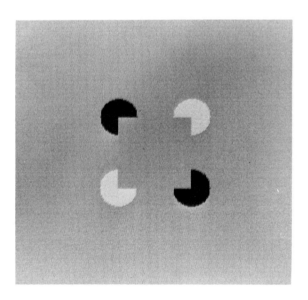

FIGURE 11.6. An illusory square produced by inducing figures that alternate in the signs of contrast. The central square and the surrounding area have the same luminance, which is the mean of the luminance of the inducing black and white figures at the corners.

form must be computed separately, because mechanisms to compute brightness must conserve sign of contrast, while form-computing mechanisms must discard the sign of the contrast. This conclusion reinforces the earlier results and conclusions of Ware (1981), who observed dissociation of induced brightness and apparent contour in shifted grids of lines of variable line density, and of Petry, Harbeck, Conway, and Levey, (1983), who showed that perceived brightness and perceived sharpness judgments differ (are semi-independent) under various spatial manipulations.

Prazdny (1983) expressed the view that the existence of a demonstration like Figure 11.6 refuted Frisby and Ginsburg, and that the only alternative explanation was cognitive. We have offered another explanation, namely something like Figure 11.5. The length summation limitations of contour interpolation support our proposal and tend to refute the cognitive explanation. There are other demonstrations and measurements that also reinforce the idea of intrinsic neural circuitry and also disconfirm a strictly cognitive explanation. These include the observations of Gregory (1977) that isoluminant heterochromatic borders do not induce interpolated contours. We have confirmed this observation recently with patterns like Figure 11.1 but with isoluminant chrominance gradients. Furthermore, we have found that temporal modulation may cause failure of contour interpolation. Detailed quantitative data are as yet lacking, but we can say that above 6 Hz of background modulation it is very hard to see interpolated contours in pictures like Figure 11.1. All of these failures of contour interpolation are reminiscent of classical psychophysical limitations imposed by discrete hard-wired neural mechanisms. Though there must be some role for cognitive high-level activity in recognizing the shapes outlined by interpolated contours, we feel that the underlying basis for this fascinating perceptual phenomenon is a basic neural circuit for sensing borders, and knitting them across small gaps. This neural circuit is blind to isoluminant color borders, cannot respond to rapid temporal variation above about 6 Hz, does not preserve the sign of the contrast but only the magnitude of contrast, and can only integrate border information over a length of about 0.5° in the fovea. These characteristics should aid in locating this neural mechanism in the brain.

Acknowledgments. The authors gratefully acknowledge the excellent technical support of Norman Milkman, Michelangelo Rossetto, and Gary Schick. The authors would also like to thank Susan Petry for her helpful criticism of an earlier version of the manuscript. The research was supported by the National Eye Institute through grant R01-EY01472, and by the Air Force Office of Scientific Research grant AF 84-0278. Computing time was provided by the CUNY University Computing Center.

CHAPTER 12

The Role of Illusory Contours in Visual Segmentation

Stephen Grossberg and Ennio Mingolla

The Role of Illusory Contours in Visual Segmentation

Many paradoxical percepts are expressions of adaptive brain designs aimed at achieving informative visual representations of the external world. Paradoxical percepts may therefore be used as probes and tests of the mechanisms that are hypothesized to instantiate these adaptive brain designs. Illusory contour percepts, in particular, provide numerous clues and constraints for a theory of boundary formation and textural segmentation, because they involve subtle interactions of form and color processing. A main theme of this chapter is the role of illusory contours in perceptual grouping processes. Our theory makes precise the sense in which percepts of illusory contours—or contour percepts that do not correspond to one-dimensional luminance differences in a scenic image—and percepts of "real contours" are both synthesized by the same mechanisms. This discussion clarifies why, despite the visual system's manifestly adaptive design, illusory contours are so abundant in visual percepts. We also suggest how illusory contours that are at best marginally visible can have powerful effects on perceptual grouping and object recognition processes.

An introduction to our theory can be gotten by considering paradoxical properties of certain cells in mammalian visual cortex that were reported recently by von der Heydt, Peterhans, & Baumgartner (1984), properties which were predicted by our theory (Cohen & Grossberg, 1984; Grossberg, 1984; Grossberg & Mingolla,

1985a). By using visual stimuli that induce perceived illusory contours in humans, von der Heydt et al. measured responses in certain area 18 cells whose receptive fields were crossed by an illusory contour. They reported that the cells appeared to act as logical gates, requiring two orientationally aligned luminance contours on either side of their receptive field in order to fire. These cells also exhibited a tendency to fire in the presence of the ends of thin lines oriented *perpendicular* to the cells' preferred orientation, which was first determined by using conventional oriented luminance edge stimuli. Cells in area 17 did not possess either of these properties. Our theory predicted the existence of cells at two successive processing stages with these properties from considering how the visual system is able to perceive line ends and corners, as well as continuous sharp boundaries, despite disruption of scenic input by retinal veins and the retinal blind spot (Kawabata, 1984). The tasks of early visual processing thus demand striking adaptations, such as topologically disconnected, separately thresholded receptive fields for single cells, and perpendicular induction of certain orientationally tuned responses.

Our theory suggests that two distinct contour-sensitive processes, which obey different rules, operate in parallel to initiate the cortical processing of scenic images. We originally introduced the Boundary Contour System and the Feature Contour System to deal with paradoxical data concerning brightness, color, and form perception, including the percepts of illusory contours. Boundary Contour signals are used to synthesize the boundaries, whether "real" or "illusory," that the perceptual process generates. Feature Contour signals initiate the filling-in processes whereby brightness and colors spread until they either hit their first boundary contour or are attenuated due to their spatial spread. We have characterized these systems by identifying the different rules that they obey, and by instantiating these rules using real-time neural circuit models. In addition to predicting the von der Heydt et al. data, these neural circuits have clarified recent neural discoveries concerning parallel processing within area 17 of the striate cortex, notably by the hypercolumn and blob subsystems, of signals from the lateral geniculate nucleus (Hendrickson, Hunt, & Wu, 1981; Hortin & Hubel, 1981; Hubel & Wiesel, 1977; Livingstone & Hubel, 1982, 1984). Some of these rules are now intuitively summarized.

In Figure 12.1a, the Boundary Contour System completes a boundary between vertical edges which possess opposite direction-of-contrast, in particular, between a vertical dark-light edge and a vertical light-dark edge (Grossberg & Mingolla, 1985a; Prazdny, 1983; Shapley & Gordon, 1985). Thus the boundary grouping process is insensitive to direction-of-contrast. A color and brightness system such as the Feature Contour System must, however, remain

exquisitely sensitive to direction-of-contrast, or we would be blind. In Figure 12.1a two vertically oriented and spatially aligned scenic edges can generate an intervening boundary across a region that has no corresponding color or luminance contrast within the image. This boundary completion propagates *inward* between pairs of inducing elements, and is *oriented*. On the other hand, a host of experiments indicate that color and brightness signals diffuse *outward* away from scenic edges in an *unoriented* manner to "fill in" regions with their own featural quality (Krauskopf, 1963; Land, 1977; van Tuijl, 1975; Yarbus, 1967).

In addition to analyzing how this boundary completion process generates illusory contours, we also suggest how the same process controls the context-sensitive ability of the visual system to segment and group textured input. An important insight into how this happens derives from considering how it is that emergent boundaries can be "invisible" but still "recognizable," as in the perception of Glass patterns (Fig. 12.1b). That is, boundary signals extracted from scenic edges can under some circumstances group in ways which do not separate regions of differing color or brightness. Despite this fact, these boundaries can strongly influ-

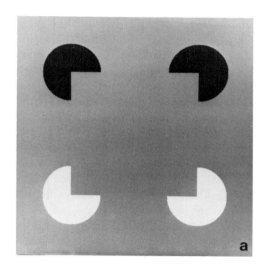

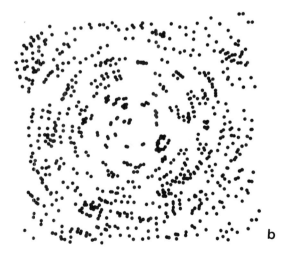

FIGURE 12.1a. A reverse-contrast Kanizsa square. An illusory square is induced by two black and two white pacman figures on a gray background. Illusory contours can thus join edges with opposite directions-of-contrast. (This effect may be weakened by the photographic reproduction process.) b. A Glass pattern. The emergent circular pattern is "recognized" although it is not "seen" as a pattern of differing contrasts. The text suggests how this can happen. (Reprinted with permission from Glass and Switkes, 1976.)

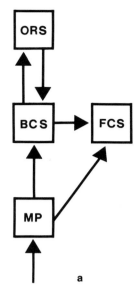

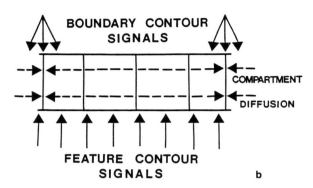

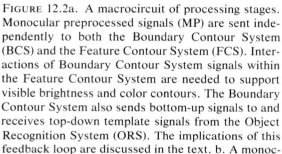

a

FIGURE 12.2a. A macrocircuit of processing stages. Monocular preprocessed signals (MP) are sent independently to both the Boundary Contour System (BCS) and the Feature Contour System (FCS). Interactions of Boundary Contour System signals within the Feature Contour System are needed to support visible brightness and color contours. The Boundary Contour System also sends bottom-up signals to and receives top-down template signals from the Object Recognition System (ORS). The implications of this feedback loop are discussed in the text. b. A monoc-

ular brightness and color stage domain within the Feature Contour System. Monocular Feature Contour signals activate cell compartments which permit rapid electrotonic diffusion of activity, or potential, across their compartment boundaries, except at those compartment boundaries which receive Boundary Contour signals from the Boundary Contour System. Consequently, the Feature Contour signals are smoothed, except at boundaries that are completed within the Boundary Contour System stage.

ence visual object recognition. In our theory the presence within the Feature Contour System of different filled-in featural signals on opposite sides of a boundary is necessary for sustaining visible figural form (Fig. 12.2b). Object recognition can, however, be based directly on boundary signals from the Boundary Contour System, whether or not accompanying featural quality is perceived (Fig. 12.2a). Such processes also underlie the perception of certain textural grouping phenomena, as we now illustrate.

Dissociation Between Visible Contrasts and Recognized Groupings

A long line of distinguished research by Jacob Beck and his colleagues has identified variables affecting textural segmentation by the human visual system (Beck, 1983; Beck, Prazdny, &

Rosenfeld, 1983). Simple displays like the ones shown in Figure 12.3 show that the slopes of small elements of color or brightness contrast are a critical determinant of grouping, with regions containing many features with similar slopes tending to group. In particular, if certain of these features are distributed in a regular manner, collinear groupings of these features can become "emergent features," capable of setting one textural region apart from another (Fig. 12.3a). A crucial aspect of such emergent features is that the collinear arrangement need not be in line with the directions of the local contrasts (Fig. 12.3b).

A remarkable aspect of displays such as Figure 12.3 is that we see a series of short lines despite the control of perceptual grouping by the long emergent features. We claim that within the Boundary Contour System a boundary structure emerges corresponding to the long lines of Figure 12.3a. This structure includes long vertical structures as well as short horizon-

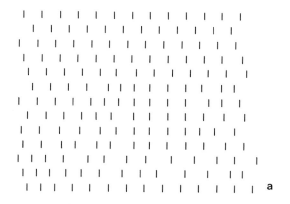

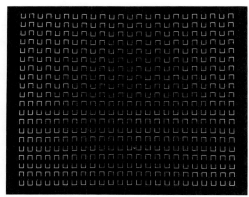

FIGURE 12.3a. Emergent features. The collinear linking of short line segments into longer segments is an "emergent feature" which sustains textural grouping. Our theory explains how such emergent features can contribute to perceptual grouping even if they are not visible (see Gellatly, 1980). b. The diagonal grouping at the top of this figure is initiated by differential activation of diagonally oriented receptive fields, despite the absence of any diagonal edges in the image. Horizontal cooperation of signals at the ends of vertical lines generates subjective contours in the bottom half of this figure. Figures 12.3a and 12.3b are reproduced with permission from Beck, Prazdny, and Rosenfeld (1983).

tal components near the endpoints of the short scenic lines. Within the Feature Contour System, these horizontal signals prevent featural filling-in of dark and light contrasts from crossing the boundaries corresponding to the short lines (Figure 12.2b). On the other hand, the output from the Boundary Contour System to an object recognition system reads out a long line structure without regard to which subsets of this structure will be seen as dark or light (Fig. 12.2a).

Hierarchical Resolution of the Boundary Uncertainty Induced by Orientational Sensitivity

The short horizontal Boundary Contour System signals that are generated in response to the ends of vertical lines (Fig. 12.3b) are related to the cortical data reported by von der Heydt et al. (1984). These horizontal signals illustrate another remarkable adaptation of the visual system, which leads us to assert that *the ends of all thin lines are illusory*. We grant that the perceived line ends correspond to actual luminance differences and so are not illusory by usual definition. However, the boundary signals indicating the position of any thin line end are necessarily weak or absent at an early stage of Boundary Contour System processing (Fig. 12.4a), and are synthesized in response to the spatial patterning of output signals from this early stage by a later stage of Boundary Contour System processing (Fig. 12.4b). We call the responses at the line end in Figure 12.4b *end cuts*.

The early stage in Figure 12.4a models how complex cells in area 17 of the striate cortex respond to a line end. These complex cells have elongated receptive fields in order to detect which orientations have scenic contrasts at given receptive field locations. At the ends of thin lines, these cells become insensitive to all orientations due to the very receptive field elongation that enables them to be sensitive to the orientations of scenic edges and bars. Compensatory processing by later Boundary Contour System stages is needed to generate end cuts, so that color signals cannot flow from every line end within the Feature Contour System (Fig. 12.2b), or for that matter from every scenic corner. Despite these precautions, colors can sometimes be seen to flow, as during the percept of neon color spreading (Redies & Spillmann, 1981a, van Tuijl, 1975).

Spatially Short-Range Competitive Interactions

Within our theory (Cohen & Grossberg, 1984; Grossberg & Mingolla, 1985b) the transformation from Figure 12.4a to Figure 12.4b is ef-

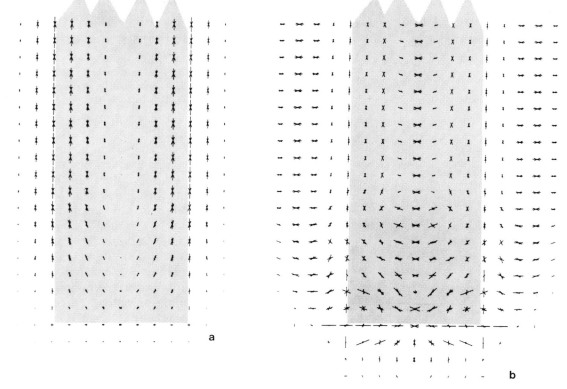

FIGURE 12.4a. An orientation field. Lengths and orientations of lines encode the relative sizes of the activations and orientations of the model-oriented cells (complex cells) at the corresponding positions. The input pattern, which is a vertical line end as seen by the receptive fields, corresponds to the shaded area. Each mask has total exterior dimensions of 16×8 units, with a unit length being the distance be-

tween two adjacent lattice positions. b. Response of Boundary Contour System cells at the competitive stage to the orientation field of Figure 12.4a. End cutting generates horizontal activations at line end locations that receive small and orientationally ambiguous input activations, but preserves the vertically oriented activations at the line edge locations.

fected by two successive stages of short-range inhibitory, or competitive, interactions (Fig. 12.5). These interactions are competent to generate the perpendicular reactions to line ends that were measured by von der Heydt et al. (1984) in area 18 of the prestriate cortex, and have been used to explain neon color spreading. In addition, they provide a new understanding of hyperacuity, or how the visual system achieves a spatial acuity finer than that of its receptive fields; for example, the end cuts in Figure 12.4b are localized in space at finer resolutions than the nominal spatial scale of the receptive fields of the cortical cells.

Figure 12.4 illustrates a general property of

the visual system that might profitably be introduced into computer vision algorithms. The uncertainty of retinal information is not progressively reduced by each successive stage in cortical processing. Each stage may eliminate one uncertainty while it generates yet a new uncertainty, much as in the Heisenberg uncertainty principle. For example, elongated receptive fields are needed to generate "orientational certainty" in response to scenic edges and bars, but thereby generate a new type of "positional uncertainty" at line ends and corners (Fig. 12.4a). The next processing stages resolve this positional uncertainty by generating end cuts (Fig. 12.4b).

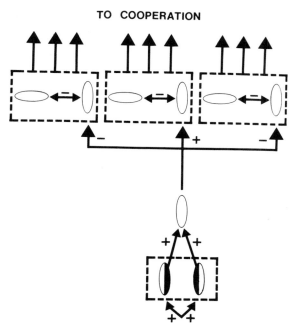

TO COOPERATION

FIGURE 12.5. Early stages of Boundary Contour processing. At each position exist cells with elongated receptive fields of various sizes, which are sensitive to orientation, amount of contrast, and direction of contrast. Pairs of such cells sensitive to like position and orientation but opposite directions of contrast (lower dashed box) input to cells that are sensitive to orientation and amount of contrast but not to direction of contrast (white ellipses). These cells, in turn, excite like-oriented cells corresponding to the same position and inhibit like-oriented cells corresponding to nearby positions at the first competitive stage (upper dashed boxes). At this stage, cells corresponding to the same position but different orientations inhibit each other via a push-pull competitive interaction.

Spatially Long-Range Cooperative Interactions

Once perpendicular boundary signals are generated at line ends, they are processed by subsequent Boundary Contour System stages according to the same rules as boundary signals originating in direct response to scenic luminance contrasts. Thus, in the texture displays of Figure 12.3, boundary completion and grouping can occur either along the direction parallel to thin line segments or in a direction perpendicu-

lar to line ends. End cuts thus increase the number of potential boundary groupings for any scene. Moreover, because oriented receptive fields are local *contrast* detectors, rather than *edge* detectors per se, certain combinations of local contrasts from disconnected scenic elements can at times trigger responses along orientations where there are no local edges. Such is the case in Figures 12.1b and 12.3b.

The complexity of the Boundary Contour System reaction to even a line end in Figure 12.4b illustrates that many "potential groupings" of parts into wholes are activated during preperceptual processes. In a final percept, a single global grouping is typically chosen and sharpened, while all other possible groupings are actively suppressed. This process of rapid preattentive boundary synthesis introduces its own remarkable geometric properties.

To understand why this is so, we first observe that the competitive interactions which generate end cuts are insufficient for choosing a global grouping, if only because their spatial interactions are of short range. We suggest that the competitive stages activate yet another stage at which a spatially long-range cooperative process occurs. Due to this process, like-oriented and spatially aligned contrasts within a scene can cooperate to form an intervening boundary, as in Figure 12.1a. Such a cooperative interaction is needed, for example, to complete boundaries that are occluded by retinal veins and the blind spot (Kawabata, 1984). Figure 12.6a schematizes our model of this cooperative process. Figure 12.6b embeds this cooperative process into the total architecture of the Boundary Contour System.

Within this cooperative process each cell can fire only if it receives sufficiently large inputs from paired populations of similarly oriented and spatially aligned cells at the competitive stage. These cooperative cells thus behave like the logical gates which were reported by von der Heydt et al. (1984). Activated cooperative cells feed back excitatory signals to the competitive cells, as in Figure 12.6a. The activated competitive cells, in turn, feed excitation backward to the cooperative level. In this way, boundary completion can rapidly propagate inwards in a spatially discontinuous manner.

The competitive cells whose orientations and

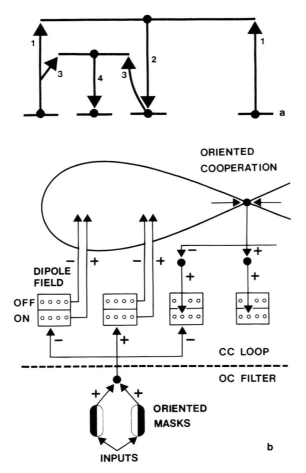

positions receive the largest cooperative signals win out over less favored cells within the final perceptual grouping. Thus the competitive stages do double duty: They generate end cuts in response to bottom-up signals and they help to choose the final segmentation in response to top-down signals. We call the cooperative–competitive feedback network which acts to choose the final segmentation a *CC loop*. Using the CC loop as a basis for synthesizing a percept of lines and curves is radically different from applying the axioms of geometry for lines and curves. In particular, the boundary corresponding to a line need not even be a connected set until the boundary completion process equilibrates. Boundary segments emerge at those locations and orientations that possess enough "statistical inertia" to survive the cooperative–competitive feedback exchange. These boundary segments may be generated, for example, by signals (almost) parallel to oriented scenic contrasts, by signals (almost) perpendicular to contrasts at the ends of thin lines or corners, or by signals generated by logical gates. In any event, perceptual lines are not merely local aggregates of points, but are rather coherent structures which emerge from several types of dynamical interactions.

FIGURE 12.6a. The pair of pathways 1 activates positive boundary completion feedback along pathway 2. Then pathways such as 3 activate positive feedback along pathways such as 4. Rapid completion of a sharp boundary between pathways 1 can thereby be generated by a spatially discontinuous bisection process. b. Circuit diagram of the Boundary Contour System: Inputs activate oriented masks, which cooperate at each position and orientation before feeding into an on-center off-surround interaction. This interaction excites like-orientations at the same position and inhibits like-orientations at nearby positions. The affected cells are on-cells within a dipole field. On-cells at a fixed position compete among orientations. On-cells also inhibit off-cells which represent the same position and orientation. Off-cells at each position, in turn, compete among orientations. Both on-cells and off-cells are tonically active. Net excitation of an on-cell excites a similarly oriented cooperative receptive field at a location corresponding to that of the on-cell. Net excitation of an off-cell inhibits a similarly oriented cooperative receptive field at a location corresponding to that of the off-cell. Thus, bottom-up excitation of a vertical on-cell,

All Boundaries Are Invisible

Unless a connected boundary can be synthesized by the Boundary Contour System, it cannot separate the Feature Contour System into domains capable of supporting different filled-in color or brightness signals. Thus if a later event can inhibit the cooperation before a connected boundary structure can emerge, no percept may be visible. This insight clarifies how later events

by inhibiting the horizontal on-cell at that position, disinhibits the horizontal off-cell at that position, which in turn inhibits (almost) horizontally oriented cooperative receptive fields that include its position. Sufficiently strong net positive activation of both receptive fields of a cooperative cell enables it to generate feedback via an on-center off-surround interaction among like-oriented cells. On-cells which receive the most favorable combination of bottom-up signals and top-down signals generate the emergent perceptual grouping.

can block the percept of earlier events during metacontrast (Breitmeyer, 1980; Gellatly, 1980; Reynolds, 1981). In our theory boundary signals are *always* invisible within the Boundary Contour System. Visible percepts emerge within the Feature Contour System. Thus the contrast-sensitivity of cells within the Boundary Contour System does not imply visibility of the final percept. Only the generation within the Feature Contour System of different filled-in featural contrasts on the opposite sides of a completed boundary (Fig. 12.2b) can lead to a visible percept.

The rules of the Boundary Contour System, first and foremost, prevent flow of color signals from line ends and corners, and complete occluded boundary segments over the retinal veins and blind spot. We now describe computer simulations which illustrate how these Boundary Contour System rules can also generate many properties of preattentive perceptual grouping, notably of the textural segmentation into regions which do not necessarily correspond to visible featural contrasts (Figs. 12.1b and 12.3).

Computer Simulations of Boundary Segmentation by the CC Loop

The segmentation and grouping of visual input into regions based on distribution of textural qualities, such as orientation, density, shape, or color, have been among the most puzzling and demanding of visual phenomena, involving a host of context-sensitive effects. A given texture element at a given location can be part of a variety of perceived groupings, depending on what surrounds it. Indeed, the determination even of what acts as an element at a given location can depend on patterns at nearby locations. We suggest that adequate grouping rules have not been previously described because the distinction between the Boundary Contour System and the Feature Contour System was not sharply made before, so their distinct rules and their interactions could not be articulated.

Computer simulations illustrate the ability of the Boundary Contour System to generate perceptual groupings akin to those seen in Figures

12.1 and 12.3. Numerical parameters were held fixed for all the simulations; only the input patterns were varied. As the input patterns were moved about, the Boundary Contour System sensed relationships among the inducing elements and generated emergent boundary groupings among them. In all the simulations, we defined the input patterns to be the output patterns of the oriented receptive fields, as in Figure 12.4a, since our primary objective was to study the segmentation properties of the CC loop. All possible oriented groupings generated inputs to the CC loop. Only the favored groupings survived. Thus the ability of the network to suppress the many incorrect local groupings is as important as its ability to choose the correct global grouping.

Figure 12.7a depicts an array of nine vertically oriented input clusters. We call each cluster a Line because it represents a caricature of how a field of oriented complex cells respond to a vertical line. Figure 12.7b displays the equilibrium activities of the cells at the second competitive stage of our model. The length of an oriented line at each position is proportional to the equilibrium activity of a cell whose receptive field is centered at that position with that orientation. The input pattern in Figure 12.7a possesses a manifest vertical symmetry: Triples of vertical Lines are collinear in the vertical direction, whereas they are spatially out-of-phase in the horizontal direction. The Boundary Contour System senses this vertical symmetry, and generates emergent vertical lines in Figure 12.7b. In addition, the Boundary Contour System generates horizontal end cuts at the ends of each Line, which can trap the featural contrasts of each Line within the Feature Contour System. Thus the segmentation simultaneously supports a vertical macrostructure and a horizontal microstructure among the Lines.

In Figure 12.7c the input Lines are moved so that triples of Lines are collinear in the vertical direction and their Line ends are lined up in the horizontal direction. Now both vertical and horizontal groupings are generated in Figure 12.7d. The segmentation can, however, distinguish between Line ends and the small horizontal inductions that bound the sides of each Line. Only Line ends have enough statistical inertia to activate boundary completion via the CC loop.

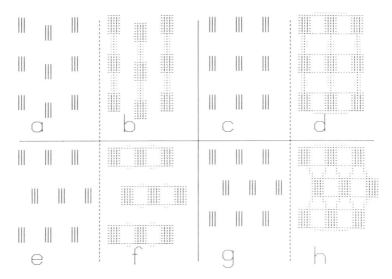

FIGURE 12.7. Computer simulations of processes underlying textural grouping. The length of each line segment is proportional to the activation of a network node responsive to 1 of 12 possible orientations. Parts a, c, e, and g display the activities of oriented cells which input to the CC loop. Parts b, d, f, and h display equilibrium activities of oriented cells at the second competitive stage of the Boundary Contour System. A pairwise comparison of a with b, c with d, and so on indicates the major groupings sensed by the network.

In Figure 12.7e the input Lines are shifted so that they become noncollinear in a vertical direction, but triples of their Line ends remain aligned. The vertical symmetry of Figure 12.7c is hereby broken. Thus in Figure 12.7f the Boundary Contour System groups the horizontal Line ends, but not the vertical Lines.

Figure 12.7h depicts a more demanding phenomenon: the emergence of diagonal groupings where no diagonals exist in the input pattern. Figure 12.7g is generated by bringing the three horizontal rows of vertical Lines closer together until their ends lie within the spatial bandwidth of the cooperative interaction. Figure 12.7h shows that the Boundary Contour System senses diagonal groupings of the Lines. These diagonal groupings emerge on both microscopic and macroscopic scales. Thus, diagonally oriented receptive fields are activated in the emergent boundaries, and these activations, as a whole, group into diagonal bands.

Von der Heydt et al. (1984) used illusory figures to discover differences in the response characteristics of area 17 and area 18 cells of the visual cortex. Our theory suggests that these same area 18 mechanisms are used to generate segmentations of a textured visual scene. It would be of great interest to directly test whether grouping properties such as those in Figure 12.7 can be measured physiologically at the area 18 cells which von der Heydt et al. discovered.

Related Concepts

A variety of other workers have developed concepts based on their data that support our conception of boundary completion, although no one of them has explicitly posited the properties of the Feature Contour and Boundary Contour processes. Petry, Harbeck, Conway, & Levey (1983) write, for example, that "apparent brightness is influenced more by number of inducing elements, whereas apparent sharpness increases more with inducing element width. . . Theoretical accounts of subjective contours must address both perceptual attributes" (p. 169). Day (1983) writes that "illusory contours . . . are due primarily to the spread of induced contrast to partially delineated borders" (p. 488), in support of our concept of diffusive filling-in, but he does not describe either how the borders are completed or how the featural induction and spread are accomplished. Prazdny (1983) studied variants of the classic illusion formed by thin lines in a radial pattern. He concludes that "simultaneous brightness contrast is not a cause of the illusion" (p. 404) by replacing the black lines by alternating black and white rectangles on a gray background. In this way, he also demonstrates that illusory contours can be completed between scenic contours of opposite direction of contrast, as in Figure 12.1a, but he does not conclude from this that distinct Boundary Contour and Feature Contour processes exist. Instead, he concludes that "it remains to be determined which of the competing 'cognitive' theories offers the best explanation . . . of subjective contours" (p. 404). Our results suggest that a cognitive theory is not necessary to explain the basic phenomena about subjective contours, unless one reinterprets "cognitive" to mean any network computation whose results are sensitive to the global patterning of all inducing elements.

We believe that our theory helps to clarify how many seemingly unrelated phenomena of illusory and real boundary detection and textural segmentation and grouping are related. The theory does this by providing a common mechanistic framework wherein issues of contour visibility and sharpness, brightness effects, and segmentation and grouping phenomena can be treated in a unified way over a variety of visual images.

Acknowledgments. Stephen Grossberg's research was supported in part by the Air Force Office of Scientific Research (AFOSR 85-0149), the Army Research Office (ARO DAAG-29-85-K-0095), and the National Science Foundation (NSF IST-8417756). Ennio Mingolla's research was supported in part by the Air Force Office of Scientific Research (AFOSR 85-0149).

The authors wish to thank Cynthia Suchta and Carol Yanakakis for their valuable assistance in the preparation of the manuscript.

CHAPTER 13

The Relationship Between Spatial Filtering and Subjective Contours

Arthur P. Ginsburg

The Kanizsa triangle represents a class of illusions that provide contours that are perceived but are not physically present in the original object. The question arises as to what visual processes, e.g., physical or cognitive, govern the visibility of subjective contours. Spatial filtering based on visual physiology has been shown to create physical intensity distributions from the Kanizsa triangle that generally correspond to the shape of the subjective contour (Ginsburg, 1975), which suggests that the basis for subjective contours may be physical rather than cognitive. This view was questioned by Tyler (1977), who noted that an outline version of the Kanizsa triangle also exhibited a subjective contour. However, examination of computer plots of the digitally filtered subjective contours of both the solid and outline triangles reveals a less well-defined subjective contour and reduced low spatial frequency energy from the outline triangle (Fig. 13.1). Both the reduced magnitude spectra and the less well-defined subjective contour predict a decreased perceived subjective contour for the outline triangle. This prediction is confirmed by noting that the solid triangle produces a stronger subjective contour than does the outline triangle at any viewing distance (Ginsburg, 1978).

The previous findings suggest an experiment. If the visibility of the subjective contour is primarily due to visual mechanisms that filter a range of low spatial frequencies, then the subjective contour of the solid triangle, having greater spectral energy at the lower spatial frequencies than that of the outline triangle, should be more visible under limiting visual conditions such as contrast threshold. This no-

tion was tested by comparing the contrast thresholds of just visible subjective contours from both solid and outline Kanizsa triangles whose sizes ranged from 0.5 to 20 cycles per degree (cpd). The contrast of the triangles was increased from below threshold until any part of the triangle was just detected. That value constituted the triangle contrast threshold. The contrast was then increased until the subjective contour was just detectable. That value made up the subjective contour threshold. The results from one subject are shown in Figure 13.2. The data from three subjects in this study generally decreased monotonically from 0.5 to about 3 cpd for the solid triangle and about 5 cpd for the outline triangle, after which the data from the solid triangle, but not the outline triangle, curve generally asymptoted.

The difference in the psychometric functions between the subjective contour contrast thresholds for the solid and outline triangles suggests that different ranges of spatial frequencies are mediating the appearance of the subjective contours even when the particular features making up the original triangles are well above threshold. Further, the contrast required to detect the presence of the subjective contour for the outline triangle for all sizes is always greater than that for the solid triangle, in agreement with the previous observations based on the greater spectral energy of the solid triangle at the lower spatial frequencies. These data show that the strength of the just detectable subjective contour for Kanizsa triangles viewed at threshold is a function of size and pattern features. In this case, the different pattern features are solid versus outline. The differences between the detec-

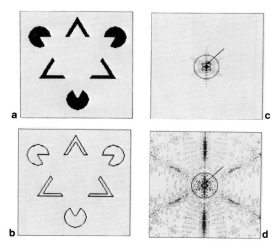

FIGURE 13.1. Solid and outline versions of the Kanizsa triangle: (a) solid triangle, (b) outline triangle, (c) Fourier magnitude spectra of the solid triangle, (d) Fourier magnitude spectra of the outline triangle. The arrows in the magnitude spectra point to the third harmonic. Although the magnitude of the low spatial frequencies is greatly reduced in the outline triangle, the highest magnitude is at the third vertical harmonic, having 28% of the same value in the solid triangle. The decreased magnitude of the perceived subjective contour of the outline triangle as compared with the solid triangle is predicted by the decreased magnitude spectrum of the outline triangle.

tion thresholds of the features of the subjective contour and those of the solid and outline triangles suggest that the visibility of the features of the subjective contours alone do not account for the differences in the perception of their subjective contours. Rather, these data suggest that the features of each triangle must reach a certain level of visibility, or contrast, in order to provide sufficient contrast energy to visual mechanisms with which to elevate the subjective contour to threshold visibility.

In order to further determine the degree to which spatial filtering based on biological data could be contributing to the visibility of subjective contours, a number of experiments using digital image-processing techniques were conducted. Solid and outline Kanizsa triangles and two versions of an Erhenstein illusion were filtered into 1.0, 1.5, and 2.0-octave bandwidth channel-filtered images whose center frequencies ranged from 0.5 to 128 cycles per picture

width (cpw) in one-octave steps. The effects of the filtering on the solid and outline Kanizsa triangles are shown in Figures 13.3a and 13.3b. The channel-filtered images provide smoother subjective contours in comparison to the earlier ideal-filtered images (Ginsburg, 1975).

Examination of the filtered images, especially those obtained from the 2-octave filter, reveals the physical existence of subjective contours in the low to mid-bandpass spatial frequency regions. The 1 cpw filtered images show increased contrast for the subjective contours. The 2 cpw, 2-octave filtered image reveals a well-defined subjective contour triangle. These filtered images were also added linearly and examined after each addition. However, linear addition did not produce a filtered image that contains a sharp subjective contour fully agreeing with the perception of the original figure. These findings suggest that other mechanisms and/or nonlin-

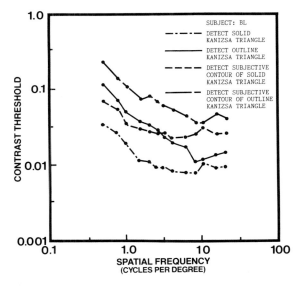

FIGURE 13.2. Contrast thresholds for the detection and identification of the original and solid Kanizsa triangles (subject BL). The parallel, generally monotonically decrease and asymptote of the contrast thresholds, between the original triangles and subjective contours suggest that the visibility of the subjective contour is mediated by contrast energy to visual mechanisms that elevate the subjective contour to visibility. The greater contrast required for the detection of the outline subjective contour as compared with the solid subjective contour is predicted from the decreased magnitude spectra at the lower spatial frequencies of the outline Kanizsa triangle.

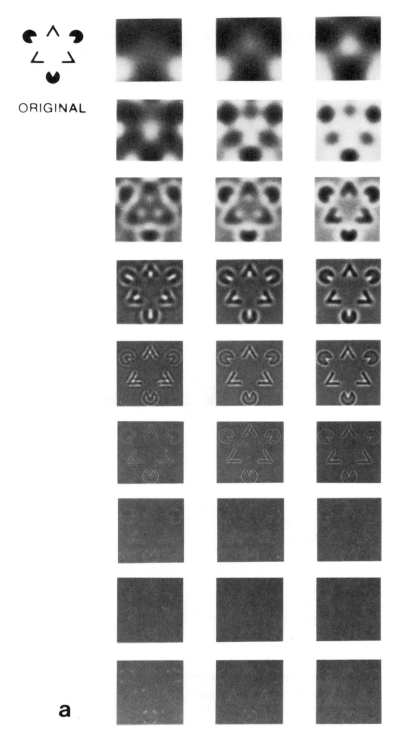

1.0 OCTAVE   1.5 OCTAVE   2.0 OCTAVE

ORIGINAL

a

FIGURE 13.3. Channel-filtered images of the solid (a) and outline (b) Kanizsa triangles. The bandwidths of the filters were 1.0, 1.5, and 2.0 octaves. The center frequencies were 0.5 to 28 cycles per picture width (cpw) in 1-octave steps from top to bottom. The in- creased contrasts of the subjective contours are seen in the 1 cpw images, especially from the 2-octave filter. A well-defined subjective contour triangle is seen in the 2-cpw, 2-octave filtered image. The en- ergy contained in the high spatial frequencies (bot-

1.0 OCTAVE   1.5 OCTAVE   2.0 OCTAVE

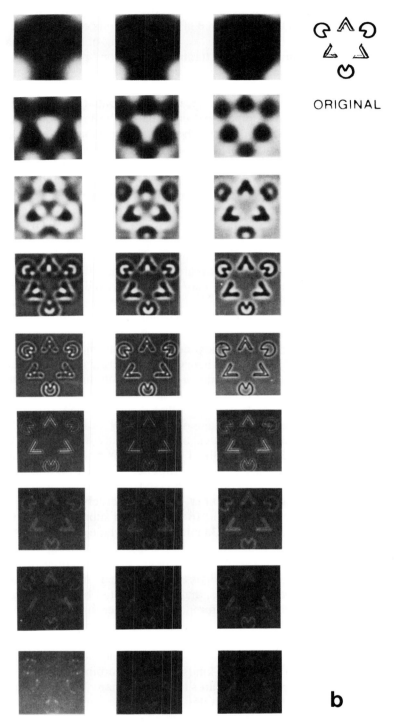

ORIGINAL

b

tom two rows) is so minimal that it cannot be adequately reproduced. These data provide further evidence for the existence of subjective contours from the low spatial frequencies of subjective contour patterns.

earities in channel image summation are needed to fully explain the sharp appearance of subjective contours.

There has been much activity attempting to determine if subjective contours are active, top-down or passive, bottom-up processes. One recent attempt to argue against a passive, bottom-up approach has been to compare patterns that cause subjective contours, some of whose features have reverse contrast (for examples, see Prazdny, 1983; Shapley & Gordon, 1985). Supposedly, the reversed contrast rules out simultaneous brightness contrast as the primary cause of subjective contours because opposite contrasts cannot spread to features of opposite contrasts and interact with features of the same contrast. The main problem with that approach is that it assumes certain rules for simultaneous brightness contrasts that may or may not be particularly relevant to how the visual system processes such patterns. These notions assume that the visual system processes the original image in a unitary manner. That is most certainly not the case. For example, if the theory of the hierarchy of filtered images is accurate as representing a central stage of visual processing of any image, then there is not one image that is present at cortical levels at any stage of visual processing but several images, such as those shown in Figures 13.3a and 13.3b. The low-bandpass filtered images may be quite different between objects composed of contrast reversed features, but the high-pass filtered images would be quite similar, such as the 16 cpw filtered images shown in Figures 13.3a and 13.3b. Other low-level filtering could then create the kind of subjective contours seen, for example, in the outline Kanizsa triangle of Figures 13.3a and 13.3b. It is suggested, therefore, that experiments created to determine differences between cognitive theories of subjective contours should first include the implications of possible internal visual images.

Shapley and Gordon use similar kinds of patterns having reversed contrast features to argue for a nonlinear type of filtering (Shapley & Gordon, 1985). Unfortunately, their argument sets up a straw man—it requires other vision models they criticize to behave linearly. They seem to confuse the use of linear filtering for demonstrations of visual models with positing linear filtering of visual mechanisms (see Shapley & Gordon, p. 84). At least one of the models they assume to be composed of linear spatial filters attempts to put linear and nonlinear aspects of spatial filtering in perspective (Ginsburg, 1978). The main point is, however, that as discussed previously, linear filtering can create quite similar images from reversed contrast features, and those internal images must be considered as possible candidates for generating subjective contours. The dichotomy that Shapley and Gordon have set up between nonlinear and linear processes seems quite premature at our present understanding of vision.

In sum, these data provide further evidence that fundamental visual filtering mechanisms are a prime candidate for why we see subjective contours. There are generally three properties of subjective contours: depth, brightness enhancement, and contours without intensity or chromatic gradients. The biologically based filtering discussed here offers first-order explanation for all these phenomena. [The depth associated with brightness differences and patterns has been discussed elsewhere (Ginsburg, 1978).] However, further research is needed to fully understand how these filtering mechanisms combine to create the images that we see.

Thus, on a first approximation a filtering approach accurately predicts the existence of a perceived contour and an enhanced brightness in subjective contours. Does this mean that the whole phenomenon is reducable to this basic physiological interpretation? No. Even from the beginning of this filtering approach, it has been suggested that set and selective attention must be used in conjunction with the filtering mechanism to achieve meaningful visual perception (Ginsburg, 1971, 1978). Further, the existence of set factors (see Coren, Porac, & Theodor, chap. 26), and the amodal work (see Gerbino & Kanizsa, chap. 27, and Minguzzi, chap. 7) would argue against this. But the possible contribution of such top-down mechanisms cannot be adequately evaluated unless the role of "low" spatial frequency mechanisms is acknowledged and controlled for.

CHAPTER 14

A Dynamic Model
of Anomalous Figures

Marco Sambin

The purpose of this chapter is to present the main features of a dynamic model of anomalous figures.[1] I shall utilize a language and terminology to describe a field theory like the one developed by Gestaltists (Koffka, 1935; Koehler, 1940) and introduce quantitive measurements whenever the situation allows it.

I shall present below the three major constructs or assumptions of the model: field activation, induced inhomogeneity (or field gaps), and intrafigural polarization. These concepts will be described, and related to perception in general and anomalous figures in particular, and in the final section, the interaction between these factors will be discussed.

Section 1: The Field Activation

The first assumption is that any perceptible presence activates the field or visual region beyond the stimulus itself. In other words, a field activation occurs along the stimulus contours in addition to the field differentiation given by the physical presence of the stimulation. This activation forms a sort of transition or connection between the stimulated area which appears as a figure and the stimulated area which appears as a ground. Let us consider in Figure 14.1 some simple patterns—lines or surfaces, straight or variously bent—to schematize the field activation found in such patterns. The arrows are a two-dimensional representation of the field acti-

---

[1] I prefer to use the term *anomalous* since the figures considered here, though different from normal ones, are neither subjective nor illusory.

vation. A three-dimensional representation as in Figure 14.2 allows us to better visualize the underlying assumptions of this dynamic model.

Shown in Figure 14.2a is the section A–A of the line l. The shaded rectangle a represents the peak energy distribution due to the stimulation given by the physical line itself which is perceived in the visual field; the horizontal line b indicates the ground energy level; the line c indicates the field activation, i.e., the energy transition between the excited zone (the area represented by the rectangle a and the state of rest indicated by b. The height of segment i represents the activation field intensity at that point in visual space.

The form of the line c is assumed; the extent $d–e$ (the "spread of activation") has been estimated psychophysically (see section 2 and Sambin, 1985); the $d–f$ value is unknown, i.e., we do not know the energy magnitude produced by a line, but it is, of course, to be expected that lines with different physical parameters (e.g., width, contrast) are associated with different amounts of energy.

There is little direct evidence for the concept of field activation, and most of the evidence comes from work concerned with chromatic features of the stimulus. This evidence includes the brightness assimilation work of Musatti (1953), and of Jory and Day (1979); the fact that in isoluminant conditions (Liebman effect, 1927) thin, tiny stripes give rise to the perception of a homogeneous veil (Buzzati, 1974); and Pastore's observations (1971, personal communication and demonstration) on the appearance of a diaphanous form or presence between two phosphorescent rods observed in the dark.

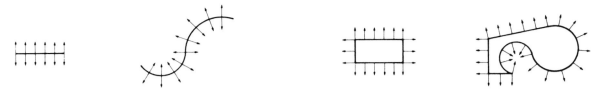

FIGURE 14.1. A schematic representation of field activation by a straight line, a curved line, a straight surface, and a curved surface.

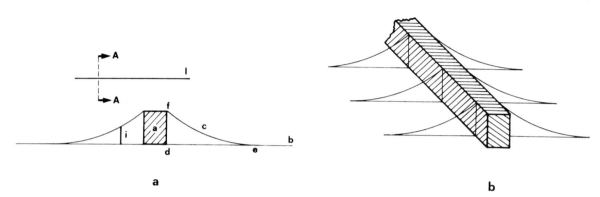

FIGURE 14.2. Field activation represented in the third dimension.

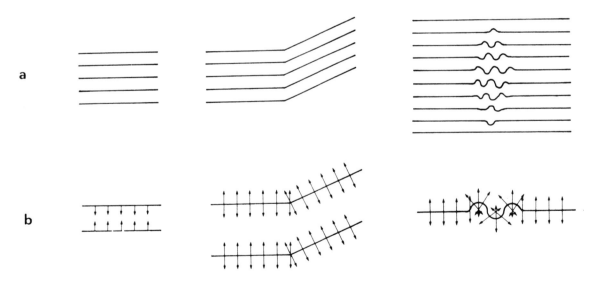

FIGURE 14.3. Some different patterns of lines (a) and their respective field activation conditions (b).

More perceptually evident are the functional effects that result from field activation. Functional effects can be observed on the perceptual level from the different organization of field activation due to the configuration of the pattern. Lines having different organizations (such as in Fig. 14.3a) are seen as having a different phenomenal appearances, a result that can be explained by the different directions of field activation diagramed in Figure 14.3b (Sambin, 1979).

The figure-ground phenomenon, at least in

some paradigmatic cases, can be described in terms of the functional effects of a more or less dense distribution of field activation (Fig. 14.4). We will see as figure those parts of the field which are more dense, i.e., those parts of stimulus or visual field which result in greater field activation. Density may depend on either form or distance (stimulus elements which are more separated yield weaker field activation and so are less likely to be seen grouped as figure) (Sambin, 1986).

Stronger functional effects are to be found with anomalous figures. We treat these in the following sections.

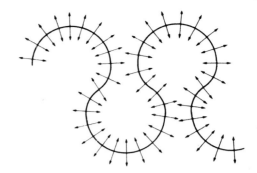

FIGURE 14.4. Figure—ground diagramed as field density.

Section 2: The Field Gaps

A second assumption, tied to the first, is that the areas of visual space in which field activation is not present (since they are perpendicular to the stimulus lines or areas) can form a gap in the field. These gaps are the hypothetical con-

structs I have referred to as induced inhomogeneity in my previous papers. We can represent the gaps (or induced inhomogeneity) as in Figure 14.5a in two dimensions and as in Figure 14.5b in three dimensions. Since such induced inhomogeneities can serve as an explanation for the anomalous figure (Sambin, 1980b), we will assume that anomalous figures are functional effects of the field activation. Now, an anoma-

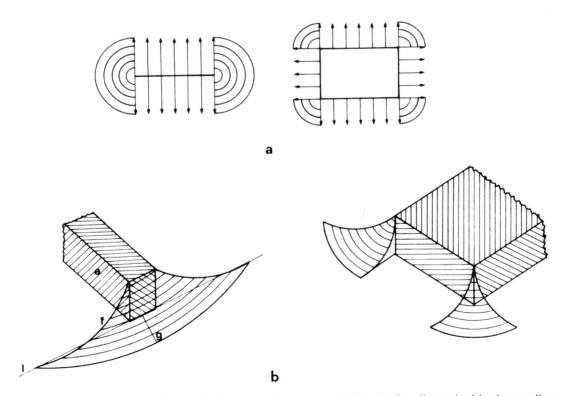

FIGURE 14.5. Diagram of gaps (induced inhomogeneities) due to field activation discontinuities in two dimensions (a) and in three dimensions (b).

lous figure is more complex than an induced inhomogeneity; an induced inhomogeneity is an explanatory hypothesis generated by the prior analysis that gives rise to the dynamic interaction which leads to the anomalous figure organization. The hypothetical construct, induced inhomogeneity, which has been used to explain anomalous figures, is inferred from observed facts of the features of the construct to be demonstrated. In the following paragraphs, I list facts that can support the reality of induced inhomogeneity.

Two classes of anomalous figures can be described: anomalous figures induced by lines and those induced by surfaces.

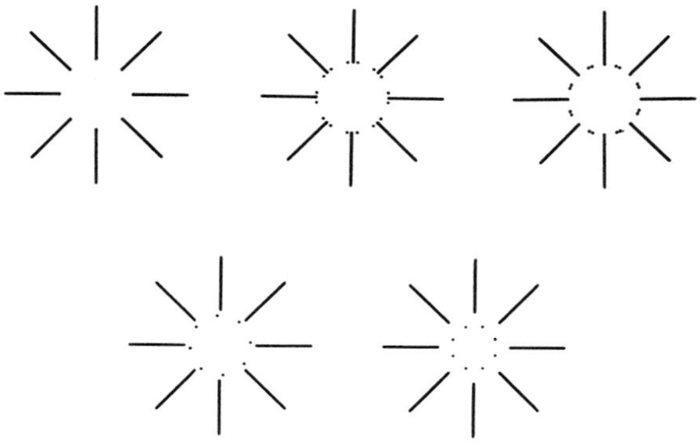

Anomalous Figures Induced by Lines

Length of an Induced Inhomogeneity

It has been possible to measure experimentally the length of an induced inhomogeneity (d–e in Fig. 14.2a). This depends on the parameters of length and thickness of the inducing line; a line 0.8-cm long and 0.4-mm thick will induce an inhomogeneity 1.17 cm in length (Sambin, 1985). A similar result can be obtained by using the method of determining the threshold of appearance of an anomalous figure as a function of number of inducing lines, and assuming that the threshold indicates the inducing inhomogeneity extent (Sambin, 1981a).

Height

The height value (d–f in Fig. 14.2a) is a graphical representation of the strength value. An inhomogeneity induced by stimuli of lower contrast should have a lower strength and thus should be represented by a shorter height. At present, the height value is known only relatively but not absolutely.

Form

The influence of small dots on the strength of the anomalous figure decreases as the distance from terminal point of the inducing line increases. A few examples are shown in Figure 14.6. From this observation, we can infer that the activation field value is also decreasing. The measurement of the form of this part of the field is the aim of a work now in progress.

FIGURE 14.6. The effect of extraneous dots, which vary in distance from the center of the stimulus, on the strength of the anomalous contour is a way to measure the field intensity.

Interaction

As we have seen, induced inhomogeneity is an *entity*, crystallized by analysis, which interacts with other induced inhomogeneities to form an anomalous figure. The interaction takes place following the Wertheimer's law of grouping (1923): we shall have a better grouping, and thus observe a better perceptual result, when the induced inhomogeneities are closer to each other, more continuous, more similar, or have a better form (prägnanz). This means that the interaction between induced inhomogeneities follows phenomenological laws (Sambin, 1985). It is too early to describe these interactions from a dynamic point of view; we can only presume that the final outcome is given by the linear sum (or other summation criterion) of the values of the activation fields which are present at the point considered. This topic is reconsidered, from another point of view, in Section 4.

Direction

The direction of perceived brightness and contour produced by the induced inhomogeneity is the more important perceptual fact, exactly the one highlighted in the literature with the terms *subjective, illusory* or, here, *anomalous contours*. In the majority of cases, the contour appears oriented orthogonally to the inducing line, and deviations from this direction result in a weaker anomalous figure (Kennedy, 1979). On the representational (diagramatic) level, this fact can be indicated by the tendency of the contour to appear along the line *l* (Fig. 14.5b), which is the area of major separation between the inducing line (plus field gap) on one side and the remaining stimulus on the other. This fact is connected to the plasticity of the induced inhomogeneity discussed below.

Plasticity

This term refers to the hypothesis that induced inhomogeneity is not rigid; the induced inhomogeneity can undergo changes that depend on field conditions. The direction assumed by the anomalous contour can be used as data that give evidence to induced inhomogeneity's plasticity. The plasticity may be thought of as a perceptual counterpart to the field intensity (*i* in Fig. 14.2a) and it is related to the anomalous contour direction. A large value of *i* will produce a low degree of plasticity, i.e., a low probability of deviation from the canonical direction, and vice versa.

This is a corollary to the assumption that, other things being equal, a variation is more likely in cases where the field is weaker. In Sambin (1974a), figures have been presented in which the anomalous figure has a form that ranges from square to circle, depending on the induced inhomogeneity plasticity. Sambin (1980b) and Sambin and Rocco (in press) have investigated the plasticity of induced inhomogeneity as it is affected by the presence of small dots.

Anomalous Figures Induced by Surfaces

The gap fields activated by surfaces have slightly different features than those activated by lines. They seem to be smaller and vary as the angle of the surface varies.

Direction

An inhomogeneity induced by a surface seems to undergo a rivalry between the fields activated by the two sides that form an angle in the surface. The final result, the prevalence of one direction of anomalous contour, depends on the general organization of the anomalous figure. There are, however, some exceptions. It can be observed that there is a tendency for a contour to appear along the direction given by the bisector of the angle; this happens as a "compromise" in particularly weak anomalous figures, as can be seen in Figures 14.7a and 14.7b.

The rivalry between directions of the anomalous contour becomes stronger as the similarity of the two direction increases (Fig. 14.8). In the Figure 14.8a, the direction of the anomalous contour is close to that of the short side of the angle, thus it does not cause a sufficient functional differentiation (see Section 4: the unilateral function of the contour) and the result is weaker; Figures 14.8b and 14.8c differ only in the orientation of the side of the angle arms and give better results since the orientation difference is increasing.

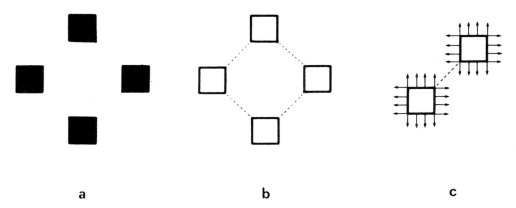

a   b   c

FIGURE 14.7. A case in which the anomalous contour direction does not follow the real contour direction.

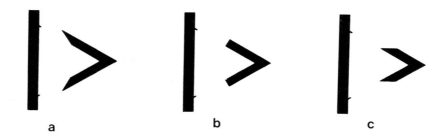

FIGURE 14.8. The strength of the anomalous contour increases as the terminus of the inducing part changes in orientation.

Intensity

In the majority of cases, anomalous figures induced by surfaces are weaker than those induced by lines as, for instance, can be seen by comparing Figures 14.9a and 14.9b. Notice the considerable difference in amount of stimulation (total black stimulus area). The field gap induced by a line is more extensive than the gap generated by a surface. As can be seen in Figure 14.5, the inhomogeneity (field gap) induced by a line extends over 180°, the induced inhomogeneity by a rectangle or square extends over only 90°; a line introduces a more extensive field gap.

Plasticity

Plasticity in surface induced inhomogeneities is less pronounced in comparison with the plasticity of anomalous figures induced by lines. In Figure 14.10a, one can observe an anomalous figure having a starlike form. In Figure 14.10b, the same form is more difficult to see (the dots are located at the same distance): the plasticity is not the same. The way in which surfaces activate the field is different from the way lines activate.

The Lack of Gaps

What is happening in the case in which the terminations of the inducing patterns do not, on this model, generate gaps (inhomogeneities) in the field? It would be expected that the lack of gaps is accompanied by an absence of an anomalous figures. An example is shown in Figure 14.11a, in which the terminations are rounded. Thus (see Fig. 14.1), there are no field gaps and thus, as expected, no anomalous figure.

An anomalous figure can be obtained easily when the terminations of every inducing part have straight contours, but this is almost impossible when the terminations have rounded surfaces (Figs. 14.11b, 14.11c).

Section 3: The Intrafigural Polarization

With the assumptions so far adopted, we have been able to consider the anomalous figure and the transition between the inducing parts and the background. However, there is something

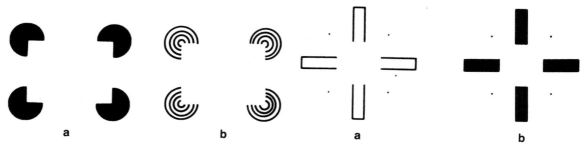

FIGURE 14.9. Difference in strength of anomalous figures depends on the nature of inducing parts: lines vs. surfaces.

FIGURE 14.10. An anomalous figure induced by lines is more plastic than an anomalous figure induced by surfaces.

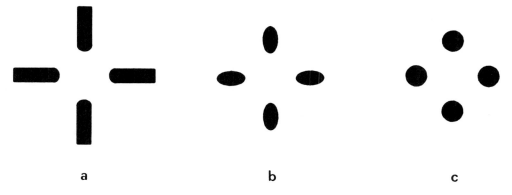

a   b   c

FIGURE 14.11. Rounded inducing part terminals do not induce anomalous figures.

more specific to be discussed about the dynamic organization assumed by the inducing parts. The inducing parts themselves are characterized by an internal organization of forces in a particular (biased) direction. We can call this condition *polarization of intrafigural forces* (Sambin, 1981b). Figure 14.12 is a representation of (Fig. 14.12a) a black rectangular surface which is not polarized, (Fig. 14.12b) the same surface polarized when in proximity of an anomalous contour, (Fig. 14.12c) a inducing line that is not polarized, and (Fig. 14.12d) a polarized one.

In Figure 14.12b, the polarization is indicated by the direction of the arrows, which represent the intrafigural forces toward the anomalous figure. In Figure 14.12d, the polarization is represented by two small arrows, which would be located on the inducing line itself.

Existence

The existence of polarization can be inferred from the comparison of the data given by Figures 14.13a–e (Sambin, 1981b). The strength of the anomalous figure decreases from 14.13a to 14.13e. Notice that the rectangles in 14.13a and 14.13e and in 14.13b and 14.13d are identical in length and width (but not orientation), and also that the form of the gaps remains constant: an-

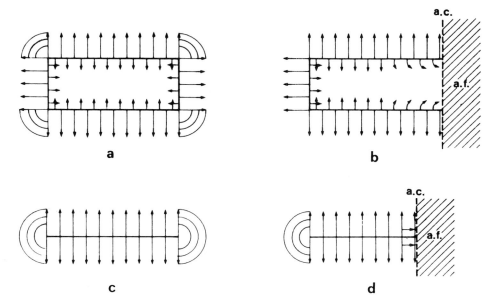

a   b

c   d

FIGURE 14.12. Graphic representation of the hypothetical construct: polarization of intrafigural forces.

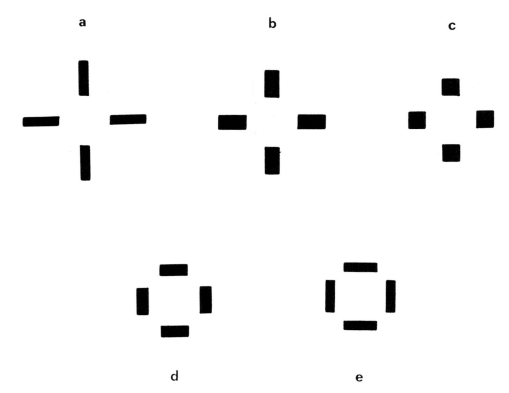

FIGURE 14.13. The strength of the anomalous figure decreases from a to e, demonstrating the effect of intensity of the intrafigural polarization.

gles of 90° in all the cases. The only difference must be due to the orientation of the inducing rectangles; therefore, intrafigural polarization is playing a role.

Strength

The polarization varies in strength. Some figures show a different reaction of the polarization to a test object as a function of distance (Sambin, 1974b). In Figures 14.14a and 14.14b, the obstruction due to the presence of a white rectangle or to a dot on the inducing part more or less varies as a function of their distance from the critical point: the anomalous contour.

Distribution

The intrafigural organization has its own distribution. In Figure 14.15a (to be compared with 14.14a), the same interior white rectangle has been rotated by 90°, in such a way the polarization along the outer contours of the inducing rectangles is not obstructed and the anomalous

figure is easily perceivable (intermediate tilts give intermediate results, Sambin 1981b). In Figure 14.15b, the test object (white rectangular notches) is much more influential. Thus, polarization seems to be more active along the outer contours of the inducing forms.

Section 4: Interaction Between Activation, Inhomogeneities, and Polarization

The general process involved in anomalous figure organization is more complex than the sum of the single constructs so far considered. A sequential scheme of the interaction between features of the dynamic model could be as follows: (1) The field activation originates the (2) field gaps (induced inhomogeneities); (3) the induced inhomogeneities are distributed so that they form an anomalous figure; then (4) the anomalous contour assumes a unilateral function. (5) The anomalous figure contour, by uni-

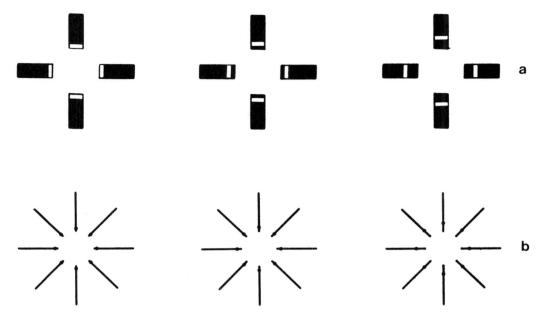

FIGURE 14.14. Test objects, rectangles (a) and dots (b), obstruct the polarization.

laterality, incorporates the margin of the inducing part. The inducing part thus has a contour that is less strong; the anomalous figure polarizes in the direction of this weak contour (6). The inducing part seems to continue beyond the anomalous figure; in some cases, it seems to have a completion beyond the anomalous figure. As a result, there is (7) a spatial and depth segregation toward the observer and, thus, a strengthening of the anomalous contour (with possible feedback and eventual recursivity starting from point 3).

The anomalous figure organization may be considered to be the result of an interactive occurrence of all the subprocesses 1–7. The inter-

action can be stated as follows: a subprocess is considered, and if a variation in the condition is introduced, it will be observed that the whole anomalous figure organization is affected. This type of procedure suggests that the whole process is interactive. By disturbing one subprocess the general phenomenon is affected; the conditions present at a given step (subprocess) are always influencing the main phenomenon. The hypothetical constructs proposed here represent a differentation introduced only for analytical purposes. Let us briefly consider the seven subprocesses. (1) The role of field activation has been discussed in Section 1. (2) The induced inhomogeneities (gaps) have been

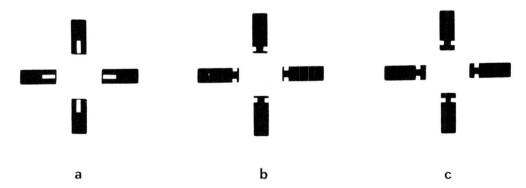

a   b   c

FIGURE 14.15. The test objects (rectangles, squares) in inducing parts variously affect the polarization.

treated in Section 2. (3) To demonstrate the role of the spatial distribution of induced inhomogeneity in the formation of anomalous figures, it would be necessary to find conditions in which induced inhomogeneities can be observed before they interact in the anomalous figure organization. But it is exactly this interaction of induced inhomogeneities, field activations, and polarizations that makes the anomalous figures perceivable.

Observe that in the cases of poorer interaction between induced inhomogeneities, the anomalous figures are less strong. The induced inhomogeneity organization follows, in the main lines, Wertheimer's law of grouping. Thus by varying the effects of grouping principles we can obtain perceivable strength differences in the anomalous figure. A very crude example can be seen in Figure 14.16 (more details in Sambin, 1980b). Figure 14.16a is weaker than Figure 14.16b; the induced inhomogeneities interact to a lesser extent because they are more distant (proximity). Figure 14.16b is stronger than Figure 14.16c; the same induced inhomogeneities are distributed on different surfaces (closure). In Figure 14.16d, the continuity (good continuation) is not present. In Figures 14.16e and 14.16f, closure is realized only partially. Figure 14.16g provides an example of good form (prägnanz).

Unilateral Function

In the literature (Rubin, 1921), it is known that a contour tends to delimit only one side of the stimulus. The classical reversible figures (Rubin, Köhler) are striking examples of the unilateral function of the contour. Since the contour is not delimiting two zones, what occurs is a reciprocal exchange of reversible anomalous figures (Sambin, 1978). From this we infer that unilateral function occurs also with anomalous contours (Fig. 14.17).

Figure 14.18 is another example of unilateral function in anomalous contours. In Figures 14.18a and 14.18b, anomalous figures can be observed; the same figures are less perceptible in Figure 14.18c. They cannot appear simultaneously since they have in common the anomalous part of the contour.

Figure 14.12b is a diagram of a rectangle whose right side coincides with an anomalous contour. The result of unilateral function of this side is an incorporation by the anomalous contour that prevails. Given these unequal conditions, the internal organization in the inducing part (rectangle) will be unbalanced in the direction of the weaker element (internal shorter side of the rectangle). This is an example of the concept of polarization and of energy flow in direction of the weaker side. The concept of polar-

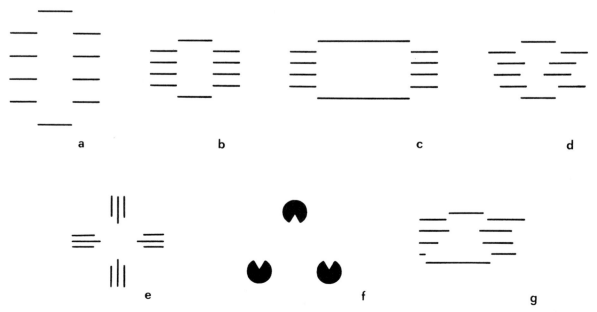

FIGURE 14.16. The interaction of induced inhomogeneity follows Wertheimer's laws of grouping.

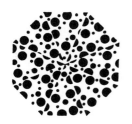 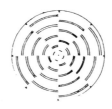

FIGURE 14.17. Two cases of reversibility of anomalous figures.

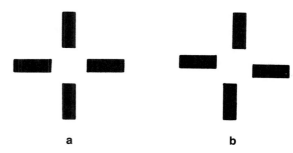

a   **b**

FIGURE 14.19. The anomalous figure strength varies, affecting perceived completion of inducing parts.

ization has also been briefly treated in Section 3.

The phenomenal aspect of the dynamic process described in Section 4 is given by the tendency to continue and to be completed shown by inducing parts (amodal perception; Michotte, 1962). In any anomalous figure, there are parts that tend to continue (incompletion; Kanizsa, 1955a).

We shall describe in more detail the idea that the inducing parts have an intrafigural organization that flows toward the weaker side. This generates the tendency to continue also in those

inducing figures that flow toward the weaker side. This also generates the tendency to continue in those inducing figures which per se would be complete (e.g., rectangles, lines, other geometrical forms). In those cases in which the tendency to continue is associated with completion beyond an anomalous figure, the flow will be facilitated and result in a more salient anomalous figure. Compare the results of Figures 14.19a and 14.19b.

Figure 14.20 shows that the completion of the inducing parts beyond the anomalous figure is not a necessary condition. The inducing lines tend to continue, but not all can be completed. Moreover, the anomalous figure is not affected by this lack of completion.

The segregation into apparent depth toward the observer is a perceptual fact first observed in 1955 by Kanizsa. The apparent depth can be measured by superimposing binocular (test) and monocular (stimulus) cues (Pandora's box; Gregory, 1966). Coren and Porac (1983) demonstrated that anomalous figures segregate into depth toward the observer. Micella, Pinna, and Sambin (1985) have found that the amount of

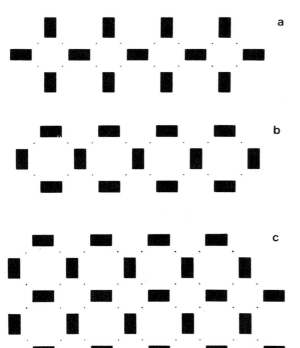

a

b

c

FIGURE 14.18. The unilateral function of the anomalous contour.

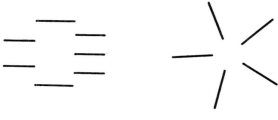

FIGURE 14.20. Perceptual completion of inducing lines is not necessary for anomalous figure organization.

segregation depends on the strength of the anomalous figure. Even this final perceptual outcome is tied to the entire dynamic of the process.

Concluding Remarks

Although a dynamic model of anomalous figures has been given here in its main features, many questions of detail have only been raised. Although many of the concepts discussed here are based on experimentally derived data, others indicate, for the moment, only possible directions of research. My opinion is that, even with these limitations, this model can economically and heuristically account for many of the features presented by the anomalous figure or, at least, is able to provide a working framework within which to ask questions.

CHAPTER 15

The Resonance Theory of Kinetic Shape Perception and the Motion-Induced Contour

Victor Klymenko and Naomi Weisstein

Perceptual Illusions and Confusions

In the last century William James described the primal perceptual world as a "blooming, buzzing confusion." In this century James Gibson observed that the confusion was only in the mind of the theorist. The term *perceptual illusion* is an ontological oxymoron. Traditionally, illusions were thought to provide insight into the nature of perceptual mechanisms by indicating when and how they are in error, the error being with reference to one's preconceptions of the ideal perceptual response. Instead, one could modify one's analysis of the nature of the effective stimulus to which the perceptual system is responding. Consider the geometric illusions in which straight lines appear curved. When analyzed in Euclidean terms the perceived curvature of the lines is illusory; however, if the lines are instead defined as geodesics, the perceived curvature provides the appropriate description of the visual space in which they occur (see Watson, 1978). The ecologically salient variables, to which a perceptual system resonates, may not correspond to the variables appropriate to a particular physical discipline (Gibson, 1961). This is explicitly acknowledged in psychophysics, where the correspondence function itself constitutes much of the subject matter. Often, however, when perceptions do not directly correspond to predetermined physical variables, the perceptual response is classified as an illusion, although it is only a matter of convention as to which of the noncorrespondences are referred to as illusions. In terms of one's preconceptions, a perceptual system may be registering aspects of the physical world which have variously been described as higher-order, emergent, abstract, or complex (Gibson, 1966; Pomerantz, 1978; Runeson, 1977; Weimer, 1982). We will describe a theory to account for a particular "illusory" contour in which the perceptual invariants are defined in visual space–time.

The term *perceptual illusion* is also sometimes used to describe perceptual decoupling (from other perceptions and/or cognitions). The simulation of motion in depth known as the kinetic depth effect (Wallach & O'Connell, 1953) has been thought of as an illusion because the distal stimulus event happens to occur on a two-dimensional surface. Here the problem is often defined in terms of "recovering" the third dimension (Ullman, 1979). The third spatial dimension need not be recovered, since it was never lost; the experience of depth simply corresponds to the visual registration of certain image events. The problem is instead the appropriate ecological description of those image events. The resonance theory, which can account for kinetic depth, will be described after the following review of the motion-induced contour, a type of moving illusory contour seen under stimulus conditions similar to those which produce the kinetic depth effect.

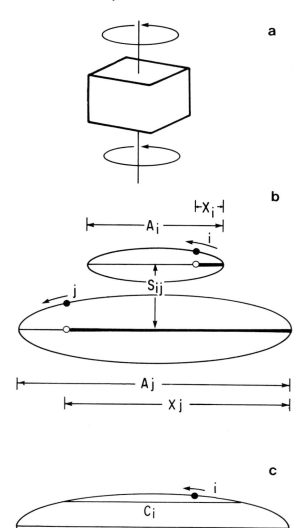

a

b

c

The Motion-Induced Contour and Structure from Motion

The stimuli reviewed here refer to computer-generated animations of virtual objects.

The motion-induced contour is an illusory contour seen in the image of an object undergoing the figural transformations associated with rotation in depth (Klymenko & Weisstein, 1981), see Figure 15.1a. It is seen where a dihedral edge would normally be located in a variety of rotating virtual objects (parallel or polar projection) under a variety of stimulus conditions; Klymenko & Weisstein, 1981, 1983, 1984; Klymenko, Weisstein, & Ralston, in press). The contour seen in rotation conditions is more salient and gives more of the impression of an edge than the contour seen in static views of the object. Observers describe the percept as a convex or concave edge which appears when the object is set in motion. Neither rigid image motion nor flicker, which can produce moving or flickering phantoms (Genter & Weisstein, 1981; Tynan & Sekuler, 1975) was as effective in producing a contour as rotation in depth (Klymenko & Weisstein, 1981). The contour is not seen if the rotation in depth sequence specifies a flat figure rather than a solid virtual object (Klymenko & Weisstein, 1983).

Since this contour is seen only when there is kinetic shape information which specifies the spatial structure of the virtual object, a number of other object transformations were tested (Klymenko et al., in press). The looming transformation, which simulates an object moving in depth along the line of sight, did not produce the contour. This was surprising, since the looming transformation contains geometric in-

FIGURE 15.1a. An example of an object which produces a motion-induced contour. The illusory dihedral edge is seen separating the two lower surfaces of the object during rotation in depth. b. The rotation ellipses of two image points, i and j, projected from two points on a rotating object. The amplitude (A) is the length of the major axis of an ellipse. Trajectory separation (S) is the distance between the major axes of any two ellipses. Converting A to S units is done by dividing A by sin(arccos (R)), where R is the ratio of lengths of the minor axis over the major axis of any ellipse. The phase angle (ϕ) between any i and j is given by the following equation:

$$\phi_{ij} = \left| \arccos\left(1 - 2\left(\frac{X_i}{A_i}\right)\right) \mp \arccos\left(1 - 2\left(\frac{X_j}{A_j}\right)\right) \right|$$

where X is defined as the distance on the major axis

to one side of the imaginary point (open dots) which is closest to the image point. The sign between the two terms is determined by whether i and j are both in the same semicycle ($-$), where X_i and X_j are both increasing or both decreasing, or in opposite semicycles ($+$), where one X is increasing and the other decreasing. c. Under parallel projection the longest dimension of the rotation ellipse (A) represents the orbital diameter of an element on a rotating object. Under perspective projection, the orbital diameter is instead represented by a diameter chord (C).

formation corresponding to the spatial structure of the virtual object. Braunstein (1966) reported that observers could distinguish between looming flat and looming solid virtual objects. However, Ullman (1979) generated animations of two coaxial random dot cylinders and noted that observers could perceive their specific spatial structure only during rotation in depth, but not during looming. Why can't observers pick up looming spatial structure? During looming the 2D image undergoes both a global size change (uniform radial motion) and a figural, or form, change (nonuniform radial motion). In terms of image distances traversed, most of the image motion is due to the size change, which specifies motion in depth, and not the figural change, which corresponds to the 3D shape of the object (see Klymenko et al., in press). The effect of radial image motion was tested in the zooming rotation in depth transformation in which the image of the object expanded and contracted as the object rotated; in each successive frame of this motion sequence there was both an orientation and a size change. The zooming motion component did not disrupt the perception of the motion-induced contour, and in addition the shape of the virtual object was perceived; it appeared to change size and/or move in depth as it rotated. A zooming object, in which shape is unrecoverable, where the image simply expanded and contracted, did not produce a contour. Thus, there appears to be a parallel between kinetic shape perception, what Ullman (1979) calls structure from motion, and the perception of the motion-induced contour (Klymenko et al., in press). Next we briefly describe a new model to account for these data.

The Resonance Theory

Consider the image resulting from the parallel projection of a rotating object. Each point on the rotating object traverses a circular orbit, which is projected into an elliptical trajectory, or "rotation ellipse" (Eriksson, 1974) in the image plane (also see Johansson, 1974b; and Todd, 1982). Three image parameters—amplitude, trajectory separation, and phase angle—based on the geometry of these rotation ellipses, specify the 3D shape and motion of the object (definitions in Fig. 15.1b). The ampli-

tudes specify the (relative) lengths of the orbital diameters of the object points in space. The trajectory separations specify the (relative) distances in space between the orbits. The phase angle between any two image points specifies the 3D angular separation between the corresponding object points with respect to the rotation axis.

Consider Johansson's (1974b) observations concerning one, two, or three dots traversing an elliptical trajectory: one dot presented alone is seen following an elliptical trajectory; however, two or more dots are spontaneously seen as rigidly connected and rotating in depth. This is because, in terms of the resonance theory, the phase angle parameter is undefined in the single dot display.

Under parallel projection the major axes of the rotation ellipses (the amplitudes) correspond to the diameters of the orbits of the object points in space. If perspective is introduced into the image, the orbital diameter is instead represented by a chord of the ellipse parallel to the major axis (see Fig. 15.1c); the displacement of this diameter chord from the major axis is monotonically related to the magnitude of perspective in the image. The major axis is a salient feature of an ellipse. Without introducing artificial constraints, such as constant angular velocity, there is no salient procedure for locating the diameter chord. Since the phase angle parameter is geometrically based on the major axis as projected diameter, variability, or perturbations, are introduced into the phase angles by perspective. The magnitude of the phase angle perturbations is correlated with the magnitude of perspective in the image. Thus, the findings reporting increasing attenuation of rigidity by increasing perspective (Braunstein, 1962; Caelli, Flanagan, & Green, 1982) are not surprising.

The resonance parameters are immune to variations in rotational velocity and display observation distance. Todd's (1982) solution to kinetic shape perception, also based on rotation ellipses, is constrained by the requirement that the object rotate at a constant angular velocity. This is because the diameter chord, from which he derives other image parameters, is located by dividing an image point's trajectory into equal temporal intervals (Todd, 1982). In a series of demonstrations in which pairs of random objects were generated, one rotating at a constant angular velocity and the other at an irregular velocity, it was observed that the differences in angular velocity were simply seen as such and had no effect on the perceived shape of the objects. Many analyses of motion perception implicitly require the observer to be situated at the computed viewpoint when the kinetic display employs polar projection. If observers took account of viewpoint by performing the inverse projective transform (see Johansson's 1974a projective decoding hypothesis), then the deformations in perceived shape would be enormous when viewing a rotating object at, say, one half or twice the computed distance. Fortunately for the movie industry, kinetic shape schemes which require the observer to be at the correct viewpoint are invalid, because the predicted deformations in shape and size are not perceived.

Perceptual Organization in Three Dimensions

Objects rotating in depth are ambiguous; a given spatial orientation or its reflection can be seen. Consider a rotating random dot sphere viewed under parallel projection. It may be seen in one spatial orientation rotating clockwise, or in the reflective spatial orientation rotating counterclockwise. It is notable that individual dots are seldom simultaneously seen in opposite spatial orientations. This is explained by applying a version of Restle's (1979) information load concept to one of the resonance parameters. Restle's model accounts for the 2D perceptual biases of ambiguous moving images; the perceptual interpretations most often seen are the ones which correspond to the minimal information load on the image parameters. In Restle's model, information load takes on various integer values, which correspond to the different perceptual organizations. The resonance theory accounts for why 3D rather than 2D motion is perceived, as well as the particular 3D biases of kinetic images, by considering the continuous variation on the phase angle parameter.

The information load on the phase angle between any two image elements is defined as the total amount of variation in this parameter over

time. Consider two dots on the sphere just described. The two perceptual interpretations usually seen are the ones where the phase angle variation is a minimum (zero), where the two dots are seen both rotating clockwise or both rotating counterclockwise. In the nonrigid interpretations less often seen (see Gillam, 1972), where the two dots are rotating in opposite directions, the phase angle between the dots is constantly varying. For parallel projection, the two rigid interpretations are equally likely. If perspective is introduced into the image, then due to the displacement of the diameter chords from the major axes of the rotation ellipses (see Fig. 15.1c), variability is introduced into the phase angle. Now the two most rigid interpretations, where phase angle variability is minimal—all dots clockwise or all counterclockwise—are no longer equal. In terms of projective geometry, the direction of rotation with the lower information load is the correct one. The discrepency in phase angle information load between these two interpretations monotonically increases with increases in the magnitude of perspective in the image. Thus, it is not surprising that "accuracy" of perceiving rotation direction increases monotonically with increases in perspective (Petersik, 1980). One can, with attentional effort, force a perceptual reversal from the preferred orientation; the "incorrect" orientation will appear less rigid. The visual system resonates to the lowest phase angle variation compatible with the event, which is also the most rigid interpretation (see Hatfield & Epstein, 1985). Thus there is no need for internal constraints such as Ullman's (1979) rigidity assumption.

Consider again the parallel projection of the random dot sphere, rotating about a vertical axis. Each dot simply moves back and forth along a linear image trajectory, yet the spatial structure of the sphere is spontaneously perceived. This is the interpretation where the phase angle variations are minimal. Lappin, Doner, and Kottas (1980) reported that the structure of a random dot (polar projection) sphere with 512 dots can be perceived in as few as two frames, differing by only 5.6° of rotation. Again, this is the perceptual interpretation, where the total information load on the phase angles is a minimum (see discussion of element numerosity and elliptical vector fields in Todd,

1982; also see Donner, Lappin, & Perfetto, 1984).

The tendency to see interpretations with minimal phase angle variation may also account for the "pausing" illusion (Harris, Schwartz, Patashnik, & Lappin, 1978; Mace, 1971). When two square arrays of dots move at a constant (image) velocity in opposite directions, they appear to pause or stick when the dots coincide. If neighboring dots are interpreted as having a constant phase angle between them (i.e., as being rigidly connected) then the linear image velocities will correspond to rotational acceleration (dots departing) and deceleration (dots approaching). The moments in time when the dots appear to pause correspond to the moments when the (phase angle specified) angular velocity is a minimum. Thus the apparent pause appears to be due to the visual system resonating to the lowest phase angle variation compatible with theis stimulus event (see Goldberg & Pomerantz, 1982 for a different view).

The Edge of an Event

The resonance theory accounts for the motion-induced contour as follows. In rotating virtual objects, the shape and motion can be geometrically derived from rotation ellipses as described above. Image elements undergoing the figural transformations associated with rotation in depth can perceptually specify a surface, or surfaces, such as is seen in a virtual sphere demarcated by random dots (see Braunstein, 1976, 1983, for reviews). In the virtual objects where the motion-induced contour is seen, there is salient information which indicates that the physical contours demarcating the two image regions to either side of the illusory contour lie in different depth planes. These two delineated image regions are seen as two oriented surfaces, and the boundary between them is seen as a dihedral edge—the motion-induced contour. The edge is not perceived in the conditions where the resonance parameters are unavailable. The perceived shape and illusory edge seen in the zooming rotation in depth condition may be accounted for in one of two ways. Either the visual system extracts the elliptical image trajectories by motion vector analysis (see Johansson, 1973) and then registers the three

resonance parameters, or the zooming motion component is transparent to kinetic shape mechanisms. The trajectory separations and the amplitudes change at the same rate, so the object relative dimensions specified by these parameters remain invariant. The phase angles are unaffected, since the two variables on which they are based, X and A, change at the same rate, see equation in Figure 15.1b caption. The visual system appears to be strongly biased towards interpreting a complexly transforming optic array in terms of minimal phase angle variation. The motion-induced contour appears to be the reuslt of visual kinetic shape mechanisms.

Perceptual Ecology

If everything in the real, nonsimulated world is seen in perspective, then why is parallel projection canonical, and why aren't real rotating objects seen as nonrigid? Normally, there is an overabundance of converging information available to specify shape. Except for unusually large magnitudes of perspective, the inaccuracies introduced into kinetic-shape by perspective are exceedingly minor. The enhanced rigidity of parallel compared to perspective projections is only noticeable in kinetic displays decoupled from other sources of information. In the real world, if the magnitude of perspective is large, then the visual angles of the rotation ellipses are necessarily large, which means that most of the transforming optic array will be registered in the visual periphery, where resolution is lower.

In terms of evolutionary tradeoffs there is greater survival value in perceiving the kinetic-shape of an object to a very close approximation despite variations in the rotation rate and the viewing distance than in perceiving the shape perfectly only for constant rotation rates, where the visual mechanisms would have to be recalibrated for each change in viewing distance. This recalibration could have been accomplished by taking into account the absolute sizes (visual angles) of rotation ellipses, since for real objects the size of a rotation ellipse is coupled with the magnitude of perspective. However, the scaling of kinetic shape parameters would then differ for different rotation ellipses on a single object, thus again increasing the informational complexity.

Why is rotation special and why were looming shape mechanisms passed over by evolution? All potential sources of kinetic shape information involve observer-relative object orientation changes (rotation), with the one exception of looming. There probably was minimal pressure to evolve the visual mechanisms needed to accurately register the shape specifying motion component (the figural changes) in looming. Only for some limited boundary conditions, such as when flying towards a mountain in a jet, or when an object is about to hit one in the face, is this motion component well above the spatio-temporal resolving power of the visual system, and even so, it will of necessity be registered largely in the visual periphery.

The rotation ellipse parameters registered by kinetic shape mechanisms are based on geometric objects whose existence is defined only over extended regions of visual space–time. Wetware (neurological mechanisms) may operate in time in a manner overlooked by most theories of perception and cognition. The specification of event structure in terms of perceptual invariants which only exist in visual space–time has epistemological implications for cognition in general. Indirect perception theories assume that perception is the handmaiden of memory. However, if wetware resonates to structure in space–time, then the opposite may be the case. The perceptual registration of events, which happen not to be in the present, may well be what we call memory. The special ontological status we psychologically attribute to the "specious present" might after all be a cognitive illusion.

Acknowledgments. The authors wish to thank the editors and James R. Pomerantz for thoughtful comments.

SECTION IV
Brightness and Spatial Factors

The chapters in this section are psychophysical in approach. They have as their primary concern the roles of basic configurational and luminance manipulations on illusory contour salience. Each chapter presents new data on this problem, as well as a discussion of theoretical implications.

In Chapter 16, Kellman and Loukides describe the results of two experiments investigating minimal conditions necessary for illusory contour perception. Their results strongly implicate the role of occlusion in illusory contour formation.

Chapter 17 by de Weert and van Kruysbergen presents a brief review of the transparency literature. Through a series of examples and experiments, they interrelate transparency and illusory contours.

In Chapter 18, Halpern presents experiments measuring illusory contour brightness enhancement. Results are discussed from a theoretical standpoint and are related to practical and historical applications.

In Chapter 19, Warm, Dember, Padich, Beckner, and Jones summarize the well-known work on the inverse relationship between illusory contour strength and luminance. The authors also present new data describing the unusual results when such measurements are made under restricted and controlled viewing conditions.

The final chapter in this section, Chapter 20 by Jory, investigates sensitivity changes along the border of an illusory contour. With this novel analysis, he integrates illusory contours with the real contour lateral inhibition work.

CHAPTER 16

An Object Perception Approach to Static and Kinetic Subjective Contours

Philip J. Kellman and Martha G. Loukides

Subjective contours are among the most fascinating of perceptual phenomena. Although subjective contours and figures have often been considered isolated curiosities in perception, they have received considerable attention, both empirical and theoretical. In this chapter, we suggest that this attention has not been misallocated, and that subjective contours are not a peripheral curiosity. Specifically, we claim that subjective contours are examples of a process of unit formation that is pervasive in ordinary visual perception. This process underlies both subjective figure perception as well as a more common ability: the perception of the unity and boundaries of partly occluded objects.

The organization of this chapter parallels the development of our own thinking about subjective contours and object perception. In the first section (Direct Tests of Brightness and Configural Factors), we report empirical results on the persistent theoretical questions of the causal status of brightness and configural factors in subjective contours. These results, along with others, have led us to dispense with brightness factors in explaining subjective contours. In the second section (Subjective Figure Perception Across Space and Time: Kinetic Subjective Contours and Related Phenomena), we focus on the time dimension in subjective contour perception, introducing some new motion phenomena and noting older phenomena that a general theory should encompass. In the third section (Prospects for an Object Perception Theory: The Identity of Subjective Figure Perception and Ordinary Perception of Partly Occluded Objects), we present the fundamental

claims of a new object perception theory, asserting that an identical unit formation process underlies subjective figures and perception of partly occluded objects in ordinary perception. In the fourth section (A Discontinuity Theory of Unit Formation in Subjective Figures and Partly Occluded Objects), we sketch a computational model of this unit formation process. Finally, in the last section (Prospects and Problems for a Discontinuity Theory), we note some prospective empirical tests of the theory, some relations to other theories, and some unresolved issues.

Direct Tests of Brightness and Configural Factors

Much debate about subjective contours has concerned the causal status of processes of brightness perception as opposed to configural factors (see Parks, 1984, for a review). By *configural* we mean factors having to do with the shape and/or arrangement of inducing elements; we will not distinguish for now among theories emphasizing simplicity, probability, local depth cues, and so on. A general strategy of research has been to try to produce subjective contours from brightness factors alone (Jory & Day, 1979; Kennedy, 1978a), or to produce subjective contours from configural effects in the absence of facilitating brightness factors (Halpern, 1981; Kanizsa, 1979; Kellman & Cohen, 1982; Parks, 1979; Prazdny, 1983). Suggestive findings on both sides of the issue have emerged but have not generally been regarded

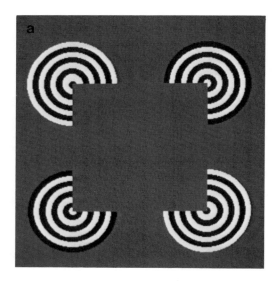

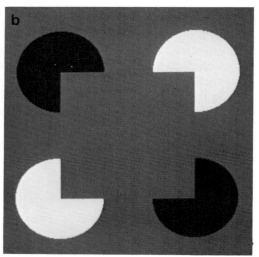

FIGURE 16.1. Subjective figures in physically and perceptually homogeneous space. (See text.)

Configural Factors: A Direct Test

Our early research on this topic (Kellman & Cohen, 1982) attempted to test configural factors in the absence of induced brightness effects, using displays of the sort shown in Figure 16.1. The display in Figure 16.1b was also developed for similar reasons by Prazdny (1983). Using black and white inducing elements on a medium gray background, we sought to test subjective figure perception in the absence of any brightness differences across the subjective contours. Because individuals might have different luminance averaging characteristics, we tested three different proportions of black to white in the striped inducer displays (Figure 16.1a). Results were generally clear: naive subjects always reported robust subjective figures in these displays, and for every subject, at least one display was reported to have no figure–surround brightness difference. However, subjects often did report brightness differences, even with inducers containing equal proportions of black and white. Moreover, it was hard to rule out the possibility of subtle, unreportable brightness differences that might have supported contour perception.

Recently, we completed a more compelling test of contour perception in the absence of perceived brightness differences. Using displays of the sort shown in Figure 16.1a and 16.1b generated on a high-resolution computer system (Apollo DN660) with 256 gray scale values, we gave subjects precise control of the brightness characteristics of the displays. Against a constant, medium gray background subjects could simultaneously raise or lower the intensities of the black and white areas of the inducers to produce or eliminate brightness differences between the central area and the surround. For example, when these intensities were raised to their highest values, their space-averaged luminance far exceeded the luminance of the surround, inducing a darker central area. Similarly, by lowering the intensities of the black and white areas, the central area could be made to appear lighter than the surround. The black and white areas could be simultaneously raised or lowered through 100 equal brightness steps; between the extreme high and low values the brightness of the central area varied by about 3 Munsell steps. Thus, each step in subjects' ad-

as conclusive. One reason is that brightness and configuration are confounded in ordinary displays: inducing elements always have shape and normally differ in brightness or color from a background. Post hoc arguments for subtle configural or brightness effects can usually be made for any display in which subjective figures occur. Contributing to this explanatory latitude has been the imprecise specification of both configural (Coren, 1972; Kanizsa, 1974; Gregory, 1972) and brightness (Day & Kasperczyk, 1983b; Jory & Day, 1979) factors.

justments varied the brightness of the central area by a tiny amount (about 0.03 Munsell steps on average). Subjects were shown two keys on a computer keyboard that varied the brightness up or down by single steps and two others for coarse adjustment that changed the brightness up and down by 10 steps per keypress.

We familiarized subjects with the subjective contour phenomenon using pictorial displays in which subjective contours are known to occur and others in which they are known not to occur; the latter procedure may be important in avoiding guessing tendencies (Kellman & Cohen, 1984). A pretest checked subjects' individual matching tendencies. Subjects were shown a rectangle composed of alternating black and white stripes, each one pixel wide. From the subjects' viewing distance, individual stripes were not visible and the rectangle appeared as a homogeneous gray. Subjects were instructed to adjust the color of the rectangle to make it match the background and disappear. All subjects succeeded, indicating that each could match the gray surround by equal amounts of black and white somewhere in the available range of intensities.

The subjective figure displays were presented initially with brightness settings making the central square appear somewhat darker than the background. Subjects were told to adjust the brightness of the display through the entire available range and to (1) try to make the edges of the central square go away, and (2) try to make any brightness difference between the central area and the surround go away.

Results were unequivocal. Every subject was able to eliminate all brightness differences between the central area and the surround. However, subjects were in general unable to eliminate clear subjective contours at any point in the adjustment range,[1] despite the fact that

every subject was able to adjust the central square from appearing darker to appearing lighter than the surround by very small steps. Subjects were asked to rate contour strength for the initial version of the display (with central area darker than the surround), using an ordinary Kanizsa triangle display (black inducing elements on a white background) as a standard of 10. Subjects were also asked to rate the contour strength again after they had adjusted the brightness of the central area and surround to be an exact match. For the striped displays (Fig. 16.1a), ratings of the 11 (out of 12) subjects who could never eliminate the subjective figure ranged from 4 to 10, and averaged 6.8. This was slightly lower than their rating prior to brightness matching of 7.5. For the other display (Fig. 16.1b), ratings ranged from 5 to 10 and averaged 7.1 at the point of matched brightness, compared to initial ratings of 9.5.

The existence of robust subjective contours in the total absence of surface quality differences indicates configural causation. The results provide strong evidence for edge perception in both physically and perceptually homogeneous space. While abrupt surface quality differences across perceived boundaries may ordinarily be causes or consequences of those boundaries (Kanizsa, 1979; Koffka, 1935), they are not necessary for the visual perception of edges.

Our data suggest that brightness differences between center and surround can enhance the strength of perceived contours. This observation does not support a causal role for brightness factors in producing contours in physically homogeneous space. In these displays, local brightness differences due to contrast are confined by edges that also exist in their absence. These differences can serve to emphasize those edges.

---

[1] The single subject who reported contour disappearance seemed anomalous in several respects. His contour strength ratings were unusually low throughout the experiment. For the initial versions (before brightness matching) of the striped and solid inducer displays, he gave contour ratings of 3 and 3, respectively, while no other subjects gave ratings less than 7 and 6. Moreover, his reports of contour disappearance were not restricted to the range in which he reported that the brightness of the center matched the surround.

Brightness Factors: A Direct Test

The existence of examples of configural causation of subjective contours does not logically exclude the possibility that induced brightness effects can also be causal. Can subjective edges ever be initiated by pools of induced brightness? Many have suggested that such brightness factors are in general the cause of subjective contours (Brigner & Gallagher, 1974; Day

& Kasperczyk, 1983b; Frisby & Clatworthy, 1975; Jory & Day, 1979). Subjective contour-inducing elements, it is asserted, enhance or decrease the brightness of adjacent regions by retinal brightness contrast (perhaps along with some other local brightness effects). Regions of altered brightness are joined by the spreading of brightness, perhaps according to configural rules, across the areas between inducers. These claims have been difficult to evaluate directly. Many purported examples either contain configural confounds or appear to be somewhat different phenomena. For instance, displays may contain clearly enhanced brightness but rather diffuse edges (e.g., Kennedy, 1976a).

Recently, we completed a direct test of the causal status of brightness factors. Using a high-resolution CRT display, we created pools of enhanced brightness by "seeding" pixels of higher intensity in certain display areas, to see if these could then be assimilated into subjective figures. Individual pixels were undetectable and were spaced so as to create no abrupt boundaries. We used displays that do not normally give rise to subjective contours but contain the same amount of real contour, bounding a central square area, as do displays that ordinarily do give strong subjective contours. Specifically, we used four inducing elements in the shape of a cross or plus sign; such displays have previously been shown to be poor inducers of subjective contours (e.g., Kanizsa, 1979; Kellman & Cohen, 1982). We also used the same seeding patterns in the absence of any inducing elements. As control displays we obtained judgments about subjective figures and edges using the cross displays with no seeding. The seeding patterns were arranged to mimic the pools of brightness that would obtain in a subjective figure display with very effective inducers. We used seeding patterns that might arise from partial circle elements, as in Figure 16.1b, if all four inducers were black on a white background. To determine the induced brightness gradient, we developed a simple model of lateral inhibition in which inhibition of each retinal element was proportional to the luminance of the display point projected to that element, and inhibition declined quickly with inter-element distance. We also "cheated" in favor of brightness causation in two ways. First of all, we did not seed enhanced brightness anywhere

outside of the central square area. Second, we seeded more than predicted by the model along the unspecified boundaries of the central square area. (This enhancement was added after no subjective contour induction was observed without it.)

The results showed very few reports of a subjective square or of subjective edges in the seeded displays, with or without the corners being specified by real contours. More frequent were uncertain reports from a few subjects of a "fuzzy diamond," "a circle," or a "plus sign." All of these reports occurred equally or more often with the unseeded cross-shaped inducing elements. There was no evidence in this experiment that subjective figures can be initiated by diffuse pools of enhanced brightness.

Some caution is required, however. Negative results such as these do not rule out that under some other conditions, induced brightness could lead to subjective contour perception. Our primitive lateral inhibition model may not have provided appropriate patterns of seeding. Nevertheless, we believe that the brightness seeding method does isolate the central claim of brightness-based theories of subjective figures. Such theories must predict the existence of a class of brightness seeding patterns that do not contain abrupt luminance changes and are sufficient to produce subjective figures. On this point, it must be added that our informal manipulations of brightness seeding, apart from the specific model we tested, have been no more successful at producing subjective contours.

Taking these results at face value, we are very pessimistic about the possibility that subjective contours and figures are initiated by areas of altered brightness.

Overview of Configural and Brightness Factors

The results of our parallel investigations of configural and brightness causation of subjective contours and figures are clear and complementary. Certain configurations produce subjective figures in the total absence of physical and perceptual differences in surface qualities. Conversely, it has not been possible to obtain direct evidence that diffuse brightness alteration can initiate the phenomenon. Subjective contours seem to demand explanation in terms of the shapes and arrangements of visible areas. So far we have said little about what properties of shape or arrangement are relevant, a matter which itself has been controversial. After examining some other phenomena relevant to a theory of subjective figures, we consider this question later on in this chapter.

Subjective Figure Perception Across Space and Time: Kinetic Subjective Contours and Related Phenomena

Recently discovered phenomena indicate that unit formation processes operating across space in subjective figure perception have analogues in the temporal domain; subjective figures can be specified by figural information given over time by motion. Some of these phenomena have been reported previously, whereas others are described here for the first time. They provide additional evidence that subjective figures are only peripherally related to brightness perception. More importantly, they suggest connections to ordinary object perception, in which the important role of information given over time is well known (e.g., Gibson, Kaplan, Reynolds, & Wheeler, 1969; Kellman & Spelke, 1983).

Kinetic Subjective Contours

Kellman and Cohen (1984) reasoned that if information separated in space is used by the visual system to create subjective figures, then such interpolation across time might also be possible. Figure 16.2 shows how such "kinetic subjective contours" might be produced. When the inducing elements are partly occluded in sequence as by a rotating figure (of the same color as the surround), the figure is clearly seen. These percepts occur despite the design of the displays so that no subjective figure can be detected in any stationary view. In the most robust version of this phenomenon, the inducing elements rotate around the central area, and the subjective figure is seen in a constant position. No explanation in terms of brightness contrast, assimilation, etc. seems remotely plausible with these moving displays. It is more likely that ki-

netic subjective contours are related to the ordinary perception of moving objects or stationary objects by moving observers (see below).

Specification of Inducing Elements Outside of the Luminance Domain

The possibility that configural factors are causal but brightness factors incidental in subjective contours has led to the attempt to specify inducing elements outside of the luminance domain. Prazdny (1985) reported failure to obtain subjective contours when the inducers were specified only by stereopsis or by motion characteristics. In his displays, both the inducing elements and the surround were covered with black and white random dots. When the inducers were defined stereoscopically, they appeared in front or in back of the surrounding surface, and when defined by motion, the streaming of random dots in the inducing areas differed from the motion characteristics of the background. Although Prazdny concluded that his results were consistent with the need for subjective contour-inducing elements to be defined in the luminance domain, he noted that certain incidental properties of his displays may have prevented subjective contour formation (for example, streaming of random dots made inducing circles appear as holes in a surface).

We have recently produced robust subjective figures in which the inducing elements were specified outside of the luminance domain. We also used motion to indicate the boundaries of the inducers, but they were designed to accrete and delete background texture as they moved. They thus appeared in front of the background surface (Gibson, Kaplan, Reynolds, & Wheeler, 1959). Figure 16.2b illustrates the displays. The three square elements had the same random dot surface as the surround and were not visible when stationary. As they rotated, they became visible atop the surrounding surface, because the points of the square progressively occluded and disoccluded elements of the background. The inducers were themselves progressively occluded as they moved behind the points of a central triangle. A complete triangle with crisp boundaries was seen, although the displays were constructed so that none is physically present.

These subjective figures demand explanation

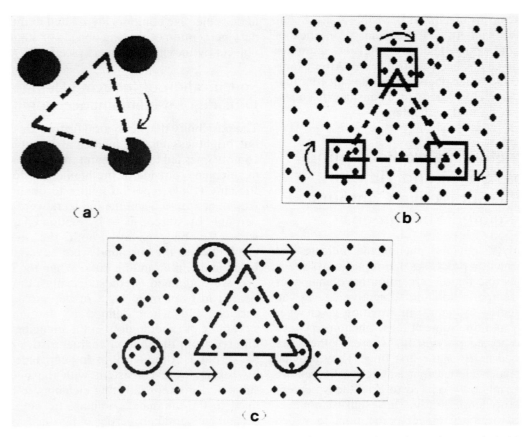

FIGURE 16.2. Schematic illustrations of subjective figures dependent on information given over time. a. A kinetic subjective figure. The black circles are partially occluded at different times as they would be by a triangle of the background color rotating in the plane. A clearcut subjective triangle is perceived. b. Kinetic specification of inducing elements. When stationary, a single surface with random-dot texture is seen. When the three squares rotate around their centers, they progressively occlude and reveal background texture, and are themselves occluded by vertices that could be part of a central triangle. A central triangle with clear edges is perceived. c. A kinetic subjective figure with kinetically specified inducing elements. Again the field is seen as a single surface when stationary, but when the circular areas translate back and forth, they become visible, and from their sequential occlusion, a central triangle is perceived.

in terms of configural factors, perhaps, as we argue below, in terms of relationships of figural discontinuities over space and time. Unless subjective figures given by kinetic specification of inducing elements are a wholly different phenomenon, it appears that the definition of inducers in the luminance domain as well as concomitant brightness effects in subjective figures are thoroughly incidental.

Although motion is involved in this new display, it is more of a static subjective figure, rather than a kinetic one, as we have used these terms. The reason is that all of the inflection points of the boundary of the subjective figure are specified simultaneously.

Kinetic Subjective Contours with Kinetically Specified Inducers

Can kinetic subjective figures also be produced using inducing elements specified outside of the luminance domain? We recently answered this question in the affirmative, using displays such as the one diagrammed in Figure 16.2c. Once again, the inducing forms had the same random dot surface appearance as the surround and were thus invisible when stationary. As the three circles translated laterally across the display, they accreted and deleted background texture and were themselves progressively occluded at different times by the corners of a central triangle. A clearly bounded, central triangle was seen, although once again, these boundaries did not exist in the actual display.

Implications of Motion Information in Subjective Figure Perception

These motion phenomena significantly extend the domain of discourse for attempts to explain subjective figure perception. The many similarities between static and kinetic subjective figures (Kellman & Cohen, 1984) suggest that a unified theoretical treatment might be possible. Moreover, taken together, they seem less likely to be incidental or isolated phenomena, and more likely to be indicators of a general unit formation process that functions in ordinary perception. In the next section, we suggest what that process might be.

Prospects for an Object Perception Theory: The Identity of Subjective Figure Perception and Ordinary Perception of Partly Occluded Objects

The wealth of previous research on subjective contours has produced few clear connections to ordinary perception. Subjective contours have remained primarily a laboratory curiosity; we almost never encounter them apart from our encounters with perceptionists.

Here we propose a new theory of why subjective contours exist and what more pervasive phenomena they can help us to understand. The central claim is this: Subjective contours are produced by the processes of unit formation that enable us to perceive objects despite occlusion.

The Problem of Occlusion

Perceiving objects and surfaces despite partial occlusion is a basic and ubiquitous aspect of normal perception. Consider the photograph of a simple scene in Figure 16.3. Although the scene is not especially cluttered, most of the objects are partly occluded by other objects. Light is reflected to an observer from only some of any object's surfaces, both because objects occlude parts of themselves and because occlusion of objects by others is pervasive. Many objects reflect light from spatially separated areas; in the photograph, this is true of each of the subject's feet, as well as the chaise lounge on which he is seated. We nevertheless perceive proximally separate light-reflecting areas to be part of a single distal object, with clear boundaries and shape. An additional complication is that adjacent light-reflecting areas that are parts of the same object may not be adjacent parts of the object. In the photograph we are able to detect that the subject's left leg does not merge with his right ankle but continues behind it.

The visual perception of objects and surfaces despite occlusion has been the subject of considerable study (Gibson, 1979; Kanizsa, 1979; Kellman & Spelke, 1983; Michotte, Thines, & Crabbe, 1964). Michotte et al. termed the perception of partly occluded areas *amodal completion,* meaning that the occluded areas are phenomenally present but do not possess the attributes of a sensory modality. For example, in the photograph, although one perceives the subject's left shoe as continuing behind the table leg, one would be unable to answer questions about whether there are scuff marks on the part of the shoe behind the table leg. Subjective figures, in contrast, are considered to be examples of modal completion, because the surface qualities of the completed surface are apparent to the perceiver.

Some have pointed out relationships between modal and amodal completion (Kanizsa, 1979; Michotte, Thines, & Crabbe, 1964). For example, it has often been observed that whereas subjective figures are examples of modal completion, the inducing elements are seen to continue behind them, i.e., the inducing elements are completed amodally (see Minguzzi, chap. 7; Sambin, chap. 14). Despite these connections,

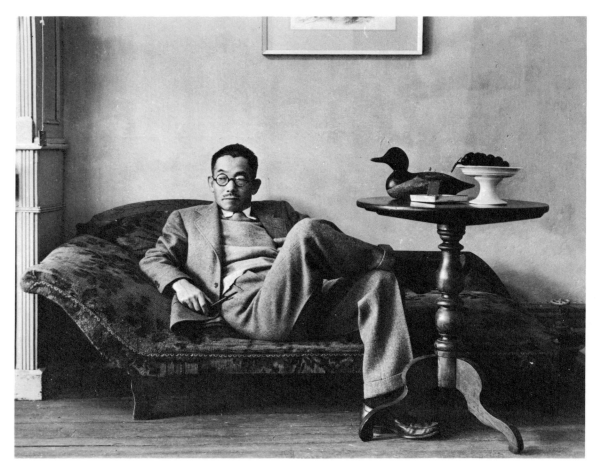

FIGURE 16.3. *Portrait of Yasuo Kuniyoshi.* New York, Metropolitan Museum of Art. Copyright by Arnold Newman; reproduced by permission. (See text.)

perception of partly occluded objects and subjective figures have usually been considered as separable phenomena and studied independently. In the present analysis, we assert that subjective figure and partly occluded object perception are not simply connected in interesting ways, but that they are in fact identical phenomena. In particular, we suggest that the process of detecting a unit visually is the same in the two cases; whether a detected unit appears modally as a subjective figure or amodally as a partly hidden object depends on an additional and independent step having to do with the arrangement in depth of detected units.

Some Illustrative Phenomena

Two phenomena illustrate this claim. First, it has occasionally been pointed out (e.g., Brad-

ley & Petry, 1977) that subjective figures can sometimes be seen as amodally, rather than modally, completed. Figure 16.4 shows a Kanizsa-type triangle, ordinarily seen as a modally completed triangle overlaying three black disks on a white background. It can also be seen as three points of a triangle *behind* the white surface showing through three windows or holes in the white surface. The black areas are then seen through the holes as a more distant surface. In Figure 16.4b some lines have been added to emphasize the "windows" interpretation. An especially vivid and intriguing example of this alternative appearance is the subjective Necker cube created by Bradley and Petry (1977). Once noticed, the two appearances tend to alternate in time. This bistability is also characteristic of kinetic subjective figures (Kellman & Cohen, 1984).

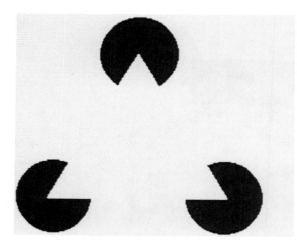

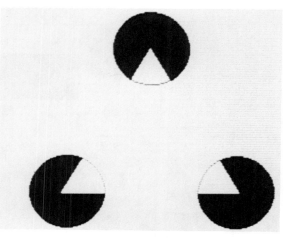

FIGURE 16.4. The bistability of ordinary subjective figures. a. A standard subjective figure display; after Kanizsa (1955a). b. The display in (a) with lines added to emphasize an alternative appearance: a uni-tary triangle is seen as partly hidden behind a nearer white surface, and the triangle's points are visible through "windows" or holes.

Before considering an interpretation of this bistability, consider another phenomenon, or rather, a set of three phenomena. Figure 16.5a depicts an occluded object; the unity of the triangle is easily seen. Figure 16.5b shows a subjective figure of the same shape. Figure 16.5c, after Arnheim (1974), shows an especially interesting intermediate case. The most fascinating aspect of Figure 16.5c is that, although it is a bounded, homogeneously colored figure, it perceptually resolves into two figures: a triangle and a rectangle. This phenomenon, the spontaneous resolving of homogeneous areas into separate entities, has received little attention. Arnheim (1974) mentions it as an indication of Gestalt tendencies toward simplicity. The second fascinating aspect of this display requires a longer period of fixation. You may notice that the triangle sometimes appears to be on top of the rectangle and sometimes behind it. In the former case, the triangle is modally completed, bounded by clear subjective contours, as in Figure 16.5b; in the latter case it becomes a partly occluded triangle, as in 16.5a, while the center part of the rectangle becomes modally present.

Separating Unit Formation and Depth Placement

If one considers modal and amodal completion to be separate phenomena, these examples of figures that alternate over time between subjective figures and partly occluded figures seem especially mysterious. We propose two complementary hypotheses that may serve to unify and clarify these phenomena:

1. The unit formation process for subjective figures and partly occluded objects is identical and is unvarying during the modal–amodal alternation. The units perceived to be in the array remain constant; in Figure 16.5c these units are the triangle and the rectangle.

2. The appearance of these units as in front of other surfaces (modal completion) or behind other surfaces (partial occlusion) depends on an independent depth placement process in which the depth relations of various units and surfaces is determined by available depth information.

When little or no depth information is available, the position of the unit relative to other surfaces will be bistable, as in Figure 16.5c, where no depth information specifies whether the triangle is in front of or behind the rectangle. When depth information is unequivocal, as in the case of most partly occluded objects in ordinary environments, an unambiguous position of the unit is perceived. The Kanizsa triangle in Figure 16.4a usually appears to be modally completed. This is probably due to the tendency of the circles to appear as figures on the white background, rather than as holes in it (Rubin, 1915). However, this fac-

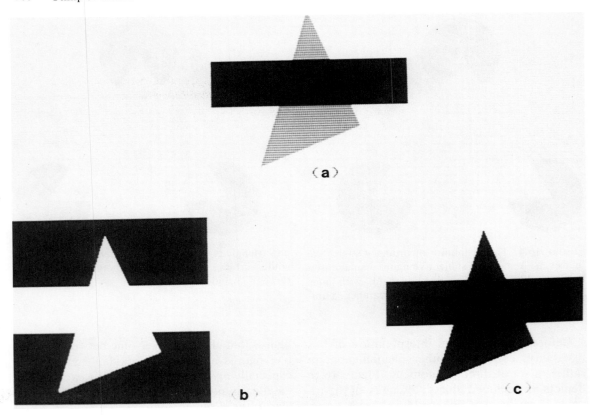

FIGURE 16.5. Equivalence of unit formation in subjective figures and partly occluded objects. a. A partly occluded object. b. An equivalent subjective figure. c. A spontaneously splitting figure. (See text.)

tor alone does not prohibit the alternative organization from being seen occasionally or with effort.

If these phenomena emerge from the same mechanisms, it remains to be determined what these mechanisms are. Recognition of a basic identity between subjective figures, partly occluded objects, and spontaneously separating figures raises many questions but also opens a number of avenues for investigating the specifics of the unit formation process. From our preliminary investigations, we believe that it is possible to specify the relevant conditions for perception of a unit. It appears that the relevant information is relatively local (i.e., it does not directly involve considerations of overall symmetry), and it involves variables of boundary shape exclusively, rather than, e.g., surface similarity.

A Discontinuity Theory of Unit Formation in Subjective Figures and Partly Occluded Objects

Because of space limitations, we present only a sketch of the model here. For convenience, we first treat static optic arrays and afterward indicate how information over time may be incorporated. The theory presented here is intended to be strictly a computational one in Marr's (1982) sense. That is, we do not even hint at a specific algorithm to accomplish the pickup of the information we describe, nor do we have any commitment to a particular realization in neural hardware. With regard to the latter, however, we have noticed with interest possible relations between our model and the neurophysiological hypotheses of Shapley and

Gordon (chap. 11) concerning nonlinear operators.

It is fairly clear how regions whose edges are defined by abrupt luminance or spectral changes may be detected (e.g., Marr, 1982). The domain of our unit formation model includes the cases where boundaries are perceived in regions where no such surface quality changes are detected. The following may roughly comprise the steps in formation of such units:

1. *A necessary initial condition is a spatial discontinuity in a luminance boundary.*

By discontinuity we mean the mathematical notion: if a boundary is described by a function, it is not differentiable at the point of discontinuity. Intuitively, this includes any abrupt change in direction of a contour. However, the relevant class of perceptual discontinuities may be larger than this, including all segments exceeding a certain sharpness of curvature (see below). An example of a discontinuity on a subjective contour-inducing element, e.g., in Figure 16.4a, is a point at which the circular boundary ends. In the homogeneously colored figure in 16.5c, the points at which the triangular section begins to extend upward from the horizontal edge are discontinuities.

A discontinuity is a necessary condition for a new unit to be formed. That is, we hypothesize that only when an abrupt change in a bounding contour is present can a figure function as a subjective contour-inducing element or as an object part that is connectable to other parts in occlusion situations. Such a discontinuity is not a *sufficient* condition for unit formation or segregation. A single subjective contour-inducing element, in the absence of others, is seen as a self-contained, irregularly shaped figure. Likewise, if the lower protrusion in Figure 16.5c is removed, the upper triangular protrusion alone does not tend to split off from the rest of the figure; again an irregular, bounded figure is seen.

2. *A unit is formed when a discontinuity is continuously relatable to others, and when the connections generated among discontinuities yield a closed form.*

More specifically, to be continuously relatable means that an edge along one side of a discontinuity may be connected to another without any discontinuity occurring between them, i.e., they may be connected via a straight line or a smooth curve. A major, and as yet untested, empirical prediction of the theory is that a determination of what a perceptual discontinuity consists of for purposes of step 1 will also provide an accurate criterion for relatability in step 2. In other words, if for step 1 a curve must change direction more sharply than some threshold in order to function as a subjective contour-inducing element, then we would expect to find, regarding step 2, that for the edges along two discontinuities to be perceptually unified, something less than that threshold of curvature sharpness must be possible at all points between them. An additional constraint here is that the connection between edges must proceed monotonically from one to the other; otherwise any two edges would be connectable without any discontinuity occurring between them.[2]

The discontinuities we have been discussing are retinally specifiable. Unit formation in our theory has the consequence that some retinal discontinuities do not correspond to discontinuities in the boundaries of perceived objects. For example, when a subjective triangle is seen in the standard Kanizsa display, two of the three retinal discontinuities in the boundaries of each inducing circle are seen as resulting from occlusion rather than from abrupt changes in the boundaries of an object. A potentially fruitful way of expressing step 2—that units are formed if discontinuities are continuously relatable to others—is that the visual system uses these rules to minimize the number of discontinuities assigned to perceived objects' boundaries.[3]

3. *A unit formed by steps 1 and 2 is positioned in depth relative to other surfaces in the array as determined by available depth information.*

In subjective figures, the unit appears in front of retinally adjacent surfaces. In the case of partly occluded objects, the unitary figure appears behind an intervening object or surface. In ordinary perception of partly hidden objects, in contrast to pictorial displays, the relative

---

[2] We are indebted to Martin S. Banks for pointing out the need for this constraint.

[3] We are indebted to Henry Gleitman for this insight.

depths of occluding and occluded objects are often very well specified.

Events as Discontinuities

When information is given over time, the unit formation process may follow the same framework, although both the initiating and relatability conditions must be broadened to include certain *events*. In the case of kinetically specified inducing elements, the application of the theory is straightforward. Initiating spatial discontinuities are specified by accretion and deletion of texture elements, rather than by changes in a luminance boundary. These spatial discontinuities function in the same way as those arising from luminance boundaries. The luminance domain per se has no special role, but serves as one way (the most common one) of specifying discontinuities.

Kinetic subjective figures and partly occluded objects detected over time raise some interesting issues, since the discontinuities are specified over time and are also separated over time as well as space. Regarding the initiating events, we propose that certain figural changes given over time function as discontinuities, analogous to abrupt changes in contour. We have not yet fully developed these ideas, but a basic parallel may hold between space and time. Continuity over time may be definable in terms of the class of projective changes on the retina that can occur from an object translating or rotating in space, or a stationary object viewed by a moving observer (Gibson, Kaplan, Reynolds, & Wheeler, 1969; Johansson, 1970). Other retinal changes that are not projectively invariant may constitute temporal discontinuities. Such discontinuities in isolation may be seen as figural deformation, although they are more likely to be seen as occlusion (Michotte, Thines, & Crabbe, 1964).[4]

Relatability of the edges forming a discontinuity to others may depend on the same requirements of smooth curvature as in the static case. When the objects' parts are changing positions in space, however, the relatability criteria must apply to the real spatial positions of these parts

at a given time, not to the retinal locations at which a part was last specified. Constraints probably exist regarding the continuity of figural motion necessary for temporally separated discontinuities to form kinetic subjective figures (Kellman & Cohen, 1984). This problem is minimized when kinetic subjective figures are specified in a stationary position by moving inducing elements, which may account for the slightly more robust subjective figures in this case (Kellman & Cohen, 1984).

As in static arrays, the formation of units from relatable discontinuity events minimizes the number of discontinuities—spatial and temporal—that must be assigned to perceived objects.

Prospects and Problems for a Discontinuity Theory

The present theory accrues some large burdens but also points toward a number of interesting predictions and some new approaches to problems in object perception. Space permits only brief mention of some of the main empirical and conceptual lines being pursued.

Much of our recent work has examined the hypothesis of identical unit formation mechanisms in subjective figures, partly occluded objects, and "spontaneously splitting" homogeneous figures. In our view, any subjective figure display should be transformable by certain simple rules into an equivalent partly hidden object display, and vice versa. Likewise, either of these displays should be transformable into a homogeneously colored display that spontaneously resolves into more than one figure. Our investigation of these equivalences has been highly confirming of these predictions. The transformation rules are readily discoverable by the reader; computer-generated displays are helpful for making rapid changes and comparisons.

These equivalences furnish convergent measures for empirical study of the initiating configurations and events in unit formation. A major challenge is to develop a measure of abruptness of curvature and find some range of values of such a variable that defines a spatial discontinuity with the explanatory power we hypothesize. Another source of convergence will be compar-

---

[4] Another possibility is that the important effects of temporal changes may be to introduce momentary spatial discontinuities in the inducing figures.

ison of data on initiating contour formation with data about relatability. There are also questions about whether the abruptness of curvature can be defined in purely retinal terms. While a mathematical discontinuity in an object boundary consistently projects a retinal discontinuity, the sharpness of certain curved contours may depend on their distance, projected size, and orientation.

Initial attempts to refine the discontinuity notion are focusing on stationary arrays. If precise characterization of the spatial discontinuity notion proves possible, a further challenge will be incorporating it with information about the spatiotemporal constraints on event-specified discontinuities. One intriguing hypothesis is that the spatial discontinuities in the static case may simply be limiting (or mildly degenerate) cases of more fundamental event-specified discontinuities. Such a view would fit with theories emphasizing the primacy of optical transformations in human visual perception (Gibson, 1979; Johansson, forthcoming).

Relations to Other Perspectives

The present theory bears important resemblances to previous views of object and edge perception. Because we are treating both subjective contour phenomena and perception of partly occluded objects, these ideas intersect with many older accounts. As noted above, however, few discussions have explicitly connected these domains. Kanizsa (1979) treats these phenomena separately for the most part, although he repeatedly notes similarities in the perceptual tendencies operating in the two domains. Michotte, Thines, & Crabbe (1964), while not explicitly discussing subjective contours, consider examples of modal along with amodal completion, suggesting that both follow Gestalt principles. The claim that subjective contours and partly hidden objects arise from the same unit formation process and differ because of an independent depth-placement step is, as far as we can determine, novel.

The specifics tentatively proposed for this common unit formation process have much in common with certain traditional Gestalt principles, especially good continuation (Michotte, Thines, & Crabbe, 1964; Wertheimer, 1923a). This is reassuring, since we believe that the older accounts and demonstrations concerning good continuation and simplicity tendencies identified important aspects of the problem. However, these notions have remained vague and have shown little predictive utility. Moreover, determining how such principles may be realized in a visual system, human or artificial, has been problematic. How might a rapidly functioning system consider all possible arrangements of an array and choose the simplest or best? Our tentative computational ideas have the virtues of suggesting precisely definable and relatively local stimulus attributes as the basis for unit formation. By developing a mathematically specifiable and local notion of contour discontinuity it may be possible to give precision to more elusive notions such as "good" continuation. Such a theory differs from a list of contributing principles, (e.g., Michotte, Thines, & Crabbe, 1964); for example, similarity of surface color and texture have no role in our model. Because our approach emphasizes local boundary properties, it contrasts with any approach emphasizing global symmetry, e.g., in the overall shape of subjective contour-inducing elements (Kanizsa, 1979). Along with others, this would seem to be a clear difference from coding theories (Leeuwenberg, 1981; Restle, 1981) which have been applied to occlusion cases. Some of the most heartening results of our investigations so far have been cases in which more global attributes such as symmetry and overall simplicity turn out to be the consequences of the application of local rules (cf. Marr, 1982).

Among subjective contour theories, our approach is perhaps closest to Coren's (1972) view that certain boundary configurations function as implicit interposition cues. We see our work as extending Coren's insights in several ways. We have suggested specifically what the initiating stimulus variable (a contour discontinuity) might be and we are developing some ways of determining its scope. Moreover, we hypothesize a relationship between the characteristics of the initiating discontinuities and the conditions that govern their connections to one another. Furthermore, we are not sure that the discontinuity notion must be characterized as initially involving depth, although its outcome certainly has consequences for the units that must be segregated in depth. While clarifying these basic notions, we are also generalizing the theory to the problem of partly occluded objects and to perception based on discontinuities given over time as well as in space.

Much remains to be learned, but we see great promise in assimilating the subjective contour phenomenon to visual processes whose main function is the ordinary perception of unitary objects in a visual world pervaded by occlusion. By considering boundary discontinuities across space and time, a comprehensive understanding of occluded object perception, encompassing objects and observers both moving and stationary, may be possible.

Acknowledgments. This research was supported by NSF Grant BNS-10110 and a Swarthmore College Faculty Research Grant to Philip J. Kellman. The authors thank Tim Shipley, Kirk Swenson, Henry Gleitman, Elizabeth Spelke and Martin S. Banks for helpful discussions. The authors also thank Steve Platt for generously lending computer facilities, George Flickinger for expert photographic assistance, and James Crowell and Marian Staats for general assistance. Reprint requests should be addressed to Philip J. Kellman, Department of Psychology, Swarthmore College, Swarthmore, Pennsylvania 19081.

Subjective Contour Strength and Perceptual Superimposition: Transparency as a Special Case

Charles M. M. de Weert and Noud A. W. H. van Kruysbergen

According to Kanizsa (1979), "The modification of brightness in the typical subjective contour stimuli is not the cause, but a consequence of the particular spatial configuration that the perceptual field is forced to assume" (p. 204). Recent data from Cavanagh (1986) expresses an alternative viewpoint. Although Cavanagh is not particularly arguing against Kanizsa's point of view, his finding that isoluminant stimuli do not evoke subjective contours can be used as a valid counter argument against the view of brightness change as a consequence rather than a cause. The lack of strong subjective contours with isoluminant stimuli has been reported several times (Brigner & Gallagher, 1974; Brussell, Stober, & Bodinger, 1977; Frisby & Clatworthy, 1975; Gregory, 1977).

This is not the place to give all the arguments and counterarguments of the cognitive versus other approaches. These issues are discussed elsewhere in this volume. The issue of the role of brightness change will be pursued in this chapter by investigating the interaction of subjective contours, perceptual transparency, and superimposition to help unravel the different processes involved in the formation of illusory contours.

The Italian Gestalt psychologists, e.g., Kanizsa and Metelli, were very influential both in the fields of subjective contours and transparency. Kanizsa (1979) presented beautiful examples of the combination of transparency and subjective contours. In a very recent paper, Metelli (1985) gave an excellent overview of the development of his transparency ideas.

The Gestaltist's concept of phenomenal splitting of a stimulus into two colors, each belonging to different surfaces, was the starting point (Heider, 1933). Metelli (1985) quantified this idea of scission in an elegant manner. "Since the phenomenon of chromatic scission is the inverse of the phenomenon of chromatic fusion, the same equation can be used to describe chromatic scission in phenomenal transparency." This equation, based on Talbot's law, describes a weighted combination of reflectances of the component surfaces, the weights being determined by the sector widths of the two components, if the two surface colors are combined by using a sectored rotating disk over a background. This concept is still used by Metelli, but in his recent paper his formulas were applied using perceptual quantities instead of physical quantities as parameters: i.e., the physically defined reflectances have gradually changed to transformed values of the same parameters, no longer indicating the physical characteristics but rather their psychological equivalents of judgmental values, related probably to lightness judgments. The work of Beck (1978) and of Beck, Prazdny, and Ivry (1984) certainly has been instrumental in this change. The argument given by Metelli for this change is that subjects are not able to judge the physical quantities directly. If anything, they have access only to the psychological measures of these parameters.

Our point of view reflects more or less the opposite. It is puzzling indeed, how subjects manage to find out the physical relations, but despite this problem we would still like to propose that the judgment of transparency by observers rests on the "testing" of physical constraints in local stimulus relations. With this information we would also like to make sure that this testing of relations is not a process at a high cognitive level. To the contrary, it is, in our view, still a rather peripheral, low-level process, and of a local character. This local testing of conditions could quite well be at the level where acceptance of parts of impossible figures occurs, just as in, for example, Escher's pictures, Penrose's triangle, or testing of corners in the Necker cube.

The basic assumptions (de Weert, 1984) underlying the experiments to be described below and ideas to be tested by the experiments are as follows:

1. Transparency and subjective contour formation have a strong relationship.

2. Transparency rules are sets of relations, based on physical rules, between brightnesses (and/or colors) in neighboring areas in the picture.

3. Brightness (or darkness) enhancement occurring in subjective contours is not a consequence of seeing contours. The brightness differences are peripherally generated data, due to two fundamental, low-level effects: simultaneous contrast and assimilation.

4. At a more central level, but still perhaps relatively low, implicit physical relations are tested in restricted areas in the image, which nonetheless involve more than one contour.

5. If physical relations for transparency (or more generally, for superimposition of light or matter) are fulfilled, only then are sharp contours seen as boundaries of the areas with enhanced brightness (or darkness).

Thus, we decouple perceived brightness difference and the perception of the contours. The difference in brightness only leads to a sharp contour if hierarchically higher-order conditions, i.e., those of perceptual transparency, are fulfilled.

Contrast and Assimilation

The picture shown in Figure 17.1a is a rather complex one, which shows how dramatic assimilation effects can be. Assimilation has, unjustifiably, been neglected in literature, in comparison with simultaneous contrast. This picture shows how the gray within the "diamonds," which is physically the same through-

out, is shifted into a darker gray when surrounded by a black line, and shifted towards a brighter gray when surrounded by a bright line. This is, of course, completely the opposite of what would be expected if simultaneous contrast is the prevailing mechanism. As a matter of fact, the effect is rather robust, not critically dependent upon the width of the black and white rings. Only three levels of luminance are present in this picture.

In Figure 17.1b to 17.1f, simpler examples of contrast and assimilation effects are given. In Figure 17.1b it is clear that assimilation is the basis for the perceived change in brightness. The whole area looks darker than the surround, due to assimilation. In Figure 17.1c, the lines are lighter than the surround and as a consequence the whole area looks slightly brighter. In Figures 17.1d and 17.1e the complementary figures are given. Here it is contrast which makes the central area look brighter or darker than the surround, depending on the values of the inducing lines. Figure 17.1f offers a striking demonstration of the combined effects: assimilation from the dark lines in the center, and color and brightness contrast due to the blue lines. Assimilation occurs along lines, contrast occurs at endpoints of lines.

In Figure 17.1g, both darkness and brightness induction are present due to the presence of both dark and bright lines in the induction field. When luminance values of the dark and bright lines are properly chosen, compensation of the two induction effects can be obtained.

The experiment to be reported here is based on combinations of stimuli presented in Figures 17.1b to 17.1e. If the lines in the two stimuli to be combined have different luminance values, and if all values are different from the background, transparency can occur. See also Van Tuijl and de Weert (1979) for the stimulus conditions which evoke the so called neon effect and come very close to the conditions for the occurrence of transparency. What has to be shown among others is that the brightness difference is still present, even when no subjective contour is reported. For that purpose some straightforward experiments were performed. The first thing investigated was whether a relations exists between subjective contour and transparency (Experiment 1a and 1b) and second, whether every induced brightness differ-

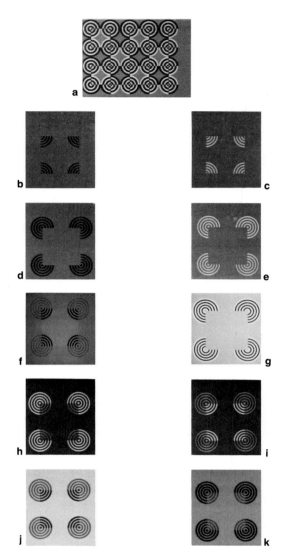

ence leads to the perception of subjective contours. It is most important that the experiments are carried out with stimuli which do not differ from each other in a structural sense. In this respect this study differs from some previous studies in which structural variation was used to demonstrate the "cognitive" character of subjective contour formation.

Experiment 1: Subjective Contour and Transparency

Apparatus

A color television monitor with separate RGB inputs was used. The stimuli were generated by computer (PDP 11/23; see Wittebrood, Wansink, and de Weert (1981) for a more detailed description of the equipment). Color and luminances of the different parts of the stimulus could be varied in very fine steps.

Experiment 1a. Subjective contour strength as a function of brightness contrasts of stimulus parts *a* and *b* (see Fig. 17.2).

Experiment 1b. Judged transparency as a function of brightness contrasts of stimulus parts *a* and *b* (Fig. 17.2).

FIGURE 17.1a. Example of the combined effects of assimilation and contrast. The background level is the same everywhere. Note that the area adjacent to the white lines looks brighter than the area adjacent to the dark lines. b, c, d, e. Examples of assimilation and contrast effects. f. The assimilation of the dark lines in the inner square makes conditions optimal for color induction in the center due to outer lines. A color plate of this figure appears on page xv. g. Simultaneous brightness induction and darkness induction, which allows complete cancellation with the proper luminance values. h,i,j,k. Combined effects of assimilation and contrast.

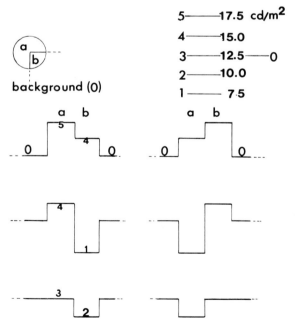

FIGURE 17.2. A sketch of luminance relations in different parts of the stimulus field.

Stimuli

For the "contrast" generating part (*a*) and for the "assimilation" generating part (*b*) five possible luminance levels were chosen. The values of these levels were: 1 = 7.5, 2 = 10.0, 3 = 12.5, 4 = 15.0, 5 = 17.5 cd/m². The background level was equal to level 3 in the main experiments. The color of the stimuli was green (color television primary; *x* = .285, *y* = .606).

In principle, 5 × 5 luminance combinations could be presented, but stimuli in which a and b are equal were omitted, so 20 combinations remained. The visual angle of the induced square subtended 2.5°.

Procedure

Both for Experiment 1a and Experiment 1b a pairwise comparison experiment was carried out (see Fig. 17.3 for examples of pairwise presentations). Each stimulus was compared with all others. The stimuli were presented side by side on the screen. This resulted in 20 × 19 = 380 presentations for the subjective contour experiment. In the transparency experiment, all those combinations in which stimulus *a* or stimulus *b* was equal to the background were omitted; this means that superimpositions of opaque squares were not included. Thus (12 × 11 =) 132 pairs remained. These were presented three times each, which resulted in 396 presentations.

Instructions

For Experiment 1a the subject was instructed to choose the stimulus with the sharper subjective contour in each pair; subjects were explicitly told to ignore (induced) brightness differences. For Experiment 1b the instruction turned out to be slightly more problematic. Initially subjects

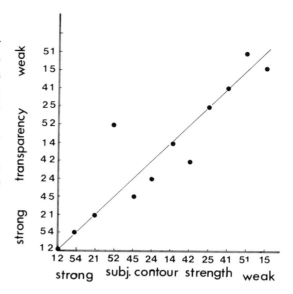

FIGURE 17.4. Rank order of transparency vs. rank order of subjective contours.

were asked to judge transparency, but gradually it turned out to be better to circumscribe the task as follows: choose that stimulus which you think can be best conceived of as being the result of physical superposition of two types of stimuli, either extra light or shadow or superimposition of translucent layers or any combination.

Subjects

Five naive subjects were used in the transparency experiment, six in the subjective contour experiment.

Results

The correlation between judged transparency and subjective contour strength is very high (Spearman's rho = .930, *p* < .001). The results are presented in Figure 17.4.

Experiment 2: Matching of Brightness Differences

An important part of our statement is that the perception of the contour is not necessarily related to the existence of a brightness difference. The prediction is that in those cases where con-

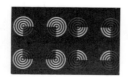 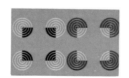

FIGURE 17.3. Examples of the pairwise-presented stimuli for the subjective contour and the transparency comparisons.

trasts of *a* and *b* are reversed there is still a considerable brightness change in the center of the figure, due to contrast and assimilation effects, but there is hardly a perception of a subjective contour.

In order to test, these brightness matches had to be made. The rank order of these brightness induction strengths had to be correlated with the rank order obtained in the subjective contour measurements.

Stimulus

In the stimulus for the brightness match, a square in the right part of the screen could be modified in luminance by the subject until a brightness match was obtained to the central part of the subjective contour figure. Luminances of the *a* and *b* parts of the figure were the same as those in the subjective contour experiment, i.e., 20 combinations of luminance values were presented to the subject. Each combination was presented five times in random order.

Procedure

The subject was asked to fixate at a point between the two squares and to change the luminance of the right square until a brightness match was obtained. The instruction was given not to judge the quality of the contour at all.

Results

The results for two naive subjects are represented in Figure 17.5 and Tables 17.1 and 17.2. The results for positive and negative luminance matchings as compared to the background level are presented separately, and for each of them the rank orders are represented and compared with the rank orders of the subjective contour strengths for corresponding stimuli.

The rank orders are systematically different. The overall rank order correlation is low. Stimuli which have a high score on the matching order, have a lower place in the subjective contour order. The effect is stronger in the case where the luminance of *a* is lower than that of *b*, but it is certainly also present in the reverse case.

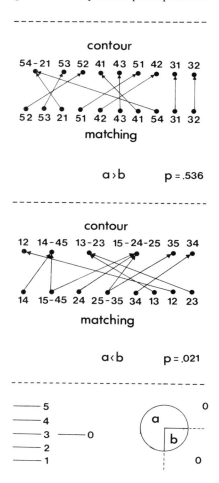

FIGURE 17.5. Rank order of the luminance differences necessary for the match compared with the rank orders obtained in the subjective contour experiment for the same two subjects. Detailed data are presented in Table 17.1.

Summary

Stimuli were used in which only brightness contrasts are manipulated without changes in figural characteristics. Our belief is that assimilation effects and contrast effects are rather simple, probably relatively peripheral effects. The accompanying brightness differences do not necessarily lead to the perception of sharp contours. In the first experiment the strong relationship between subjective contour perception and transparency was reconfirmed. As to the latter, we think that the relationship must be generalized to judged likelihood of a physical superimposition of matter, light, or shadow, or

TABLE 17.1. Luminance differences with respect to the background necessary to obtain brightness matches to the area included by the subjective contour.

Ranking of combinations for subjective contour; $n = 6$

Rank	1	2	3	4	5	6	7	8	9	10		
Combination	12	13	23	53	54	21	45	43	52	14		
Sum	180	167	165	161	149	148	138	136	125	118		
Rank	11	12	13	14	15	16	17	18	19	20		
Combination	24	42	41	25	15	51	35	31	32	34		
Sum	116	100	97	97	92	91	54	54	47	45		

Ranking of combinations for transparency; $n = 5$

Rank	1	2	3	4	5	6	7	8	9	10	11	12
Combination	12	54	21	45	24	42	14	52	25	41	15	51
Sum	311	282	280	244	185	157	153	131	81	64	55	37

Correlation of subjective contour and transparency rank orders

Rank	1	2	3	4	5	6	7	8	9	10	11	12
Contour	12	54	21	45	52	14	24	42	41	25	15	51
Transparency	12	54	21	45	24	42	14	52	25	41	15	51

Spearman's rho $= .930$; $p < .001$.

a combination of these. The second experiment demonstrated that induced brightness differences are not a sufficient condition for the perception of subjective contours.

TABLE 17.2. Brightness matching.

Combination		Subject 1		Subject 2	
a	b	Delta lum.	SD	Delta lum.	SD
1	2	+.35	.045	+.39	.005
1	3	+.39	.081	+.39	.118
1	4	+.86	.180	+.47	.127
1	5	+.64	.241	+.46	.079
2	1	−.56	.096	−.44	.107
2	3	+.33	.064	+.30	.079
2	4	+.71	.253	+.41	.077
2	5	+.54	.105	+.39	.101
3	1	−.34	.130	−.24	.073
3	2	−.25	.102	−.19	.080
3	4	+.39	.082	+.41	.045
3	5	+.36	.142	+.42	.090
4	1	−.49	.125	−.26	.143
4	2	−.56	.143	−.32	.071
4	3	−.49	.088	−.28	.093
4	5	+.45	.118	+.59	.102
5	1	−.79	.337	−.32	.071
5	2	−.83	.139	−.38	.117
5	3	−.75	.147	−.44	.066
5	4	−.23	.055	−.30	.038

These data are supported by previous experimenters. Kanizsa (1979, Figs. 9, 13a & b, pp. 168–169) demonstrated that unless the stimulus configuration was in accord with transparency, a subjective surface was not perceived. Meyer and Senecal (1983), using a chromatic subjective contour, found that strength of the illusory color contour was predicted by the probability of transparency in the various configurations.

Similarly, Smith (1983) tested a subject who, because of brain damage, was unable to interpret interposition in two-dimensional drawings. This individual was unable to perceive transparency-based subjective contours. This supports a finding by Meyer and Dougherty (1986) that flicker-induced depth will eliminate transparent illusory contours even though contrast relationships remain the same.

Although some studies disregard the role of transparency in illusory contour formation in favor of assimilation (Ware, 1980) or contain demonstrations that are incompatible with transparency (Gerbino and Kanizsa, chap. 27), our work that indicates transparency can be a major determinant of illusory contour strength. Brightness differences are not likely to be the sole factor.

CHAPTER 18

The Functional Equivalence of Objective and Illusory Brightness Enhancement

Diane F. Halpern

Illusion is the perceptual rule, not the exception.
—Geldard (1972, p. 144)

The research literature on the processes and mechanisms underlying illusory contour perception has been proliferating in recent years. Yet, what exactly do we know about illusory contour perception, and how much have we learned since Schumann first introduced it in 1900.

An optimist would conclude that we have learned a great deal about illusory contour perception and, by extension, the operating properties of the human visual system. In the overwhelming majority of stimulus displays that give rise to illusory contours, observers perceive a figure that is bounded by the illusory contour as well as illusory brightness and illusory depth. Although these perceptual attributes covary in the majority of illusory contour configurations, none of these is a necessary condition for illusory contour perception (Halpern & Salzman, 1983). Illusory contours can be perceived in three-dimensional displays (Ware & Kennedy, 1977), in the absence of apparent depth (Bachmann, 1978), and even without the perception of brightness differences (Parks, 1980a; Prazdny, 1983; Ware, 1981), an anomalous effect that contradicts the definition of a contour. It even seems that under appropriate conditions, illusory contours remain visible when the physically present portions of the stimulus display are not (Gellatly, 1980; Halpern & Warm, 1980, 1984).

The answer to the question of illusory contours is really quite simple. The answer is, "It all depends!" All we need to do is know what it

depends on, and the phenomenon is explained. One of the most important variables in understanding how and why illusory contours are perceived is the stimulus configuration. Assimilation and dissimilation operate with line end stimuli (Day & Jory, 1978). Large dark inducing areas usually create simultaneous contrast effects, and stimuli that provide monocular depth cues operate, at least in part, via Gestalt and interposition principles. Illusory contours that reliably appear only in peripheral viewing can be explained by appeals to antagonistic properties of receptive fields (e.g., Spillmann, Fuld, & Neumeyer, 1984). It is no longer fruitful to argue over which of these perceptual effects is generative because the answer must depend upon the specifics of the stimulus display, as well as viewing (e.g., size, illumination), retinal locus, measurement, and subject conditions (e.g., set).

Much of the current research is concerned with determining the way selected manipulations, such as the number of inducing elements or stimulus size or level of illumination, affect the various perceptual concomitants of illusory contours. The impetus for most of the research in this field is either to test predictions derived from a particular theory or to explore systematically an anomalous visual effect. The impetus for this study came from thinking about brightness enhancement.

At our college, all faculty received a memo from our physical plant director requesting that we cut back on lighting whenever possible. Humorously, I proposed that we could use illusory brightness enhancement to augment lighting, and then I began to wonder exactly how much brightness enhancement would be perceived under conditions that were known to yield strong brightness effects. Illusory brightness enhancement has been studied in numerous other investigations, but the dependent measure is almost always a magnitude estimate in which illusory brightness is compared to its background or some other modulus or the frequency of a "brighter than" or "darker than" response. While we might never read by the light of illusory contours, how does the brightness enhancement compare in cd/m²?

The purpose of the present study was to compare the illusory brightness enhancement found in strong illusory contours displays with objective brightness enhancement. A double level illusory contour was used in addition to two single illusory contours that varied in size. The double level contour, which I have previously dubbed an illusory tower (Salzman & Halpern, 1982), was included in this research in order to determine the extent to which the illusory brightness of a large illusory figure could alter the brightness properties of a smaller figure centered upon it.

Report of the Research

Twenty female and 20 male students from introductory psychology classes participated for class credit. All subjects had normal or corrected-to-normal vision.

A specially constructed viewing box was employed for stimulus presentation and threshold measurement. It consisted of a black light-tight box which measured about 250 cm long and sat on a table. Subjects were seated in front of the box, and binocularly viewed the stimuli within through an eyepiece centered on the front wall of the box.

The box was divided into a front and back compartment by a partition. Two square windows were cut into the partition. The windows were each rear illuminated with Sylvania Tungsten Halogen lights which provided relatively white light at low illumination levels. The center or outer portion of each window could be independently adjusted for illumination via four dials located on a panel in front of the subject (two on each side, corresponding to the inner and outer portions of the right and left viewing

windows). When subjects turned a dial (calibrated in arbitrary units), a polaroid filter in the rear compartment of the viewing box was rotated relative to a stationary filter. When the filters were 90° opposed, no light from the rear portion of the viewing box was visible to the subject. When the polaroid filters were parallel, maximum rear illumination was transmitted through the windows into the front compartment. In addition, the front portion was illuminated by a Kodak projector, which was concealed from the subject's view. All light sources were adjusted with dimmer switches to preset levels at the start of the experiment.

The 20 subjects were assigned at random to either an experimental or control group. The subjects in the experimental group viewed the three stimulus displays shown in Figure 18.1.

Illusory squares created from four wedge-shaped inducing areas were selected for this investigation of illusory brightness because previous work has shown that this configuration yields extremely strong illusory contours (Halpern, Salzman, Harrison, & Widaman,

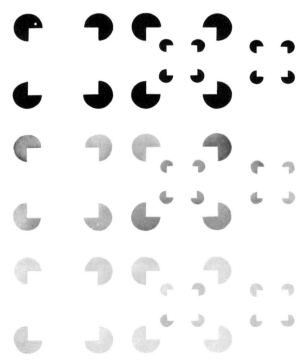

FIGURE 18.1. Large, small, and double-level illusory squares drawn to simulate their appearance under varying conditions of inducing area lumination.

1983), with the illusory figure appearing approximately 68% brighter than its background when measured with magnitude estimation procedures (Halpern, 1981). Subjects in the control group viewed stimuli consisting of the same inducing areas (pie shaped wedges) as in Figure 18.1, but they were rotated so that the inducing areas did not define the edges of an illusory square. Previous research has shown that illusory contours are not perceived in these stimuli. The stimuli were affixed one at a time, according to task demands, to the right-hand viewing window. The first illusory contour display was a large square that subtended a 4°34' visual angle (overall size with inducing areas was 6°18'). The second illusory contour display consisted of a double level illusory contour configuration—a smaller illusory square subtending a 1°9' visual angle (1°43' with inducing areas) centered on the large square. The third illusory contour display consisted of a single small illusory square identical in size to the small square in the double illusory contour display. Bradley and Dumais (1984) reported that illusory figures of this approximate size are optimal for producing strong contours and depth stratification.

With front and rear illumination, the cut portions (inducing areas) appeared black, as in the top row in Figure 18.1. The figures bounded with the illusory contours appeared white and somewhat brighter than their isoluminant background. When a polaroid filter behind the figure was adjusted, the amount of light transmitted from the rear compartment to the subject's eyes through the cutout inducing areas was varied. In this manner, subjects adjusted the luminance of the inducing areas on the right viewing window so that the inducing areas could be made to appear in continuous shades of gray to black. Adjustments of the inner polaroid filter resulted in luminance changes of the small square's inducing fields. Adjustments of the outer polaroid filter affected luminance changes in the large square's inducing fields. Thus, the apparent darkness of the large and small square's inducing areas could be independently manipulated by rotating the appropriate dial.

Brussell, Stober, and Bodinger (1977) have shown that illusory contour clarity varies inversely with inducing field luminance. Thus, by varying the amount of light allowed to pass through the inducing areas, the illusory contours could range from clearly visible to nonexistent. Brussell, Stober, and Bodinger's results were replicated in a preliminary phase of the present study.

Subjects were dark-adapted for 15 minutes at the start of the experiment in a totally darkened room illuminated only with a small lamp for data-recording purposes. They were instructed about the use of the dials to vary luminance and had several practice trials with the apparatus. All measurements were obtained with the method of adjustment and represent the mean of five ascending and five descending trials, with the value of the starting luminance determined at random.

Task 1: Relationship Between Illusory and Objective Brightness Thresholds

This task was designed to investigate the relationship between the just noticeably brighter (jnb) thresholds for objective (i.e., physically real) changes in luminance and jnb thresholds for the illusory brightness enhancement found in illusory contour displays. With the light from the right window extinguished, subjects made the central portion of the left-hand window just noticeably brighter than its background (background was preset to 3.4 cd/m²). All subjects in both groups found this to be an easy task.

The left viewing window was then darkened and for subjects in the experimental group the large illusory square configuration was seen in the right window. Control group subjects viewed a stimulus composed of four wedge-shaped inducing areas that were misaligned. Subjects were instructed to adjust the luminance of the inducing areas until a square partially bounded by the inducing areas appeared jnb than its background. For subjects viewing the illusory contour display, the central square area appeared to brighten (or lighten) as the inducing areas grew darker by appropriate rotation of the dial. In this manner, a threshold value was obtained for each subject that corresponded to sensitivity to illusory brightness differences across homogeneous space. Brightness enhancement of the central square was not perceived for subjects who viewed the control stimulus. Subjects in this group did not seem to understand the instructions as a bright square did not appear when they darkened the inducing areas. Consequently, data analysis was performed only for subjects in the experimental group.

Inducing fields were then set for each subject to that subject's mean jnb adjustment value. Subjects adjusted the background portion of the left window until a phenomenal match was obtained with the background of the subjective figure. Given perceptually identical backgrounds, subjects then adjusted the inner portion of the left window (the circle) until it matched the perceived brightness of the illusory square on the right. Thus, two mean values were computed for each subject. One value was a perceptual match to the illusory figure, the other to its background. Subjects' mean settings for the figure and background corresponded to luminance values of 6.4 and 2.1 cd/m^2, respectively (.806 and .322 log units). These values obtained statistical significance when analyzed with a repeated measures t-test. Thus, the perception of the illusory figure involved an apparent darkening of the background and brightening of the figure across physically identical luminances, suggesting that we should really be calling this phenomenon illusory contrast.

The relationship between objective and illusory brightness enhancement was explored by correlating the jnb settings for objective luminance with jnb settings that matched illusory brightness enhancement for the 20 subjects in the experimental group. The reasoning behind this analysis is that a significant and substantial correlation between these two values would provide support for the notion that brightness disparities created by the human visual system in the absence of brightness gradients have similar psychophysical properties to those dependent on objective changes in brightness gradients. Mean threshold values in both conditions were in arbitrary units obtained from dial settings. These values were closely negatively correlated across subjects, $r = -.94$, $p < .001$. Thus, subjects who required only small increments in physical brightness to perceive a difference also tended to require small decrements in inducing field luminance to perceive enhanced brightness in the illusory square. These

data need to be interpreted cautiously, however, as the present research method does not allow the separation of possible response bias from perception.

Task 2: Comparison of the Small Square in the Double Configuration with the Small Square Alone

The purpose of this task was to compare the perceived brightness of the component squares in the double configuration with their perceived brightness in the single figure displays. Three sets of brightness measures were obtained. In the first set, the double configuration was presented with the inducing areas of the large outer square set to each subject's previously obtained setting in which it appeared just brighter than its background. Subjects were then instructed to manipulate the brightness or darkness of the small square's inducing areas until it appeared just noticeably brighter than its background, which in this case was the large outer square. They then produced brightness matches for both squares on the left-hand window. The second set of measures was also obtained with the double configuration, but for these trials the inducing areas of the large square were set to their maximal darkness—a condition which made the large square appear much brighter than its background. Once again, the subjects manipulated the inducing area luminance of the small square until the figure appeared brighter than its background and matched the perceived brightness of the two squares. In the third set of measurements, the small square was presented alone and subjects manipulated inducing area luminance and produced a perceptual match. The results of these manipulations are shown in Figure 18.2.

Data were analyzed with two separate repeated measures analyses of variance—one for the three levels of the large illusory contour (alone, double and just noticeably brighter than its background, and double and maximally brighter than its background) and one for the corresponding three levels of the small illusory contour. Main effects were significant in both analyses.

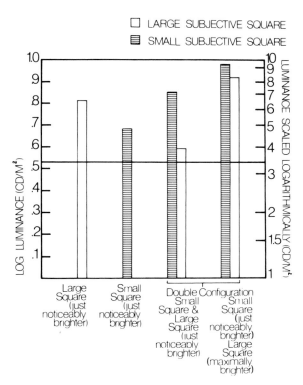

□ LARGE SUBJECTIVE SQUARE
▤ SMALL SUBJECTIVE SQUARE

FIGURE 18.2. Luminance and log luminance (cd/m²) of the large, small, and double-level illusory squares under specified conditions.

uration because the luminance setting for the large square inducing areas was based on each subject's previous response.

The present results demonstrate that, at least under limited and optimal viewing conditions, the illusory brightness enhancement in illusory contour displays is considerable as are illusory contrast effects. If these results are extrapolated to normal room illumination (120 to 130 cd/m²), the amount of enhancement seen in these displays is, on the average, equal to 5% of normal reading illumination, or in other terms, like adding a 10-watt bulb to your usual lighting.

I was recently surprised to find that using illusory brightness enhancement to augment objective brightness is a very old idea. It is found in prayer books that are almost 900 years old and in copies of *Canterbury Tales* that were written in the early and mid 1500s. Writers and scribes at this time in history commonly used a method known as illumination. Many of the fine vellum books had gilt edges and gold leaf decorations on the initial letters in each paragraph. It is important to remember that these books were read under dim illumination, perhaps, literally, one candle per square meter. The gilt edges and gold leaf were good reflectors for the low level of light. When I looked closely at the large decorated letters, known as rubrications, many of the intricate designs and historiated letters contained line end and simultaneous contrast effects. It seems that monks and scribes during the Middle Ages were aware of the possibility of illusory brightness enhancement, and the idea of utilizing this illusory perceptual effect to augment objective luminance is at least several hundred years old.

Discussion

The present results are anomalous in one respect. Previous research has shown that the small square alone should appear reliably brighter than the large square alone, a result that was not obtained in this study. Upon further reflection, however, it seems likely that this result is due to task order effects. Salzman and Halpern (1982) found that when using double configurations or illusory towers similar to the one used in this study, task order is an important variable in determining perceived depth probably because the first task focuses attention on one attribute in the display. It was not possible to randomize task order in the present study. Just noticeably brighter brightness matches for the large square alone had to be made before subjects viewed the double config-

Acknowledgments. The author wishes to thank Dr. Billie Salzman and Mr. Christopher Youngworth for technical assistance and Dr. James Rogers at California State University, San Bernardino, for helpful comments on an earlier draft of this manuscript.

Please send reprint requests to Diane F. Halpern, Undergraduate Studies, California State University, San Bernardino, 5500 University Parkway, San Bernardino, CA 92407.

CHAPTER 19

The Role of Illumination Level in the Strength of Subjective Contours

Joel S. Warm, William N. Dember, Robert A. Padich,
John Beckner, and Scott Jones

A Comparison of Real and Subjective Contours

The Functional Equivalence of Contours

Although they are not physically present in the field of view, subjective or illusory contours are nonetheless psychologically meaningful, and they also share many of the same functional properties of real contours. Geometric illusions and reversible figures can be produced with subjective contours (Bradley & Dumais, 1975; Bradley & Petry, 1977; Gregory, 1972; Meyer & Garges, 1979); these contours can be placed in apparent motion (von Grünau, 1979); they can be enhanced by kinetic depth information (Bradley & Lee, 1982); they can serve as targets or masks in visual masking experiments (Reynolds, 1981; Weisstein, Matthews, & Berbaum, 1974), and they are susceptible to motion, tilt, and color—contingent aftereffects (Meyer & Phillips, 1980; Smith & Over, 1975, 1979). In addition, like real contours, subjective contours can serve as landmarks aiding in the localization of elements in visual space (Pomerantz, Goldberg, Golder, & Tetewsky, 1981).

The Illumination Intensity Effect

While subjective contours have a functional resemblance to real contours under many viewing conditions, there is one condition in which they

This report was completed while Joel S. Warm was a National Research Council Senior Postdoctoral Fellow at the National Institute for Occupational Safety and Health Taft Laboratory, Cincinnati, Ohio.

differ considerably from their objective analogs. That condition involves the amount of light in the visual field. It is well known that visual acuity for real contours, and therefore their clarity or strength, varies directly with illumination intensity (Geldard, 1972). By contrast, Dumais and Bradley (1976) have reported that the strength of subjective contours varies inversely with illumination intensity. In that influential study observers were asked to make magnitude estimates of the strength of a subjective triangle seen in varying illumination, using as the modulus a real triangle seen in dim light. Except when the visual angle of the subjective figure was very small, the apparent strength of the figure increased with a decline in its illumination level. Thus, the strength of a triangle that was not physically present in the visual field improved as the light which bathed it declined.

Dumais and Bradley's (1976) finding has important theoretical implications for an understanding of how the visual system fabricates contours in homogeneous areas of the visual field. One mechanism that has been offered in explanation of the genesis of subjective contours is simultaneous brightness contrast (Frisby & Chatworthy, 1975; Jory & Day, 1979). According to this view, the physically present elements of the display induce the perception of local brightness differences, which spread across areas whose boundaries are defined by the line ends and the points of the inducers. A second proposed account invokes the notion of neural feature detectors. According to this view, subjective contours result from the partial activation of contour-specific cortical units by the physically present edges of the inducing areas (Jung & Spillmann, 1970; Smith &

Over, 1975; 1979; Stadler & Dieker, 1972). Both the amount of contrast produced and the number of feature detectors engaged would be expected to increase with increases in illumination intensity, and therefore the strength of subjective contours should do likewise. Clearly, Dumais and Bradley's (1976) findings do not fit with expectations derived either from a brightness contrast or a feature detector account.

In light of the unusual nature of the Dumais and Bradley finding and its theoretical importance, the effect of illumination intensity on the strength of subjective contours warrants further study. Toward this end, we pursued a methodological issue that Dumais and Bradley did not address, which we call the transitivity issue. The earlier experiment leads to the inference that in a comparison of two subjective contours, one in dim light and the other in bright light, the former would be sharper than the latter. This inference, however, is based upon a comparison of a subjective contour against a real one; Dumais and Bradley provided no direct evidence regarding the relative strength of two subjective contours seen in different illumination levels. The generality of the finding that subjective contours become stronger as illumination decreases would be considerably enhanced if this result could be demonstrated when subjective contours are compared against other subjective contours.

Figure Type

A second issue concerned the type of subjective figure used. Dumais and Bradley (1976) used only the standard Kanizsa triangle (see Fig. 19.1). However, some researchers suggest that mechanisms may differ for line-end subjective contours (Halpern, 1981; Halpern & Salzman,

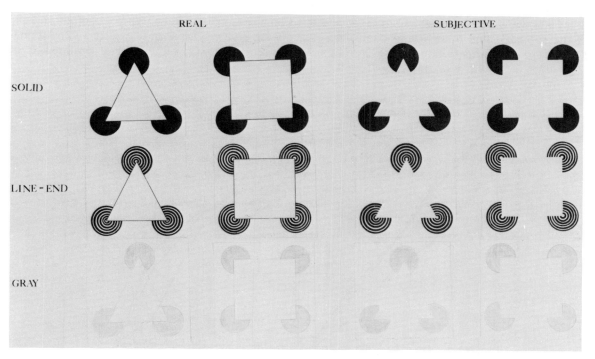

FIGURE 19.1. The stimuli used in the present experiment. Stimuli were constructed by inking black or gray inducing elements, and in the case of real figures, black or gray edges onto white posterboard (82% reflectance). In all figures, the diameter of the inducing areas was 2.5 cm. The reflectance of the black, line-end, and gray inducing areas was 7%, 40%, and 74%, respectively. With both real and subjective contours, the length of the sides of the square figure was 5.0 cm; likewise the altitude and base of the triangle. The stroke width of the physically present edges of the real figures was 0.5 mm. When presented in the viewing box, all stimuli subtended a visual angle of 2.86°.

1983; Parks, 1978; Petry, Harbeck, Conway, & Levey, 1983; Pritchard & Warm, 1983; Richardson, 1979). Accordingly, both figure types were used.

Two Experiments

Experiment 1. Tracking the Effects of Illumination

Twelve sophisticated observers viewed real contours and 12 viewed subjective contours as target luminance varied (4.0, 3.0, 2.0, 1.0, −1.0, −4.0, and −6.0 $\log_e$ cd/m^2). Contour type (real and subjective) was combined factorially within subjects with type of figure (square and triangle) and kind of inducing area (solid black, solid gray, and line end). The gray inducers were employed as a control for the effects of space-averaged luminance.

The stimuli that we employed are displayed in Figure 19.1. They were presented binocularly in a black viewing box. Light sources were out of the subject's line of sight and controlled by Munsell neutral density filters.

On each trial, the subjects were instructed to rate the sharpness and clarity of the sides of the figure that they saw on an 8-point scale ranging from 7, "the sides of the figure appeared to be very sharp and distinct," to 0, "the sides of the figure were indistinct and blended into the background." Exposure time on each trial was 3 sec.

Median ratings of sharpness/clarity were determined in all experimental conditions after appropriate practice trials. As results for the square and triangle figures were identical, we collapsed the data across these figure types.

Means of median category ratings for real and subjective contours are plotted as a function of target luminance in Figure 19.2. The most prominent aspect of the data is that the clarity of both the real and the subjective contours declined as the luminance of the visual field was reduced ($p < .001$).

This effect depended upon the type of contour and the type of inducing area involved ($p < .01$). The nature of the double-order interaction between luminance, type of contour and inducing area can be seen in Figure 19.2. Among the real contours, target clarity declined as a

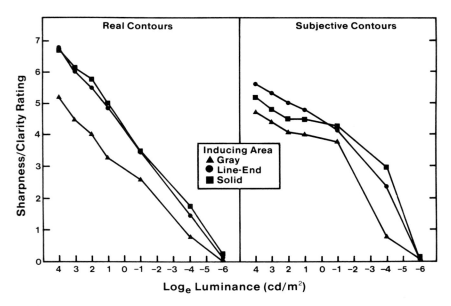

FIGURE 19.2. The perceptual clarity of real and subjective contours as a function of luminance for several inducing area conditions. The order in which each subject experienced the three inducing areas was counterbalanced by means of a Latin Square. The order of appearance of figure types was balanced within the inducing area sequences. Target luminance was varied at random for each subject across trial blocks with the restriction that each value appear once per block.

linear function of luminance. Among the subjective contours, the relation between target clarity and luminance was positively accelerated: the rated clarity of the subjective contours remained relatively stable with changes in luminance at the high levels of stimulus intensity and then declined precipitously when the luminance of the visual field reached its lowest levels. This decline may be occurring at the transition between cone and rod function.

Experiment 2. A Direct Comparison Between Real and Subjective Contours

Still another way to view the complex findings that we have just described is to consider the differences in the relative ratings of real and subjective contours. It is evident in Figure 19.2 that when the luminance of the visual field was high, real contours received higher ratings of sharpness/clarity than did the subjectives. On the other hand, as luminance declined the relative sharpness of the two types of contours reversed, with the point of reversal occurring at different luminance values among the different inducing areas. While it would be tempting to infer that subjective contours may be clearer than real contours in dim light, such an inference would not necessarily be warranted because the two types of contours were not directly compared in our first experiment. Consequently, we carried out a second study to see if subjective contours are indeed sharper than real contours in dim light when subjects are asked to make a direct comparison between the two types of contours.

We secured a second group of 24 sophisticated psychophysical observers. A mixed-factorial design varied figure type (triangle, square) as a between-subjects factor and inducing area (solid black, solid gray, and line-end) and target luminance (4,3,2,1, and -1 $\log_e$ cd/m^2) as within-subjects factors.

The stimuli and apparatus used in this experiment were identical to those of the first experiment. The subjects were instructed that each trial would be composed of two repetitions of a standard and a comparison figure. In all cases, the standard was a real contour and the comparison its subjective analog. On each trial, the subjects were to rate the sharpness/clarity of

the sides of the comparison figure (subjective contour) to those of the standard (real contour) using a 15-point scale that ranged from +7, "the sides of the comparison were much sharper and clearer than the standard," through 0, "the sharpness/clarity of the figures was the same," to -7, "the sides of the comparison figure were much less sharp and clear than those of the standard." The exposure time for each presentation of the standard and comparison figures in each trial was 3 sec each.

Median ratings of differences in sharpness/clarity between the real and subjective contours were determined. The results again led us to combine the square and triangle figures. Means of median difference ratings are plotted for the three types of inducing areas as a function of luminance in Figure 19.3.

Three aspects of the figure are most striking: (1) the relative sharpness/clarity of the subjective contours never exceeded that of the real contours, with all ratings negative; (2) the dif-

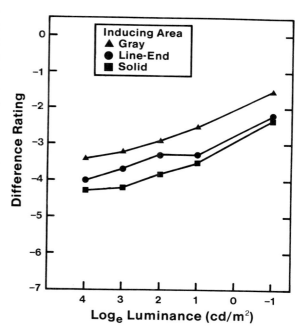

FIGURE 19.3. Differences in clarity between real and subjective contours as a function of luminance for several inducing area conditions. The order in which the subjects experienced the three inducing area conditions was counterbalanced by a Latin Square. Target luminance was varied at random for each subject in each trial block with the restriction that each value appear once per block.

ference between the two types of contours declined as the luminance of the visual field was lowered; (3) the difference in clarity between the subjective and real contours was never so great as to warrant categorization by the lowest value on the rating scale employed.

Statistical analysis of the data of Figure 19.3 revealed that both inducing area and luminance had a significant impact upon the difference ratings ($p < .01$). In order to examine the inducing area effect more fully, supplementary Newman-Keuls tests were performed on the scores for the three inducing area conditions. These tests indicated that the scores for the gray inducing area condition were significantly less negative than those for the other two conditions ($p > .05$), which in turn did not differ significantly from each other ($p < .05$). Thus, the difference in clarity between real and subjective contours was least when the gray inducing areas were used.

At first glance, the results of our second experiment seem to parallel those reported by Dumais and Bradley (1976). When compared against real contours, the clarity of subjective contours improves in dim light. Two factors must be kept in mind, however. Our first experiment indicated that the clarity of both real and subjective contours was poor in dim light, and the gray inducing area condition, where the difference between reals and subjectives was smallest, also produced the weakest figures. Therefore, rather than permitting the inference that subjective contours grow sharper in dim light, our results lead to a simpler conclusion: When real and subjective contours are hard to see, there is less difference between them than there is when they are easy to see.

A Psychophysical Conundrum

Possible Solutions

Contrary to the report by Dumais and Bradley (1976), we have found that the clarity of subjective contours does not improve in dim light. Instead, the perceived sharpness/clarity of the subjective figures in our investigation declined as the luminance of the visual field was lowered. One clue to the disparity in the outcome of the two investigations could come from the

results of our second experiment, in which differences in the clarity of real and subjective contours were minimized in dim light. Recall that in the Dumais and Bradley study, the real figure which served as the standard for magnitude estimates of the subjective figure was also seen in dim light. It is conceivable that instead of judging the strength of the subjective contour per se, Dumais and Bradley's subjects responded to the *relative* difference between the strength of the real and the subjective figure, and as in our case, when the figures were hard to see, the difference between them became smaller. This could have been reflected in the subjects' assigning to the subjective contour a value similar to that of the real contour as the light in the field declined.

Although an argument of this sort is plausible, it is challenged by a recent study in which Bradley and Dumais (1984) used the same methodology as in their earlier investigation to assess the effects of target illumination on the brightness and depth of a subjective figure relative to its background. They found that reductions in target luminance were accompanied by the subjective figure's being seen as increasingly brighter than its background and more stratified in depth. A similar result has also been reported by Parks and Marks (1985). It is unlikely that results on these aspects of the perception of subjective contours would parallel those of contour clarity in dim illumination if the latter were merely a judgment artifact.

Our study varied methodologically from Dumais and Bradley (1976) in several ways. Two of the most obvious differences, however, do not explain the disparity in outcomes. Target sizes were not identical but were in the same range as those in the earlier study which yielded the illumination enhancement effect. Furthermore, while magnitude estimation and category rating procedures are not perfectly equivalent, they usually yield very similar results (Stevens & Galanter, 1957).

In addition to the fact that subjective contours were judged against real contours in the Dumais and Bradley (1976) study but were not in our first experiment, there are other more subtle methodological differences between the two investigations that might be helpful in accounting for their disparate outcomes. For example, it is possible that the perceptual quality being judged (sharpness or clarity in our study; brightness, depth, or salience in Bradley and Dumais) made a difference since Petry et al. (1983) have shown these qualities to vary independently with configurational manipulations (see also Parks & Marks, 1983). Still another potentially important source of difference resides in the richness of the viewing conditions that were afforded subjects in the two experiments. Dumais and Bradley's subjects viewed stimuli in a perceptually rich, open-room environment. Under such conditions, both Dumais and Bradley (1976) and Parks (1986) have suggested that decreases in luminance may diminish the availability of cues that could lead subjects to disconfirm the existence of subjective contours. For example, under lowered illumination, the microstructure of the display to be examined is rendered less visible, and subjects may be less likely to notice the homogeneous textural appearance of the subjective figure and its immediate surround. Such homogeneity could cause the figure to merge with its background and become weaker. Thus, the perceptual salience or "objectness" of the subjective contour may be enhanced in dim light.

In contrast to the perceptually rich environment used by Dumais and Bradley, the apparatus employed in the present study provided subjects with a more limited viewing situation. Indeed, the Gelb effect which occurs under reduced-cue conditions was clearly evident in this apparatus. When the black surface of the box's viewing field was illuminated in the absence of any other stimuli, subjects consistently judged it to be gray or white. Thus, it is possible that the reduced cue situation in our study did not permit subjects to gain disconfirming evidence as to the presence of contours in homogeneous areas of the visual field. As a result the subjective contours remained stable until the illumination reached a level low enough to weaken them.

Whatever the explanation of the disparity between our results and those of Dumais and Bradley (1976), one thing is clear. The psychophysical relation between the amount of light in the visual field and the apparent strength of subjective contours is complex and dependent upon a variety of factors. Along these lines, it is of interest to note the observation by Parks and Marks (1983) that subjective contours with abrupt or sharp edges (such as those used in this investigation and by Dumais and Bradley) decrease in strength with increasing luminance, while those with diffuse edges increase in strength as luminance increases. Moreover, Spillmann, Fuld, and Gerrits (1976) have reported that the Ehrenstein illusion is at least as strong when viewed in a dark-adapted as in a light-adapted state.

While this inconsistent state of affairs is unsettling, it should not be surprising. As noted in a recent review by Parks (1984), there are many gaps in our understanding of subjective figures and many fundamental issues have yet to be resolved. Perhaps one reason for these inconsistencies is a lack of detailed psychophysical analysis in research on the perception of subjective contours. An attempt to provide such an analysis was one impetus for Dumais and Bradley's (1976) early study. Evidently, with regard to the effects of luminance, that analysis is far from complete.

Theoretical Implications

On a theoretical level, our results give some support to a contrast explanation of subjective contours since the gray inducing areas, which had the poorest contrast, also produced the weakest figures. On the other hand, our results also indicate that a contrast approach does not provide a completely satisfactory account of the perception of subjective figures. Because of the absence of physical edges, such figures generate less contrast than do real figures, yet they are more resistant to local luminance changes than are real contours. By the same token, our findings also challenge a feature detector account of the perception of subjective contours. Since such stimuli have fewer lines and angles to activate feature detectors, one would expect them to be less not more resistant to the degrading effects of local luminance changes than their real contour counterparts. As noted earlier, Dumais and Bradley (1976) reached a similar conclusion regarding the merits of the contrast and feature detector views. Thus, we find ourselves in the anomalous situation in which two investigations yielding opposite psychophysical results lead to the same theoretical conclusion.

Contrast and feature detector explanations of

subjective contours can be characterized as data-driven, bottom-up views, in which the perceptual system is considered to begin with raw stimuli and to work upward toward an integrated conceptual structure.

Top-down, or conceptually driven explanations, which begin with a conceptual structure and work toward the identification of a particular stimulus, have also been suggested as explanations for the ability of the perceptual system to fabricate contours in homogeneous areas of the visual field (see Pritchard & Warm, 1983). One such account has been offered by Rock (1983; Rock & Anson, 1979), who maintains that subjective contours represent a solution to a cognitively puzzling stimulus array. According to this view, discontinuities in the inducing areas, such as indentations or line ends, lead the perceptual system to formulate hypotheses as to the type of form most likely to produce them, and the configuration that best fits the stimulus array emerges as the perceived subjective figure; that is, subjective contours reflect an inferential leap by the perceptual system. Some support for this type of explanation comes from demonstrations that perceptual set

can result in subjective contours becoming visible in areas of the visual field where previously they were not (Rock & Anson, 1979) and in subjective surfaces being seen as curved when previously they appeared to be straight (Bradley & Petry, 1977), and by the fact that the perception of subjective contours is more capacity demanding than that of real contours (Pritchard & Warm, 1983).

If subjective contours are indeed less dependent on local stimulation than real contours, they may well be expected to be more resistant to local luminance changes than real contours. Once formed in "the mind's eye," subjective contours can be sustained in the absence of strong physical data (Meyer & Chow, 1984). In support of this notion, we point to the fact that subjective contours have also been found to be more impervious than real contours to local physical changes brought about by adaptation (Halpern & Warm, 1980) and backward masking (Gellatly, 1980) procedures and by the short-circuiting of early stages of information processing produced by dichoptic viewing techniques (Halpern & Warm, 1984; Spillmann, Fuld, & Gerrits, 1976).

CHAPTER 20

Increment Thresholds in Illusory Contour Line Patterns

Maxwell K. Jory

The increment threshold for a small spot of light has been used as a probe to investigate the brightness and physical intensity of stimulus patterns in terms of changes in sensitivity of the visual system. Increment thresholds have been measured in the center of a uniformly illuminated area (Cornsweet & Teller, 1965), near the borders between contrasting areas (Burkhardt, 1966; Fiorentini & Zoli, 1966, 1967; Novak & Sperling, 1963; Van Esen & Novak, 1974; Ward & Tansley, 1974; Wildman, 1974), across regions displaying Mach bands (Novak, 1969; Petry, Hood, & Goodkin, 1973), and across the apparent edge formed by illusory contours (Coren & Theodor, 1977).

The detectability of a small spot of light superimposed on an illuminated background appears to be unrelated to apparent brightness in some stimulus patterns, while in others, unrelated to luminance (Van Esen & Novak, 1974). Cornsweet and Teller (1965) noted that both apparent brightness and the increment threshold of an illuminated disk varied directly with luminance, but the increment threshold did not change when the brightness of the disk was reduced by surrounding it with an annulus of higher luminance. However, Novak (1969) noted that the shift in the increment threshold across a light–dark boundary was related to the brightness distribution near the boundary. It may be the case that Cornsweet and Teller's conclusion that brightness and the increment threshold are unrelated applies only to thresholds measured in the center of a display and does not generalize to spatial locations near an edge. Increment thresholds may reflect border changes in brightness due to lateral inhibition but not brightness changes in extended regions away from borders.

Typically, the increment threshold is elevated at a point on the light side of an edge in comparison to a point slightly away from it (Petry et al., 1973). This increase is thought to represent higher response for those neural elements at the edge due to a reduction of lateral inhibition from neighboring elements in an adjacent area of lower luminance. However, Van Esen and Novak (1974, and also Petry et al., 1973; Novak & Sperling, 1963) reported increased increment thresholds near the edge on the darker side of a light–dark boundary, a region in which greater rather than less lateral inhibition could be expected to occur. Furthermore, Fiorentini and Zoli (1966) reported that the increment threshold was lowest near the border on the light side of a light–dark boundary. In a later study (Fiorentini & Zoli, 1967) using a low-contrast bipartite field it was found that the increment threshold was elevated on the dark side of the edge and lowered on the light side. They argued that the shift in the increment threshold on either side of the boundary could be explained in terms of lateral inhibitory processes. Hence, the increment threshold data appear to be equivocal since both elevated and lowered thresholds on the light side of a border have been attributed to the same lateral inhibitory mechanism. The difference between these studies may, in part, be accounted for in terms of a differential effect of contrast; in some experiments (Novak, 1969; Petry et al., 1973; Van Esen & Novak, 1974) the contrast between field and surround was relatively high, and in others (Fiorentini & Zoli, 1966, 1967) it was low. The significance of this is not clear although Fiorentini and Mazzantini (1966) conclude that 'the mechanisms acting upon the threshold response in the case of an adapting or inducing stimulus of high contrast are probably nonlinear, and may not supply a simple and immediate picture of the elementary excitatory and inhibitory effects in the retina' (p. 747).

Novak (1969) noted the paradox of increment threshold changes near a light–dark border, commenting "that although the perception of a contour is enhanced by an increase of apparent contrast, this process also results in a reduction of detectability near the contour because of increases of increment and decrement thresholds" (p. 1384). This paradox is not in accord with the visual acuity data reported by Day and Jory (1978), who found enhanced visual acuity (1.74) in an area of enhanced contrast, the interspace between two lines lying end to end. To the contrary, the elevation of the increment threshold near an edge might explain the finding that acuity (1.29) is lower for the interspace between two lines lying side by side (Day & Jory, 1978).

It seems reasonable to conclude that increment thresholds are not reliable indicators of changes in apparent brightness in extended regions but do reflect changes in brightness in regions of local contrast activity, near borders between regions of different luminance. Perhaps changes in apparent brightness in these regions occur primarily as a result of lateral inhibitory processes. As Wildman (1974) notes, the threshold elevation on the light side of a light–dark border "represents a real change in visual sensitivity near an edge" (p. 753).

Increment Thresholds in Illusory Contour Patterns

Coren and Theodor (1977) measured increment thresholds on either side of the locus of an illusory contour in a version of the Kanizsa figure. Increment threshold elevation was found in the central region of enhanced brightness, indicating that visual sensitivity in this region is reduced. In Coren and Theodor's study increment thresholds were determined at a point distant (at least 1°) from any contrast-inducing elements, yet changes in the increment thresh-

old were obtained. This is at variance with other studies which found no change in the increment threshold with changes in apparent brightness when the increment spot is displaced more than 10–15′ of arc from the contrasting edge (Novak, 1969; Van Esen & Novak, 1974; Wildman, 1974). The threshold shifts in Coren and Theodor's study occur in extended regions beyond the spatial limits over which lateral inhibiting mechanisms operate. Hence, an explanation in terms of lateral inhibition seems unlikely here.

Often, strong illusory contours occur in line patterns in which the inducing elements are insufficient to generate strong brightness contrast. Increment thresholds hitherto have not been measured in illusory contour-inducing line patterns (end of line contrast) to determine whether lateral inhibitory processes contribute to the strong brightness enhancement and illusory contours thus generated. In the series of experiments to be reported, increment thresholds were measured in a grating pattern broken across the center to form an illusory contour (see Fig. 20.1; see also Kennedy's Mind Line, chap. 28, this volume) and at a number of locations across the Ehrenstein illusion (see Fig. 20.4).

In the first experiment, increment thresholds were measured at both the interspace between line ends and in the neighboring region offset from line ends. It was expected that if lateral inhibitory processes mediate the brightness enhancement effect in this pattern then a shift in the increment threshold would occur near the contrasting elements (line ends) relative to the neighboring region offset from line ends.

Eight subjects made increment threshold judgments for a small spot of light presented at line ends (location A, Fig. 20.1a) or in the gap offset from line ends (location B, Fig. 20.1a). The target spot of light was always presented in the center of the display field (background luminance 5.8 cd/m^2) and the pattern moved to locate it at the appropriate position. Subjects viewed the display through a 3-mm artificial pupil. The target spot subtended a visual angle of 5.2′ and, in location A, was located 2.6′ of arc from the ends of the upper and lower lines. Subjects were initially dark-adapted and then adapted to the stimulus field which was continuously visible throughout the experiment. Pre-

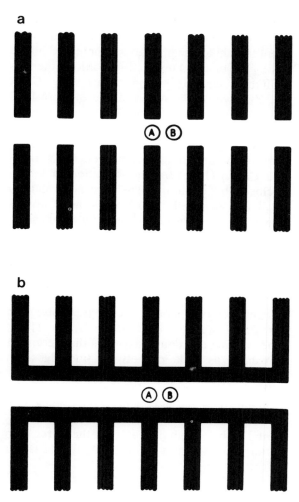

FIGURE 20.1. Illusory contour line pattern a (upper) and control pattern b (lower). In each pattern, increment thresholds were determined at the two target locations—(A) at line ends and (B) in the gap offset from line ends.

sentation of the target spot was initiated by the subject at the direction of the experimenter, and each presentation lasted 1.5 sec. Intensity of the target was varied by rotating a photometric wedge. Increment thresholds were established by adjusting the luminance of the target according to a random double staircase procedure (Cornsweet, 1962).

Mean increment thresholds and standard errors in degrees rotation of the photometric wedge are shown in Figure 20.2. It can be seen that the increment threshold at line ends (A) is significantly lower than in the gap offset from line ends (B), ($t_7 = 3.36$, $p < .02$).

This finding is consistent with the argument that the increment threshold reflects changes in brightness only in regions of local contrast activity due primarily to lateral inhibitory processes. Lower threshold at line ends suggests an increase in visual sensitivity in this region. This finding is of interest since data reported by Day and Jory (1978) showed acuity for fine detail at line ends to be markedly better than between line edges.

Increment thresholds (shown in Fig. 20.3) for the same locations in a control pattern (Fig. 20.1b) were not significantly different. In this pattern the line end contrast effect was eliminated by linking the ends of lines with a contour. The elimination of brightness enhancement at line ends by a connecting contour was first noted by Ehrenstein (1941). The increment threshold data of these two experiments supports the view that line end contrast enhancement is mediated by lateral inhibitory processes. The finding that the increment threshold

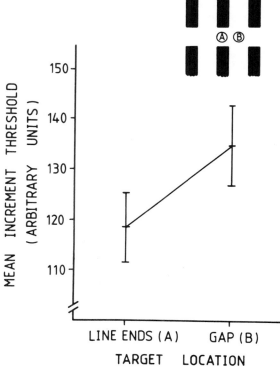

FIGURE 20.2. Mean increment thresholds and standard errors for the two target locations, line ends (A) and the gap offset from line ends (B), in the illusory contour line pattern shown in Figure 20.1a.

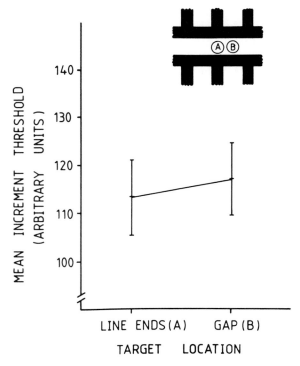

FIGURE 20.3. Mean increment thresholds and standard errors for the two target locations, line ends (A) and the gap offset from line ends (B), in the control pattern shown in Figure 20.1b.

did not change significantly between a line end position and the gap offset from line ends when the lines were linked by a contour is consistent with both the elimination of brightness enhancement in such a figure and the poorer acuity for detail between line edges reported by Day and Jory (1978).

Increment Thresholds in the Ehrenstein Pattern

The third experiment was designed to measure increment thresholds at a number of locations across the Ehrenstein pattern. While the effect of line end contrast significantly lowers the increment threshold relative to an adjacent region offset from line ends, the effect of assimilation of brightness between lines lying side by side (Helson & Joy, 1962; Helson & Rohles, 1959) has not yet been established. Since its effect on brightness is opposite to that at line ends, perhaps its effect on the increment threshold may

also be opposite, i.e., to increase the increment threshold. There is direct evidence that increment thresholds near edges are increased on the light side of the border. In addition, there is indirect evidence to support this view. Craik and Zangwill (1939) reported that the threshold for a small target enclosed between parallel lines was higher than when the target was presented alone (the enclosing contour effect). This phenomenon was confirmed by Youniss and Calvin (1961) for the detection of letters enclosed by contours. The threshold shift in Craik and Zangwill's and Youniss and Calvin's experiments can be explained in terms of assimilation of brightness which produces a suppression of brightness differences between line edges and their interspaces. This explanation is supported by Day and Jory (1978), who reported acuity, or visual sensitivity, for fine detail between two parallel lines to be poorer than for detail defined by line ends. In short, whereas line end contrast lowers the increment threshold, assimilation between line edges can be expected to increase it.

With the same procedure and apparatus, increment threshold judgments were obtained on 10 subjects at 11 target locations along a horizontal path through the center of the Ehrenstein pattern, as shown in Figure 20.4. The 11 target

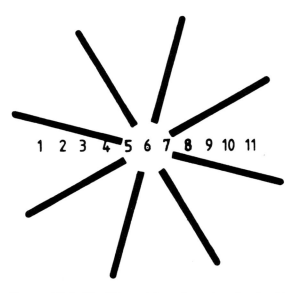

FIGURE 20.4. The Ehrenstein pattern showing the 11 target locations where increment thresholds were measured.

locations were presented in a different random order for each subject.

It was expected that the increment threshold would be low when positioned at line ends (location 6, Fig. 20.4) and high when it was positioned between line sides (locations 1–4 & 8–11). As assimilation has been shown to become progressively weaker with increasingly wider spaces between lines (Helson & Joy, 1962; Helson & Rohles, 1959), it was expected that the increment threshold would be greatest for the narrowest separation of the lines, i.e., immediately adjacent to the illusory contour (locations 4 & 8).

The radiating lines in Figure 20.4 were 5.6' of arc wide terminating on a circle 26' of arc in diameter. The target spot at location 6 was 10' of arc from the ends of all eight radiating lines.

Increment thresholds in degrees rotation of the wedge together with standard errors are shown for the 11 target locations in Figure 20.5. Target location is plotted in degrees of visual

angle from the center of the pattern, with 0° corresponding to location 6 and positive and negative values corresponding to locations on the right and left of the pattern, respectively. It can be seen that the increment threshold is markedly lower for the center position (location 6) in the center of the illusory disk compared to the adjacent locations on either side of the illusory contour locus. A slight increase in the increment threshold can be observed between line edges as the width of the interspace between them decreases. Statistical analysis showed that location 6 differed significantly from locations 5 and 7, $(F(1,9) = 20.27, p < .01)$, but thresholds for locations 1 and 11 did not differ from locations 4 and 8, $(F(1,9) = 2.18, p < .1)$.

In general, the results of this experiment are consistent with the expectation that line end contrast significantly lowers the increment threshold. Although assimilation can be expected to occur between the edges of the radiat-

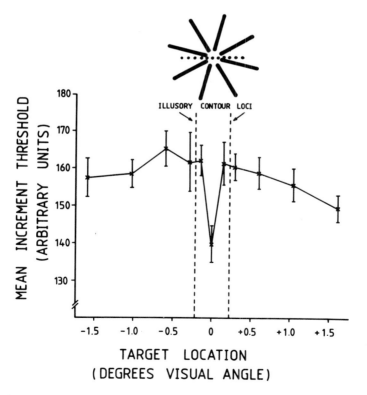

FIGURE 20.5. Mean increment thresholds and standard errors for the 11 target locations across the Ehrenstein pattern shown in Figure 20.4. Target location is plotted in degrees of visual angle from the center of the pattern. The value 0° corresponds to location 6, and positive and negative values to locations on the right and left of the pattern, respectively.

ing lines, no significant increase in increment threshold occurred as the lines converged.

The thresholds for locations 5 and 7 are significantly higher than location 6 yet all three are located within the central region of enhanced brightness. In addition, increment thresholds for locations 4 and 8 on the dark side of the illusory contour are not significantly different from those next to the illusory contour on the bright side (locations 5 and 7). Thus, the shift in the increment threshold does not correspond to the illusory contour locus. This finding is not in accord with Coren and Theodor (1977), who reported a shift in the increment threshold corresponding to the illusory contour locus. However, the results of the present experiment are entirely in accord with the findings of the earlier experiments, and possibly can be accounted for in terms of the spatial limits of lateral inhibitory activity associated with line end contrast.

A Physiological Basis of Illusory Contours?

Novak and Sperling (1963) and Van Esen and Novak (1974) commented that brightness enhancement near border regions fills in extended regions with uniform brightness. Increment threshold changes arise only in regions of local contrast activity which correspond to the spatial limits of lateral inhibitory processes. However, uniform brightness extends well beyond these limits, but the increment threshold remains invariant for a particular luminance level. Osgood (1953) noted earlier that contrast was most prominent about the borders of adjacent areas yet it affects the brightness of entire regions. Van Esen and Novak's (1974) data are in accord with Osgood's (1953) statement that "regions well beyond the distances over which lateral summation and inhibition operate are modified in accordance with what transpires at the borders" (p. 235).

Cornsweet (1970) has argued that brightness is not a simple monotonic function of the intensity of light radiating from an object but depends on factors other than the intensity of light from that region. Areas of equal physical intensity can appear to differ in brightness when they are separated by a narrow graded border, the area on the light side of the border appearing

uniformly lighter and that on the dark side uniformly darker—the Craik–O'Brien effect. The brightnesses of the two regions in this pattern do not correspond to the physical distribution of light as it is the same for both but are affected by the changes in brightness in the narrow region which separates them. Hence the brightness of an area appears to be attributable to key information to brightness in border regions.

Ratliff (1965) suggested that the visual system economizes on the amount of information it transmits by extrapolating information from select points in the visual field so that highly repetitive patterns are treated as though they covered the entire field and any gaps are "filled in." This compressed and abbreviated transmission process means that the visual reconstruction is based on scant but key information. Sekular and Levinson (1977) point out that while this information usually is adequate for veridical perception, illusions may occur as a result of this compression and reconstruction of visual information. It is this notion of visual perception based on key information which has been suggested in one form or another as the probable basis of illusory contours (Kanizsa, 1955a, 1974; Coren, 1972; Gregory, 1972). Kanizsa and Coren have claimed that the key information is incomplete elements and stimuli to depth, respectively, whereas Gregory has argued that it is information about the presence of a masking object. The essential difference between these explanations and the one being proposed is that here it is argued that the key information for illusory contour formation is brightness generated by simultaneous contrast, assimilation, and line end contrast. This view is supported by Spillman, Fuld, and Gerrits (1976), who claimed that in Ehrenstein-type patterns brightness and darkness activity originating from retinal receptive units could, at higher levels of the visual system, spread laterally and fill in brightness or darkness over distances greater than the size of retinal receptive fields. In addition, Frisby and Clatworthy (1975) argued that simultaneous contrast in Kanizsa-type patterns and brightness enhancement at line ends spreads to fill in larger areas.

The increment threshold data reported here support the view that lateral inhibitory mechanisms contribute to the formation of illusory brightness in line patterns. It remains to be seen whether increment thresholds can explain illusory brightness in Kanizsa-type patterns devoid of line elements. With the more or less simultaneous advent of the use of computers in visual perception research and spatial frequency sensitivity analysis and measurement, increment threshold measurement fell out of favor. It provides, however, intriguing and challenging data and thus further theorizing on the relationship between increment threshold, visual sensitivity, and lateral inhibition seems in order.

SECTION V

Time, Motion, and Reaction Time

The chapters in Section V are concerned with the often overlooked temporal properties of illusory-contour perception. Using temporal manipulations of inducers and/or reaction time measures, each chapter presents/describes new data and makes frequently strong theoretical conclusions.

The first chapter in this section, Chapter 21 by Petry and Gannon, presents results of experiments directly measuring the time course and role of apparent motion in illusory-contour formation. They present a somewhat philosophical discussion of illusory contours as prime examples of the necessary object quality of perception.

In Chapter 22, Bradley describes in detail the role of motion in illusory contours. Showing many examples, Bradley discusses the role of

cognition in the organization of stimuli which produce illusory contours.

In Chapter 23, Maguire and Brown review the literature on visual phantoms. They present new data on the phenomenon which ties phantoms to illusory contours.

Chapter 24 by Bruno and Gerbino describes the results of reaction time studies of illusory and real contours. They use these data to discuss the formation of illusory contours from a Gestalt viewpoint.

The final chapter of this section, Chapter 25 by Meyer and Fish, also presents new data on reaction time and illusory contours. Through these data, Meyer and Fish discuss the relationship between illusory contours and preattentive processing.

CHAPTER 21

Time, Motion, and Objectness in Illusory Contours

Susan Petry and Robert Gannon

One of the more fascinating conscious experiences one can have is the abrupt and dramatic change in awareness that takes place when an "ambiguous" stimulus somehow becomes organized into a stable and meaningful configuration. One particularly dramatic example of this can be seen in Gellatly's Figure 29.5 (this volume), and many other lovely original examples may be found in Wade (1976, and chap. 31, this volume). A prime reason for our interest in perceptual organization is a desire to discover what is happening during this organization period. Illusory contours have been treated as almost the Platonic Form of a perceptual organization stimulus. When illusory contours are perceived they are perceived quickly, unlike ambiguous or reversible stimuli which may take seconds or minutes to "become organized." Casual observation suggests that there is a short but finite period of time for the perceptual organization of illusory contours to take place. (See Rock, 1983, for a fuller discussion of this point.) Yet to date little psychophysical data exist concerning temporal parameters of illusory-contour formation.

Microgenesis of Real and Illusory Contours

Percept microgenesis is a visual system operation carried out endlessly during our daily experiences. Clearly, however, the visual system's response to any stimulus does not result in a final percept without some time delay. Ganz (1974) conceptualizes form recognition as being

multiphasic, beginning with a transient phase, in which the visual system generates representations of stimuli, and ending with storage of the representations in a nontransient form. Werner (1935), Werner and Wapner (1952), and Cheatham (1951) first suggested that the perception of any object—specifically real contours—takes a finite time to develop. Using simple metacontrast paradigms they demonstrated that the time taken for development of any percept could be observed. In these studies, the briefest test-mask asynchrony at which no metacontrast is obtained is the encoding time. Results of both these and other more current studies (e.g., Weisstein, 1966) indicate that contours take about 50 msec to be perceived. These results are in accordance with subsequent research which has shown that the time course of lateral inhibition in the human visual system is between 30 msec and 50 msec (Petry, Hood, & Goodkin, 1973.)

In our lab we have been investigating some of the temporal properties of illusory contours. Our interest in this problem is not unique. In fact, while the above studies have provided consistent information concerning the time course of real contour development, the results of studies examining the time course of illusory-contour development have been contradictory and confusing. For instance, though Gellatly (1980) has recently found that inducing element exposures as long as 1000 msec are needed to produce the effect, Spillman, Fuld, and Gerrits (1976) reported that exposures of only a few dozen msec were adequate. Parks (1983) points out that the latter results should not be taken as strong evidence that illusory contours develop this quickly, rather that they may be established later on the basis of an iconic sensory trace of the pattern.

Reynolds (1976, 1981) provided evidence that Parks's interpretation of Spillman's results is correct. Using a masking procedure in which a normally adequate 50 msec presentation of inducing elements was followed by a mask, Reynolds found that with long delays of the mask, illusory-contour formation was not inhibited. However, with mask delays of less than 50 msec illusory contours were not perceived. Reynolds suggests from his observations that illusory-contour microgenesis requires a minimum of about 150 msec.

Von Grünau (1979), looking at apparent motion of illusory contours, has shown that "long exposure times were necessary before illusory contours could contribute to stroboscopic motion . . ." (p. 208). Moreover, Meyer & Chow (1984) have found that illusory contours show longer persistence times than control figures. It may be the case that these differences are due to a two-stage process of development of illusory contours (i.e., illusory contours develop only as a result of and hence after real contours). However, in an influential paper, Ginsburg (1975, see also chap. 13, this volume) hypothesized that illusory contours are the result of responses by a low-spatial frequency sensitive system (transient system). Physiologically, such cells are known to be highly sensitive to temporal manipulations (while being relatively insensitive to spatial manipulations). The differences in time course between real and illusory contours found in the studies cited above suggest that the transient system contribution to illusory and real contour processing may differ. Thus, direct tests of the sensitivity of illusory contours to temporal manipulations would be valuable.

Some Data

Experiment 1. Duration

The first question we considered was the change in illusory-contour strength as a function of stimulus duration, since despite the stud-

ies cited above, results of this basic manipulation have never been reported.

We were interested both in the time course of the growth functions and the possible existence of temporal brightness enhancement effects as a function of stimulus duration. It is well known that real contours (luminance step functions) vary in brightness as a function of duration and typically show enhanced brightness at intermediate (75–150 msec) durations. Known usually as the Broca–Sulzer effect, the phenomenon is often analyzed as the result of differential time courses of excitatory and inhibitory components of the visual response. Under some conditions defocused real contours do not show brightness enhancement (Bobak, Reichert, & Petry, 1978; Kitterle & Corwin, 1917; and by inference Higgins & Knoblauch, 1977; but see Bowen & Pokorny, 1978). We (Petry, Harbeck, Conway, & Levey, 1983) and others have evidence to suggest that enhanced brightness and clarity of illusory contours are semiindependent of qualities. Since sharpness or clarity of illusory contours is almost never as great as of real contours, it is possible that illusory contours behave more like blurred than sharp real contours.

In separate sessions we asked subjects to rate brightness and sharpness of real and Ehrenstein configuration illusory contours as a function of stimulus duration. Stimuli are shown in Figure 21.1. Illusory-contour stimuli varied in the number of inducing elements (IEs) and in the contrast of the inducing elements, (the degraded stimuli give rise to bright but blurred illusory contours (Kennedy, 1976a). In separate sessions, seven observers made magnitude estimates of (1) the perceived brightness of the area subsumed by the real and illusory borders relative to the background field, and (2) the perceived sharpness or distinctiveness of the real and illusory edges relative to a continuously present real edge.

Figure 21.2 shows mean brightness and sharpness judgments as a function of duration for all stimuli. For clarity we have plotted 8 IE, 16 IE, and 32 IE subjective contour data together, and 8 IE degraded and 16 IE degraded also together. No significant differences between these subconditions were found.

Real contour sharpness increased gradually

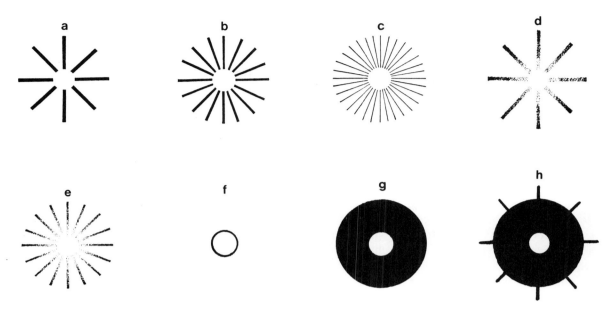

FIGURE 21.1. Stimuli used in Experiments 1 through 3: subjective contours (a, b, c), degraded subjective contours (d, e), and three real-contour control figures (f, g, h).

with duration, while illusory-contour sharpness increased slightly with duration, leveling off at a duration of 300–360 msec. Illusory-contour sharpness was never as great as real-contour sharpness, nor did it change appreciably with changes in stimulus duration.

The perceived brightness of the control stim-

uli varies as an inverted U-shaped function of duration (classic temporal brightness enhancement) with a peak at about 200 msec. Even though the stimuli are less distinct, the illusory contours are also responded to in a way which shows brightness enhancement. However, maximum enhancement is *always* at longer du-

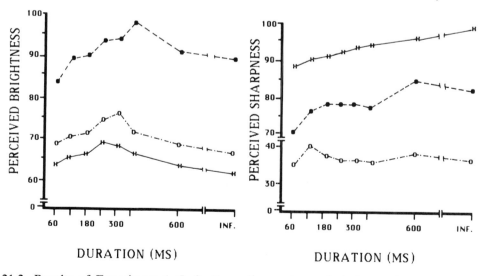

FIGURE 21.2. Results of Experiment 1. Left: Perceived brightness of subjective contours. Right: Sharpness of subjective contours. ●—●—●— = subjective contours; ○-··-○-··-○ = degraded subjec- tive contours; ⊩—⊣⊢—⊣ = real-contour control figures all as a function of stimulus duration. Infinity = 4 seconds.

rations (300–360 msec). While the increase in perceived brightness with duration is greater for illusory than real contours the subsequent decline in brightness, usually thought to be due to inhibition, is at best comparable to real contours.

These results imply that (1) brightness and sharpness are semiindependent functions of temporal manipulations, and (2) illusory-contour brightness changes more slowly than real contour brightness.

Thus it may be inferred that illusory contours have a longer "time to develop" than real contours. This is not surprising. Illusory contours are perceived only in situations in which inducing elements or edge cues (Day, chap. 5, this volume) are present. These inducing elements or edge cues (real contours) require processing time which is probably prior to and independent of the illusory contours which they induce. While lateral inhibition mediates real-contour perception, the research cited above shows that it is not sufficient for explaining illusory-contour development. Nor is it necessarily surprising that Bruno and Gerbino (chap. 24, this volume) found no difference in reaction time between real and illusory contours. Similar dif-

ferences are well known in the masking literature (cf. Fehrer & Raab, 1962).

Experiment 2. Interruption

In a second experiment we measured the effects of a brief interruption of the inducing elements on illusory-contour brightness and clarity. A trial consisted of presentation of a stimulus interrupted for 60 msec during midpresentation (X msec ON—60 msec OFF—X msec ON) preceded or followed by the same stimulus continuously ON for a period of time equal to the ON time of the interrupted stimulus. Sequence was randomized, and a two-alternative forced-choice paradigm was used in which observers were instructed to indicate which stimulus presentation was brighter/sharper: the uninterrupted or the interrupted stimulus. Ten comparisons of both brightness and sharpness of all stimulus pairs were made by all observers.

Plotted in Figure 21.3 as a function of stimulus duration are the mean percentage of trials during which the uninterrupted stimulus was judged brighter or sharper. The area defined by the illusory edges was relatively unaffected by interruption, especially of short durations.

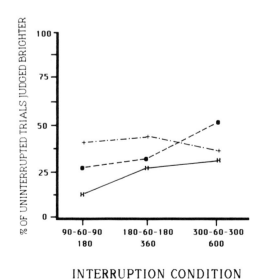
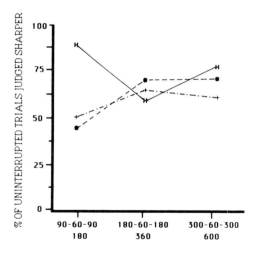

FIGURE 21.3. Results of Experiment 2. The percentage of trials during which the uninterrupted (continuous) presentation of each stimulus was judged brighter (left) and sharper (right) than the interrupted (on-off-on) presentation. Stimulus durations (inter-rupted vs. continuous) are shown along the x-axis. ●-----● = subjective contours; +-··-+-··-+ = degraded subjective contours; ‖———‖ = real-contour control figures.

Again, as was shown above, the sharpness judgments show that illusory borders approach real-border sharpness at longer durations. However, again, they are never judged to be as sharp.

Experiment 3. Apparent Motion

In a third experiment we looked at the influence of another basic temporal manipulation: inducing-element flicker and apparent motion. We and others have shown that the hypothesized response of a transient (low spatial frequency) system is enhanced when the stimulus is flickered briefly (cf. Kitterle & Beard, 1983; Petry, Grigonis, & Reichert, 1979). In addition to being flickered, the inducing elements in two of the conditions were displaced spatially as well. Depending on the time cycle used, these manipulations produced either weak or strong apparent motion of the inducing elements.

In this experiment, subjects and procedure were identical to the first experiment. Five stimuli were used (a, b, d, e, and h in Fig. 21.1) and the control stimulus (h) was modified by the addition of line segments, similar to inducing elements, protruding from its outer edge. This modification allowed us to easily produce apparent motion of a real contour. Five temporal conditions, as shown in Figure 21.4, were used. The "rotate" condition produced weak apparent motion, while the "flicker/rotate" produced strong apparent motion of the inducing elements.

Figure 21.5 presents the results of this experiment. In general, both real- and illusory-contour brightness and to a lesser extent sharpness were enhanced by stationary flicker despite its lower effective stimulus duration. This is probably analogous to the Brücke effect, the flicker equivalent of brightness enhancement. Apparent motion, on the other hand, greatly enhanced subjective-contour brightness while reducing real-contour brightness. Real-contour sharpness was unaffected by apparent motion while illusory-contour sharpness under the apparent motion condition was so great as to be indistinguishable from real-contour sharpness. Note again that in all previous experiments and conditions illusory-contour sharpness had been significantly lower than real-contour sharpness.

The results of Experiments 2 and 3 indicate

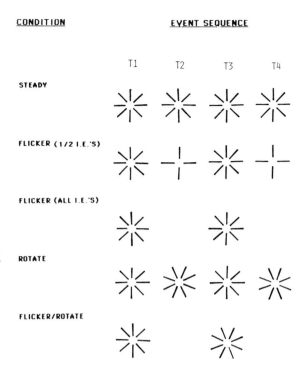

FIGURE 21.4. Sequence of stimulus events (T1 through T4) that occurred during the various temporal manifestations in Experiment 2. Sequence was identical for all stimuli.

that real contours are more enhanced by both stimulus interruption and flicker than are illusory contours. However, illusory contours are even more enhanced by temporal manipulations which produce apparent motion in the inducing elements. Real and illusory contours are both enhanced in brightness by flicker; however, while apparent motion diminishes real-contour brightness (perhaps because real contour is perceived as ground) this manipulation greatly enhances illusory-contour brightness. Based on our present characterization or understanding of peripheral physiological mechanisms in vision, the fact that illusory contour brightness is enhanced both with intermediate stimulus durations and with apparent motion of the inducing element, implicates a mechanism involving low spatial frequency detectors (i.e., a transient system).

However, the peak of the Broca-Sulzer function for illusory contours is at considerably longer durations than for reals. This and the fact

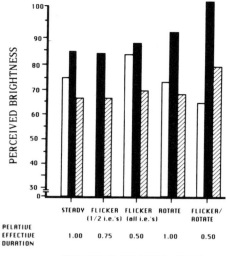

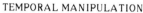

FIGURE 21.5. Results of Experiment 3. Perceived brightness (left) and sharpness (right) of subjective contours (black areas), degraded subjective contours (hatched areas), and real-contour control figures (white areas) as a function of temporal manipulations. Relative effective stimulus duration is shown under the x-axis.

that only illusory- and not real-contour brightness is enhanced by apparent motion imply that the physiological mechanisms involved are not necessarily simple and that *perceptual qualities of the stimuli are also relevant*. Manipulations which enhance the objectlike quality of illusory contours enhance *both* brightness and sharpness—especially sharpness. In fact, illusory- and real-contour sharpness are indistinguishable under apparent motion conditions.

General Discussion

Illusory contours have been used as the archetype for, and intuitive proof of several models of the perceptual organization process. Conversely, there are several theories which have been generated to account for illusory contours. Debate surrounding the role of basic neurological mechanisms, peripheral and central locus of processing, and the role of higher order cognitive variables continues. Much of our fascination with illusory contours is due to their intriguing properties: the bicamerality of their perception (Kennedy, Day, Rock, Gregory, all in this volume); the influence of factors such as set (Coren, this volume) and attention (Meyer

& Phillips, 1980) on their appearance and aftereffect; their role in transparency (de Weert, this volume) and magnification and capture (Ramachandran, this volume); and their perhaps counterintuitive sensitivity to small changes in stimulus parameters.

The striking feature of this field, however, despite the huge number of articles on the topic, is the lack of a body of parametric data on the phenomenon. We know very little about the systematic influence on subjective contour strength of such basic parameters of the inducing elements as size, intensity, contrast, hue, configuration, duration, flicker, etc., and almost nothing about their interactions. This is quite unlike the case for basic visual phenomena such as color, brightness, masking, edge, and motion perception. Without this data base, experiments tend to be hypothesis testing or even hypothesis confirming in nature. Thus, there are a plethora of theories which tend not to refer to the same sets of data—or only in the most superficial way. This is not a scientifically progressive situation (Greenwald, Pratkanis, Leippe, & Baumgardner, 1986), and the need for more parametric data on subjective contours is, we believe, very great. With this in mind, we proceed to our own speculations.

Speculations

The visual system (and of course, other sensory systems) is designed to detect change. When a stimulus (real or contrived) is homogeneous either spatially or temporally it is after a short period of time not present in our perceptual experience. Moreover, to be detected or experienced the change in stimulation must be abrupt not gradual. Abruptness is obviously relative to the spatiotemporal domain of the visual (sensory) system (e.g., receptor density, neural conduction speed, etc.). Thus, while we can immediately perceive the movement of the second hand on a watch we are not able to perceive the movements of the minute or hour hands. Students point out that this is particularly true during a boring lecture.

Now, it is reasonable to ask how this detection of change is experienced by us. We experience the external physical variables to which we are sensitive in terms of a certain perceptual form or quality (Kelley, 1986). It may be helpful to think of the doctrine of specific nerve energies in this context. For example, we are sensitive to changes in light wavelength within a certain range. The form or perceptual quality by which wavelength is experienced we call *hue*. Thus, hue is neither an intrinsic quality, contained within the physical entity, nor is it subjective, created by the organism. Rather, it refers to the experiential result of an objective relationship.

The apple sitting on the table is perceived to be red. This perception is the result of the capacities and limitations of the visual system with respect to wavelength sensitivity as well as the ambient lighting and surround conditions. The apple will look more or less red as influenced by the external and perhaps even our own internal context; however, the hue quality per se is inherent in the experience and provides a perceptual description of the entity in context.

On the basis of this formulation we would like to propose that we, as perceiving organisms, are primarily "object extractors." That is, the fundamental or primary form (perceptual quality) in which we experience the world is that of "objectness." Thus, it is not just the case that our visual system is designed to extract information about external entities. Rather, the visual system conveys information about the external world in the perceptual form of *objectness*. Objects, or objectness, is the natural, primary, and fundamental quality by which we experience reality. Our perception is not *of* objects it *is* objects. Thus, is it not surprising that we see illusory "contours" (or objects). What would be surprising, on this view, is if we did *not* see them. In this respect we argue against some cognitive accounts of illusory contours. The illusory contour is no more "added" to the percept than hue would be in the preceding example.

Illusory contours are not the only example of this *objectness* view of perception. In addition, ambiguous stimuli, reversible figures, and other multistable percepts are experienced as objects in all their perceived states. That is, although ambiguous, they are seldom if ever perceived as isolated elements. The work done on stabilized images also suggests that objectness is preserved under these conditions. Our visual system is designed to extract and process information, and to convey it in terms of (in the form of) objects with associated attributes. Our perceptual world is filled with two-dimensional objects. Pictures, numbers, words are ecologically neither rare nor artificial. The meaning and functional importance of such arrays derive from the *objectness* quality of perception.

Objectness may be considered, therefore, to be a necessary part of the perceptual experience. In fact, it seems to be the case that when objects are not present in perception (e.g., ganzfeld, spinning around, sensory deprivation) the experience has a decidedly strange quality and hallucinations may result.

This characterization of perception in general and illusory contours in particular, we believe, leaves open questions such as the roles of peripheral physiological mechanisms, hypothesis-testing procedures, learning and experience. Indeed, it may be possible that what we would think of as different types of processing may be occurring conjointly.

Our own work, presented above, indicates that temporal changes in the inducing elements produce large changes in the saliency of illusory contours. Thus, physiological mechanisms sensitive to temporal manipulations, i.e., a low spatial frequency system, are strongly implicated in illusory-contour formation. The data also imply, however, that the relatively simple low spatial frequency (transient) peripheral system discussed by Ginsburg (1975 & chap. 13, this volume) is insufficient.

The properties that characterize perceptual *objectness* are the features of the environment, the physical characteristics of entities, to which we are maximally sensitive. Our thinking, we believe, is similar to that of Ross Day's and influenced by it. In particular, these properties include the presence of a more or less distinct border or edge, a surface quality distinct from its background, and a location and separation between the object and its background (depth relation). Any manipulation which enhances the object/cues or features of the stimulus, e.g., apparent motion, will greatly enhance the saliency of illusory contours. This would lead us to conclude that certain types of temporal change, movement, or events are also attributes of the perceptual quality of *objectness* (see Prazdny, 1985).

Indeed, one might speculate that the reason that normally illusory contours and possibly other two-dimensional arrays are simultaneously seen and judged to be unreal (Kennedy, Day, Gregory, this volume) is that not all the attributes of *objectness*, in particular motion, are present.

It is only through generation of more parametric data that we can determine the environmental cues for surfaces, location, and edges that give rise to object perception.

CHAPTER 22

Cognitive Contours and Perceptual Organization

Drake R. Bradley

Contours perceived in the absence of a corresponding gradient in physical stimulation have been variously called subjective, illusory, virtual, and cognitive contours. For some time now, my students and I have been conducting quantitative and qualitative investigations of this phenomenon. While this chapter will focus on the effects of perceptual organization on subjective-contour perception, I would like to first briefly summarize our quantitative research in this general area.

As far as I know, Susan Dumais and I were the first to employ magnitude estimation as a method for assessing subjective-contour strength relative to a real-contour modulus. Using this method, we reported some time ago that decreasing the level of illumination produces dramatic increases in the strength of subjective contours (Dumais & Bradley, 1976), and this finding was later replicated with a larger sample (Bradley & Hirsch, 1987; see Parks & Marks, 1983, for an independent replication). More recently, we have reported that decreasing the level of illumination also increases the apparent separation in depth between a subjective-contour object and its background (Bradley & Dumais, 1984). These studies have also demonstrated that the strength (Dumais & Bradley, 1976) and depth separation (Bradley & Dumais, 1984) of subjective contours rapidly diminish with increases in visual angle, as manipulated by varying the size and/or distance of the figure. In research investigating the effects of eye movements, we found that observers instructed to fixate the center of the pattern experience much weaker subjective contours than those instructed to scan along the contours, across the

contours, or to freely view the display (Bradley & Pennella, 1987). Prolonged fixation also results in a steady drop in contour strength over trials, a decrement which is not found in the three conditions requiring eye movements. Finally, in research investigating individual differences, we failed to find any relationship between field dependence/independence and subjective-contour perception (Bradley & Hirsch, 1987). Although field independents did perceive somewhat stronger illusory contours, and showed larger effects due to changes in illumination level, these trends were not statistically reliable.

The research reviewed above attempted to quantify the effects of illumination level, retinal size, eye movements, and cognitive style on subjective contours. However, an equally important segment of our research has addressed the role of perceptual organization in the perception of illusory contours. Consider, for example, the map of western Long Island shown in Figure 22.1. This map was provided to the participants and guests attending the International Conference on Illusory Contours, which met at Adelphi University in November 1985. As I used it to negotiate my way from eastern Long Island (having taken the ferry to Orient Point) to the general vicinity of the conference, I remained oblivious to the subjective-contour figure cleverly embedded in the map. Perhaps it was the late hour and the fact that my wife, 10-month-old daughter, and I had been on the road for 12 hours, or perhaps my mind was simply preoccupied with the presentation I would be making the following evening. Whatever the reason, as I studied the map in greater detail I

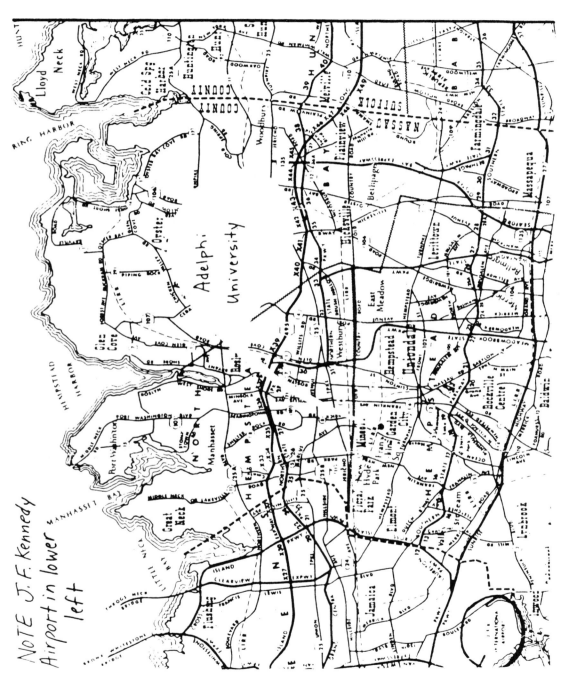

FIGURE 22.1. Map of western Long Island illustrating the effects of perceptual organization on illusory contours. A subjective contour "balloon" enclosing the name of Adelphi University points to its location in Garden City. This map was prepared by Robert Gannon of Adelphi University.

found myself amazed at the size of the Adelphi campus, seeming as it did to cover a huge chunk of the Oyster Bay section of Long Island. Nor could I fathom how major turnpikes and other roads could come to such an abrupt terminus at the "edge" of the campus. After pondering this incongruity for a moment, I experienced a sudden reorganization of the perceptual field and saw (plain as day now) the balloon enclosing the name of the university and "pointing" to its location in Garden City. The balloon, of course, is bounded by illusory contours, and provides a kind of visual pun for those of us searching for a conference on illusory contours. I was torn between feeling dense for not seeing the illusory figure sooner, and feeling thankful that providence had provided such a timely and relevant anecdote for the introduction of my paper.

My experience with the map in Figure 22.1 demonstrates the obvious but frequently overlooked fact that perceiving subjective contours reflects the selection of one of at least two possible organizations of the display: i.e., the one in which subjective contours are seen as opposed to the one in which they are not. All subjective contour patterns are ambiguous in this minimal sense. For instance, in Figure 22.2a we can see a subjective triangle superimposed on three black disks, or three pacman characters having a conversation at the International Conference on Nonillusory Contours. When naive observers are shown this pattern, about 28% do not see the subjective contours initially. We have found that these same people fail to perceive the usual center–surround brightness difference, whereas those seeing the subjective contours almost always perceive the center as brighter than the surround (Bradley & Mates, 1985). This finding suggests that the brightness effect commonly reported for subjective-contour displays requires an appropriate perceptual organization for its expression. In support of this view, we have developed a variety of subjective-contour figures in which several alternative organizations are possible. In these displays, the apparent locations of the subjective contours and the associated brightness gradients vary from one organization to the next.

To illustrate, consider Figure 22.2b which presents the first ambiguous subjective-contour figure "discovered" in our laboratory. Here, Susan Dumais and I were simply trying to produce a square subjective-contour figure to accompany the triangle of Figure 22.2a. For some fortuitous reason we elected to use square rather than circular inducing elements. This

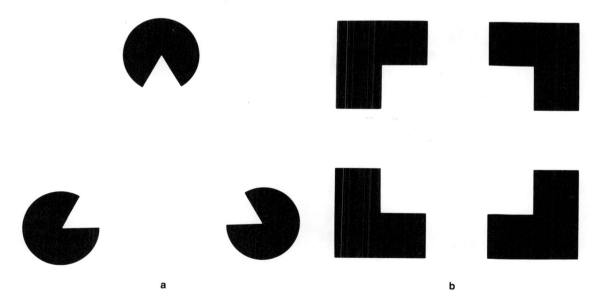

a   b

FIGURE 22.2. a. A modified Kanizsa triangle in which roughly 28% of observers initially fail to see the illusory contours of the triangle. b. An example of an ambiguous subjective contour figure, the Swiss cross configuration.

seemingly innocuous decision was critical: if we had used circular inducers the resulting figure would not have had the variety of alternative organizations that turned out to be possible. The first and most obvious organization of Figure 22.2b consists of a white square superimposed on four smaller black squares, as depicted in Figure 22.3a. However, it is also possible to see a Swiss cross superimposed on a black square border (or picture frame) that runs underneath each arm of the cross, as shown in Figure 22.3b. In both of these organizations illusory contours are seen in the locations delineated in Figures 22.3a and 22.3b, and the square and cross seem somewhat brighter than the background. Another and more difficult organization of Figure 22.2b consists of a white square rotated 45° from the vertical, as shown in Figure 22.3c. The corners of the square located between the inducing elements appear somewhat rounded and indistinct. In addition, the square appears slightly darker than the surround, just the reverse of the usual finding. Figure 22.3d

presents yet another organization of Figure 22.2b. In all the examples given, the locations of the contours and the associated brightness gradients depend on the prevailing organization of the figure.

We discovered a second ambiguous pattern while investigating binocular rivalry in subjective-contour figures (Bradley, 1982; Bradley & Dumais, 1975). While viewing an upright and inverted subjective triangle in the left and right channels of a stereoscope, we expected to see the intersecting illusory contours rival and show contralateral suppression in the manner of real contours (Fig. 22.4a, top and bottom panels). Instead, the two triangles fused to produce a six-pointed star in which the interior angles were formed by blending selected portions of the subjective contours originating from each channel of the stereoscope (Fig. 22.4b). We soon found that this star was perceptually ambiguous, regardless or whether it was produced through dichoptic presentation of two triangles or presented as a monocular stimulus. In addi-

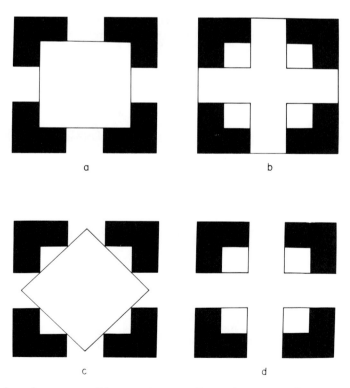

FIGURE 22.3. Examples of some possible organizations of illusory contours in the Swiss cross configuration of Figure 22.2b. a. A square. b. Swiss cross. c. Rotated square or diamond. d. A set of small white squares superimposed on larger black squares.

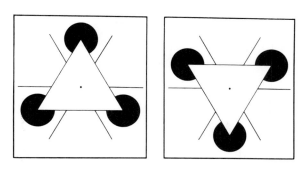

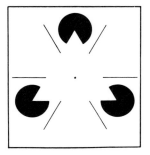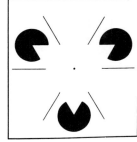

a

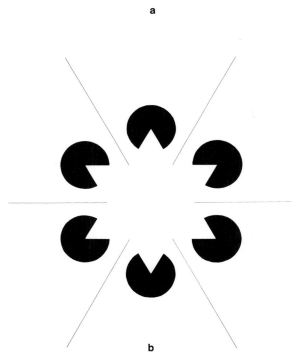

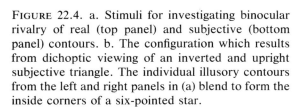

b

tion to the star, it is possible to see an upright triangle superimposed on an inverted triangle (Fig. 22.5a), or an inverted triangle superimposed on an upright triangle (Fig. 22.5b). It is also possible to see a bow-tie (Fig. 22.5c) or a diamond (Fig. 22.5d) organization of subjective contours in the pattern. Note that each of these organizations is associated with a uniquely defined set of illusory contours and brightness gradients, all or which originate from the same physical pattern.

Another good example of an ambiguous subjective-contour figure is provided by the ship's wheel configuration shown in Figure 22.6a (Bradley & Dumais, 1975). This pattern can be seen as consisting of three separate objects: +, x, and o. Since the stratification in depth of these objects is ambiguous, any one of them can be seen in the top (i.e., closest), middle, or bottom positions, thereby providing a total of six permutations of illusory contours. Depending

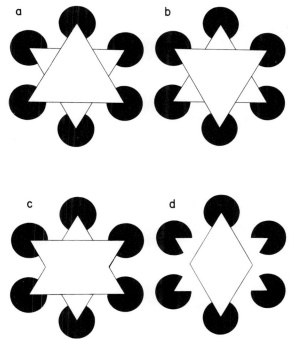

FIGURE 22.4. a. Stimuli for investigating binocular rivalry of real (top panel) and subjective (bottom panel) contours. b. The configuration which results from dichoptic viewing of an inverted and upright subjective triangle. The individual illusory contours from the left and right panels in (a) blend to form the inside corners of a six-pointed star.

FIGURE 22.5. Some possible organizations of illusory contours in Figure 22.4b in addition to those forming the inside corners of a six-pointed star: a. An upright triangle superimposed on an inverted triangle. b. An inverted triangle superimposed on an upright triangle. c. A bowtie organization. d. A diamond organization.

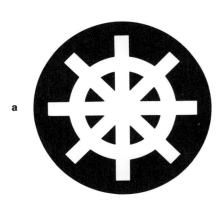
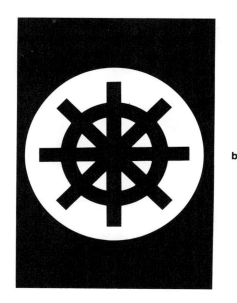

FIGURE 22.6. A positive (a) and negative (b) photographic reproduction of the ship's wheel, another ambiguous subjective-contour configuration.

on the prevailing organization, straight subjective contours bounding the arms of the + or x can be seen extending over the o, or curved subjective contours bounding the o can be seen extending over the arms of the + or x (see Fig. 22.7). Yet another organization of this figure corresponds to a ship's wheel, and since this organization does not involve the stratification in depth of separate objects, no subjective contours are seen. Finally, in both the star and ship's wheel configurations, those objects perceived on top appear somewhat brighter than those on bottom, and the brightness gradients delineating the illusory contours of overlaying objects are redistributed as the figure undergoes spontaneous reversals. Of course, in a negative photographic reproduction, such as the ship's wheel shown in Figure 22.6b, the brightness relations are reversed: objects perceived on top appear somewhat darker than those on bottom.

Another quite striking ambiguous pattern developed in our lab by Heywood Petry is the subjective Necker cube shown in Figure 22.8a (Bradley, Dumais, & Petry, 1976; Bradley & Petry, 1977). Most observers have no difficulty perceiving subjective contours connecting the corners of a phenomenally complete cube superimposed on eight black disks (Fig. 22.9b).

However, it is considerably more difficult to see one of the alternative organizations of this figure: i.e., that of a white cube suspended in a dark enclosure and viewed through the eight holes of an intervening surface (Fig. 22.9c). In this latter case, the black inducing elements are seen as holes rather than disks, and curved subjective contours can be seen demarcating the interior edges of the holes. (Fig. 22.9d illustrates an organization having a blend of the previous two.) Most observers report that the cube-in-back appears substantially brighter than the cube-in-front (Bradley & Petry, 1977). This may be due to a constancy scaling mechanism which compensates for the lower level of illumination assumed to be incident on the cube-in-back (see Coren & Komoda, 1973, and Hochberg & Beck, 1954, for similar effects and interpretation). These effects are also observed with the negative photographic reproduction shown in Figure 22.8b, except that the cube-in-back now appears darker than the cube-in-front, as again would be predicted from a constancy scaling mechanism.

Although Kanizsa (1955b) did not make note of the fact, his transparency figure (Fig. 22.10) manifests the same ambiguity as the subjective Necker cube. In this pattern, Kanizsa demon-

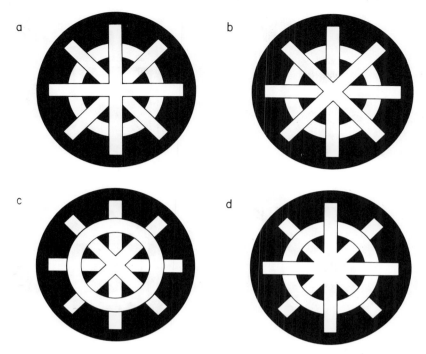

FIGURE 22.7. Some possible organizations of illusory contours in the ship's wheel configuration of Figure 22.6: a. + over x over o. b. x over + over o. c. o over x over +. d. An interleaving organization.

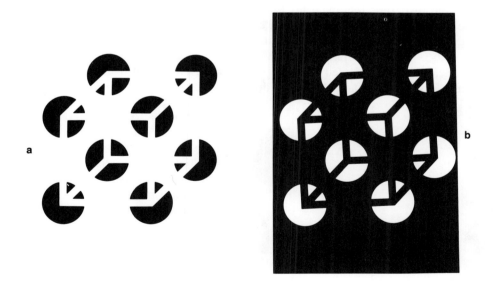

FIGURE 22.8. A positive (a) and negative (b) photographic reproduction of the subjective Necker cube.

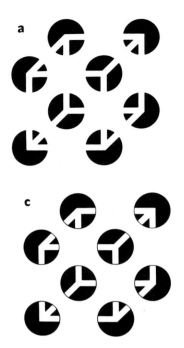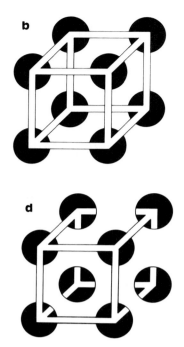

FIGURE 22.9. Some possible organizations of illusory contours in the subjective Necker cube configuration. a. The original (ambiguous) figure. b. The cube-in-front. c. The cube-in-back. d. The "straddled" organization. Most observers report that the cube-in-back appears substantially brighter than the cube-in-front, and some perceive the cube-in-back as glowing or emitting light.

strated that graying out selected portions of several black disks could produce the impression of a semitransparent rectangle floating in front of the disks. The reader can no doubt anticipate the alternative organization I will now suggest: namely, that of a rectangle suspended in a dark enclosure and viewed through the holes of an intervening surface. Note the dramatic change in the surface character of the rectangle as the organization shifts from front to back: when in front we see a semitransparent rectangle having a whitish film color; when in back we see an opaque rectangle having a gray surface color. Finally, note that when the rectangle is seen in back, the subjective contours of the rectangle in front are absent. As in the other ambiguous patterns I have illustrated, the perception of subjective contours is inextricably linked to the observer's perceptual organization of the display.

Multistable subjective-contour patterns, such as the Swiss cross, star, ship's wheel, Necker cube, and transparency figure, illustrate that illusory contours are not tied in any simple or direct manner to the luminance distribution of the display. A similar conclusion is suggested by our research on animated subjective contours, which reveals the important role played by kinetic information in facilitating the perception of illusory contours (Bradley, 1983; Bradley & Lee, 1982). We employed a figure originally developed by Kanizsa (1955a), and later discussed by Gregory (1972), which uses small

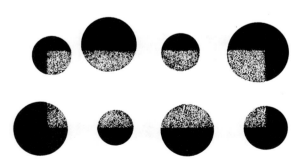

FIGURE 22.10. The Kanizsa transparency figure. A semitransparent subjective rectangle can be seen overlaying several black disks, or an opaque gray rectangle can be seen through the holes of an intervening surface (similar to the cube-in-back organization of Figure 22.9c).

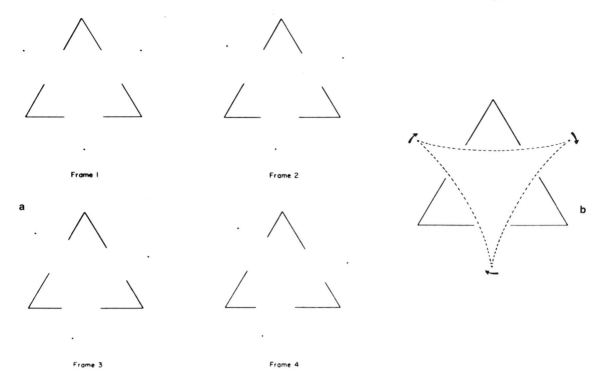

FIGURE 22.11. a. The first four frames from an animated sequence of a rotating illusory triangle. b. The apparent shape of the triangle as it rotates.

dots in place of the usual pie-shaped inducing elements (see Frame 1 of Figure 22.11a). The dots form the corners of a subjective triangle superimposed on a black outline triangle. By rotating the dots and the gaps of the outline triangle, we produced an animated film of a rotating subjective triangle (Fig. 22.11a). About 95% of the observers shown the film report that the subjective contours appear stronger while rotating, and most also report that the sides of the triangle appear bowed inward (Fig. 22.11b). Subsequent work has verified that the bowing inward of the subjective contours increases with rotational velocity, and that this effect is more pronounced with subjective than real contours (Bradley & Wood, 1987). We prepared another animated sequence in which the dots were omitted altogether, and only the gaps were rotated about the center (Fig. 22.12a). Although very few naive observers report seeing the subjective triangle while the gaps are stationary, once rotation commences virtually all report seeing a rotating triangle having somewhat

rounded corners (Fig. 22.12b). Apparently, the kinetic information provided by rotation allows observers to see subjective contours in a display that would not normally produce them.

We next investigated the effects of rotating the pie-shaped inducing elements which are often used to generate subjective contours (see Fig. 22.13a). At T1 the inducing elements are unaligned and observers do not see subjective contours. However, as the inducing elements rotate into alignment at T2, the subjective triangle pops into view. It is interesting to note that while proper alignment of the inducing elements is critical for establishing the subjective triangle, it is much less critical for maintaining the perception of the triangle as the elements continue to rotate. At T3 for example, nearly all observers report that they can still see a subjective triangle, although the sides are distorted. Some even report seeing the triangle at T4, although it is grotesquely warped by this point, and appears more like the wings of a bird than a triangle. Eventually, the rotation of the induc-

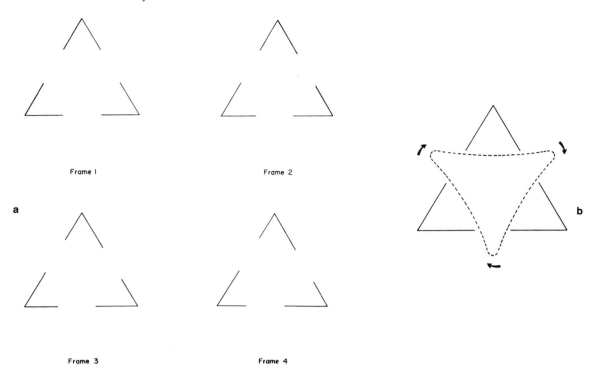

FIGURE 22.12. a. The first four frames from an animated sequence of a rotating triangle based on gaps only. b. The apparent shape of the triangle as it rotates.

ing elements exceeds some threshold, and the subjective contours "burst" or "fracture." Still, the remarkable thing about this animated sequence is the rather extreme deformations the subjective triangle will undergo before disintegrating: the triangle persists for much greater misalignments of the inducing elements than anyone would have predicted on the basis of prior research, for example, that of Mori & Ronchi (1960), which found that misalignments of only one degree destroy the subjective contours in a stationary pattern.

In another animated sequence, the shapes of the inducing elements were manipulated so as to produce the impression of a continuously distorting subjective triangle (Fig. 22.13b). Over time, the sides of the triangle appear to sweep back and forth between an extreme outward and inward bowing, creating the impression of a pulsating or breathing triangle. Both the illusory contours and the brightness gradients may be seen moving in and out from the center of the display. A few observers report that the subjective triangle appears to move back and forth in

the third dimension, much as the sail of a boat inverts with a sudden change in wind direction.

In closing, I would like to briefly consider the implications of ambiguous and animated subjective contours for sensory and cognitive theories. As noted elsewhere in this book, sensory mechanisms such as contrast, assimilation, spatial filtering, feature detection, and so on, can often provide a reasonable explanation of the subjective contours seen in "static" configurations, i.e., configurations in which only one set of subjective contours are seen. However, sensory mechanisms alone seem inadequate to account for the large variety of subjective contours seen in the ambiguous displays I have illustrated in this chapter, or to account for subjective contours seen only after movement-related cues are provided. Since sensory theories derive subjective contours from an analysis of the luminance distribution of the display, it is difficult to see how they can accommodate such findings. While the luminosity gradients of a

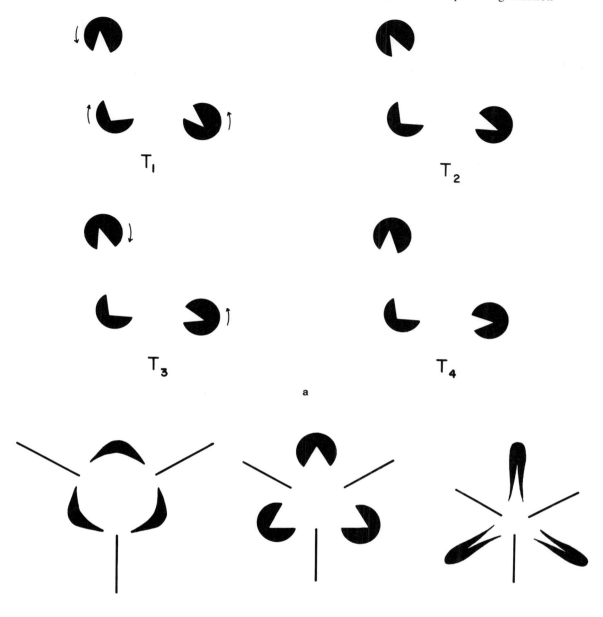

FIGURE 22.13. a. Four frames from an animated sequence in which the inducing elements rotate into and out of alignment. b. Three frames from an animated sequence in which the inducing elements are manipulated to produce the impression of a "breathing" triangle. Note that the frames shown in (a) and (b) are not adjacent in the animated sequence: frames for intermediate positions are also included.

stimulus pattern certainly set constraints as to where subjective contours might be seen, they do not necessarily determine where they will be seen. Both the perception of the illusory contours and the associated brightness effects seem to be directed by a selection process analogous to hypothesis testing, as first suggested by Gregory (1972). However, once such a process has organized the display in a coherent fashion, it is possible that local contrast and assimilation effects might be "recruited" to help give expression to the illusory-contour object (Bradley &

Mates, 1985). More specifically, Talis Bachman of the USSR has suggested that a mechanism of "cognitive inference" works in ensemble with various sensory mechanisms, and through feedback can selectively favor the extraction of certain features over others, the assimilation and contrast of certain regions over others, and the grouping and stratification in depth of certain elements in the display over others (Bachman, 1978). The novel feature of Bachman's theory is that it replaces the bottom-up processing assumption of most sensory theories with a concurrent, multilevel, processing assumption. This model allows the tentative outcomes or decisions reached at higher levels to affect the processing operations at lower levels, as well as the reverse.

The general approach taken by Bachman has great merit, and it serves to remind us that the integration of sensory and cognitive theory represents one of the greatest challenges to perceptual psychology at the present time. It is no accident that this issue should manifest itself so clearly in the theoretical debate surrounding subjective contours: the relative contribution of sensory and cognitive factors in the formation of illusory contours is more nearly equal. Furthermore, as interpolated events, subjective contours seem to provide good, perhaps even prototypical, examples of the productive operation of the visual system. Such contours arise out of the analysis of raw sensory material guided by the concurrently developing cognitive inference as to what is being viewed. Consequently, the investigation of illusory contours and other interpolative phenomena provides a necessary impetus for clarifying the interactions between sensory and cognitive mechanisms in vision.

CHAPTER 23

The Current State of Research into Visual Phantoms

William M. Maguire and James M. Brown

If a vertical square or sine wave grating drifting horizontally is partially occluded by a dark strip so that portions of the grating above and below the strip are visible, then dark bars of the grating will be seen to continue through the occluding region, appearing dim or transparent but nonetheless distinct. These illusory forms move in tandem with the grating and may alternately appear and disappear. Tynan and Sekuler (1975) called the illusory forms moving visual phantoms. The illusion, however, was noted earlier by Rosenbach (1902) and later by Fuchs (1924/1967).

Early research described a number of properties which were apparently unique to phantoms and by which they were distinguished from illusory contours (Kanizsa, 1974). Foremost, phantoms appeared to depend critically upon motion of the inducing elements, disappearing when the inducers stopped moving (Tynan & Sekuler, 1975), while illusory contours were vividly produced with stationary figures. However, although phantoms are widely regarded as being enhanced by motion or flicker (Fuchs, 1924/1967; Genter & Weisstein, 1981; Mulvanny, Macarthur, & Sekuler, 1982; Rosenbach, 1902; Tynan & Sekuler, 1975; Weisstein & Maguire, 1978), they are also visible with stationary inducing patterns (Fuchs, 1924/1967; Gyoba, 1983; Rosenbach, 1902).

This review of the phantom-contour literature shows that phantom contours share a large number of properties with Kanizsa type illusory contours. Both illusions demonstrate similar configural, spatial, and temporal constraints. Additionally, there is evidence that the mechanisms responsible for these illusions share a common neural locus and are normally involved in registration of real contours.

Phantoms have been produced with a limited number of displays. Inducing patterns have typically been square or sine wave gratings of low spatial frequency, though a single oscillating bar is sufficient (Fuchs, 1924/1967; Rosenbach, 1902). A horizontal strip, extended across the display, has typically been the occluder, but a square or trapezoidal patch that is completely surrounded by inducing forms produces good phantoms as well (Weisstein, Maguire, & Williams, 1982). The term *occluder* describes the homogeneous surface physically occluding the inducing contours or sometimes produced in an animated sequence to represent an occluding surface (Brown, 1985; Brown & Weisstein, 1985a, 1985b, 1986; Genter & Weisstein, 1981). The latter method has permitted greater control of the lightness relationships between the occluder and inducing pattern. Regardless of the method used, the occluder undergoes a unique figure/ground transformation when phantoms appear and disappear. It is seen in front of the inducing pattern when phantoms are not visible, and recedes behind the inducing surface when phantoms appear.

There have been reports of phantom completion involving illusory texture completion different from the simple edge interpolation. Both random dots (Tynan & Sekuler, 1975) and columns of Xs (Weisstein & Maguire, 1978) have been reported to fill the occluding region, when the appropriate pattern (dots and Xs) is occluded. This type of completion may be a different phenomenon from the edge interpolation effects described here. At any rate, these effects have not been extensively studied and are not included in subsequent discussion.

Phantoms and Lightness Relationships in Displays

It has been reported that phantom contours are less evident when the dark occluder is replaced by a lighter gray occluder. Under these conditions the observer may see a brightness contrast illusion produced by interaction between inducing and occluding regions. A phase-shifted grating without sharp edges is seen to move across the occluding surface in tandem with the inducing grating (Maguire, 1978). This illusion has been reported to be particularly evident with stationary displays and has been called brightness induction (McCourt, 1982).

In recent experiments the critical lightness relationships needed to produce phantoms have been examined. Brown & Weisstein (1985a) varied occluder lightness while a 0.5 cycles per degree square wave inducing pattern was flickered at 5 Hz under two types of on/off flicker. In one type (Type 1), during the off portion of the cycle, the gratings were replaced by a blank field with luminance equal to the dark bars of the grating. In Type 2 flicker, the blank field luminance was equivalent to the light bars of the grating. As a result, in Type 1 flicker the dark areas do not flicker, while in Type 2 the light areas do not flicker. Subjects indicated when phantoms were visible by pressing a timer button, and the percentage of total viewing time was calculated as an indicator of phantom strength. The results of the experiment are shown in Figure 23.1.

The percentage of time when phantoms are seen is greatest when lightness differences are minimal between the nonflickering parts of the inducing pattern (either light bars or dark bars) and the occluder. The nonflickering parts of the inducing pattern are seen to extend in front of the occluder, while the flickering parts of the inducing pattern and the nonphantom parts of the occluder become background for the completed stripes. These results illustrate two sensory influences on the phantom illusion. One influence is the lightness relationships in phantom displays; dark bars will tend to complete across dark occluders, and light bars across

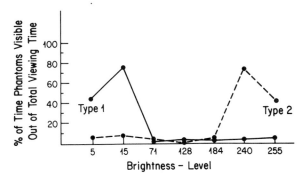

FIGURE 23.1. Flickering phantom visibility for a square wave inducing pattern using two types of flicker. The lightness of the occluder was one of seven values on a brightness continuum from black (5) to white (255), while the inducing pattern was made of dark (15) and light (240) bars. The dark inducing bars were nonflickering with Type 1 flicker, the light bars were nonflickering with Type 2 flicker.

light occluders. In fact, phantoms may be produced with an occluder of any lightness providing there are inducing regions of the same or similar lightness (Brown, 1985). The second influence is the recently reported effect of flicker rate on depth segregation. Flickering areas of a surface appear to recede behind nonflickering areas, creating depth stratification in the absence of other depth cues (Wong & Weisstein, 1984). Flicker-induced depth segregation affects phantoms by specifying the stationary bars to be completed as figures on a background specified by the flickering regions. In another study where subjects only saw Type 1 flicker (Brown, 1985), subjects reported phantoms to be visible for light bars when the occluder was light but less so than for dark bars when the occluder was dark. This result is consistent with other findings of the organizational influence of flicker on phantom displays.

A second experiment extended these findings. Maguire and Blattberg (1986) varied occluder lightness for flickering inducing gratings whose temporal frequency varied as one condition of the experiment. The observer viewed a flickering display for 10 seconds. During the off phase, the grating was replaced with a gray field of the same space averaged luminance. The observer judged whether the region of the occlusive surface below the dark bar of the grating was darker or lighter than the region below the

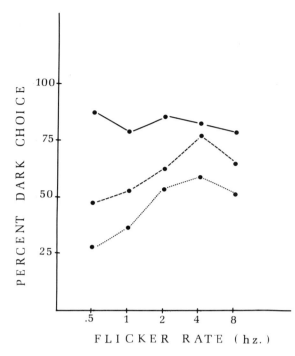

FIGURE 23.2. Percentage of dark responses. Inducing pattern, 0.25 cycle per degree vertical square wave. Light bars 10.6 cd/m², dark bars .03 cd/m². Occluder height 1°, occluder lightness (solid line) .03 cd/m², (broken line) 2.4 cd/m², (dotted line) 4.7 cd/m². Five flicker rates as shown. Fourteen observers participated. Each judged each display three times. Dark response corresponds to phantom appearance.

light bars of the inducer in a forced choice procedure. In essence the observer was forced to decide whether the appearance of the occlusive surface was more consistent with brightness assimilation (the phantom appearance and the "darker" judgment) or brightness contrast (the "lighter" judgment). The results are plotted in Figure 23.2.

Consistent with the Brown and Weisstein results, there was a dramatic decrease in the number of phantom reports when the lightness of the occluder differed from that of both light and dark bars of the inducing pattern. Additionally, the shape of the temporal tuning function appears to depend critically upon the lightness of the occluder it is measured against (when the occluder lightness is equivalent to dark bar lightness). The illusion shows no falloff at low temporal frequencies. The medium lightness occluder, however, shows a pronounced falloff

at the lowest temporal frequencies. With the high lightness occluder (lightness midway between light and dark bars) there is little evidence that darker reports are above chance level for any temporal frequencies save the optimal 4 Hz. At low temporal frequencies, however, lighter reports are well above chance, indicating that brightness contrast can be reliably elicited with this display when temporal frequency is low. This brightness induction effect would appear to be absent for temporal frequencies above 1 Hz.

Sakurai and Gyoba (1985) found similar influences of occluder lightness on stationary phantom visibility. Phantoms were perceived best when the occluder was equal in lightness to maximum or minimum lightness of the inducing grating. Brightness induction was reported when occluder luminance equaled the space averaged luminance of the grating.

The reason phantoms are not readily seen with occluding surfaces of intermediate lightness may be the presence of clear edges between all parts of the inducing grating and the occluder. These edges may act to block the assimilation of brightness across the occluding region (Grossberg & Mingolla, 1985), unambiguously defining the occluding surface (Brown, 1985). Displays that produce brightness contrast exaggerate and increase these edge effects. In this way, to the extent that conditions favor brightness contrast, the phantom illusion will be less probable. There is a piece of indirect evidence to support the disruptive effects of brightness contrast. Mulvanny et al. (1982) used a brightness cancellation technique to measure phantom strength. This consists in superimposing on the occluding surface a low-contrast grating 180° out of phase with the inducing pattern. They found that otherwise vivid phantoms were cancelled by the presence of even a just visible out-of-phase pattern on the occluding surface. This counterphase pattern mimics the perceptual effects of brightness contrast.

Spatial and Temporal Properties of Phantoms

The strength of the phantom illusion varies with the spatial frequency and motion or temporal frequency of the inducing pattern. The most consistent finding in this regard is that the phantom illusion is stronger with low spatial frequency inducers than high spatial frequencies. With an occluder 2–3° in height, there is a considerable falloff in vividness and percentage of time phantoms are seen in the 1–6 cycle per degree range (Genter & Weisstein, 1981; Maguire, 1978; Tynan & Sekuler, 1975). Investigating phantoms with stationary displays, Gyoba (1983) found phantoms were always visible with low spatial frequency inducing contours. Whether they were seen with higher spatial frequencies, however, depended critically upon the height of the occluder. The highest spatial frequency for which phantoms could be seen decreased from 4 to 1.5 cycles per degree as occluder height increased from 1° to 5°. The sole exception to the reported superiority of low spatial frequency inducers in producing phantoms is the Mulvanny et al. (1982) report that threshold inducer contrast to produce phantom contours increased for low spatial frequencies below 5 cycles per degree at some inducer velocities, but these thresholds were almost completely determined by the threshold for seeing the inducer itself. It was the inducer threshold in turn which was elevated at low spatial frequencies.

Displays which produce illusory contours generally have complex spatial frequency spectra, making direct comparison with the phantom studies somewhat difficult. Ginsburg (1975) has maintained that the information critical to the perception of illusory contours is contained in the low spatial frequencies. While new demonstrations make his specific model unlikely (Prazdny, 1983; Shapley & Gordon, 1985), his demonstrations that illusory contours survive high spatial frequency filtering remain relevant. It has also been demonstrated that illusory contours, like phantom contours, are reduced in strength when distance between inducing figures is increased (Shapley & Gordon, 1985).

Phantoms are widely regarded as being enhanced by motion or flicker (Genter & Weisstein, 1981; Mulvanny et al., 1982; Tynan & Sekuler, 1975; Weisstein & Maguire, 1978). The data, however, are not uniformly supportive in this regard. Tynan and Sekuler (1975) reported that phantoms disappeared when stationary inducers were used. Genter and Weisstein (1981), using flickering inducers, found optimal phantoms with 5-Hz flicker for a variety of spatial frequencies. Gyoba (1983), however, has reported that phantoms can be produced with stationary inducers. Maguire (1978) found little effect of grating velocity for drift rates from 0.36 to 5.8 degrees/second. With both dark and light occluding strips, Brown (1985) failed to find a low temporal frequency cutoff for flickering phantoms. A number of these studies used amount of time phantoms are seen as a measure of phantom strength. With on/off flicker, this measure can be ambiguous because the inducing contours themselves may be phenomenally absent during the off phase at low temporal frequencies (Brown, 1985).

The measure used in the Maguire and Blattberg (1986, Fig. 2) experiment avoids this ambiguity. With the darkest occluder, no low temporal frequency cutoff is evident. With the gray occluders, however, low temporal frequency rolloff is evident.

Those results suggest one way in which motion and flicker might contribute to phantom visibility. For certain displays motion or flicker may prevent brightness contrast from developing in retinal areas where the occluder is imaged. When conditions are not favorable to the development of brightness contrast, such as the use of an occlusive surface that matches regions of the inducing surface in lightness (McCourt, 1982), phantoms may be visible with stationary and slowly flickering patterns.

Figural Cues with Phantoms

Such an explanation, however, does not account for all data concerning the role of motion nor does it preclude another role for motion in the phantom illusion. Tynan and Sekuler (1975) created a display which produced phantom contours when in motion but did not when the display was stationary. When the eyes moved across the display following a moving fixation point, the phantoms did not reappear, despite the movement of the contours on the retina. This indicates that environmental motion may play a role in the phantom illusion which is distinct from the effects of retinal motion.

The role of environmental rather than retinal motion in the phantom illusion may be figural. It is known that the phantom illusion is sensitive to information about the relative spatial position of occluder and inducing contours. If binocular disparity cues are present, indicating that the opaque region is in front of the inducing contours and the display is viewed binocularly, the illusion is reduced (Maguire, 1978; Weisstein et al., 1982). Analogous effects have been obtained with illusory contours which are diminished if disparity cues contradict the depth relations implied by the configuration and are enhanced by compatible disparity cues (Gregory & Harris, 1974; Harris & Gregory, 1973; Lawson, Cohen, Gibbs, & Whitmore, 1974).

In the absence of binocular disparity cues, the depth relations in phantom displays are ambiguous. This is perhaps most evident when the inducing grating is a square which is otherwise surrounded by the inducing contours in motion (Weisstein et al., 1982). When phantoms are not seen, the grating moves clearly behind the occluding square being amodally completed. When phantoms are seen, the square is still clearly visible behind the moving bars.

There is a modification of the Kanizsa triangle which appears particularly congruous with phantom displays. The cutout portion of the inducing circles is filled with color. The resulting form sometimes appears as a Kanizsa type subjective triangle with assimilation of the wedge color by the whole triangle (Meyer & Senecal, 1983; Ware, 1980). Alternatively, the triangle may be amodally completed, viewed as through portholes in the surface. As with phantom contours the identical figure alternates between modal and amodal completion.

As discussed earlier (see Fig. 23.1), induced depth between adjacent flickering and nonflickering surfaces can also bias the perceptual interpretation and hence influence the vividness of the phantom illusion. In particular, nonflickering inducing regions are more likely to complete as phantoms than flickering inducers (Brown & Weisstein, 1985a). Recently, Meyer and Doughery (1985) found analogous biasing effects with the modified Kanizsa triangle described above. When the inducing elements were flickering, they appeared below the surface, and amodal rather than modal completion of the triangle was the dominant percept.

In a series of experiments, Brown and Weisstein (1986) showed that the vividness of the phantom illusion will be affected by manipulation of figural cues, even when these cues are relatively distant from the site of the illusion. The figures used in these studies are shown in Figure 23.3.

The first experiment found no differences in incubation time or phantom strength between patterns (a), (b), (c), and (d). In the second experiment there were no differences in the two measures for patterns (a), (b), and (f). For pattern (e), however, incubation time was nearly double and phantom strength was about half. A third experiment found phantom visibility to be significantly less and incubation time to be significantly longer for pattern (g) compared to patterns (h) and (i). Cueing the gray parts in pattern (a) as figure, in front of the white parts, did not affect phantoms, while cueing the gray parts as ground, behind the white parts, in patterns (e) and (g), reduced phantom visibility. Phantom contours imply that the inducing surface is in front of the occluder. Phantom visibility is reduced when interposition cues are present in the display that conflict with this interpretation. (Brown, 1985; Brown & Weisstein, 1986).

Similarly, when the standard phantom display is set in motion or caused to flicker, figural cues are introduced that are absent from the stationary display. In particular, when the inducing contours move or flicker, interpretations of the display that specify the top and bottom inducers as parts of the same figure are strengthened by gestalt common fate (Maguire, 1978). This type of enhancement by motion-produced figural cues is not unique to phantom contours, however. Quite vivid illusory contours of the Kanizsa type can be produced with displays that utilize motion-produced cues (Bradley & Lee, 1982; Kellman & Cohen, 1984).

Mechanisms Underlying Phantoms

Research using a variety of psychophysical methods suggests common mechanisms underlying illusory and phantom contours. It has been found that real and illusory contours interact in masking paradigms. Prior brief exposure to real contours reduces the apparent contrast of illusory contours, and vice versa (Weisstein,

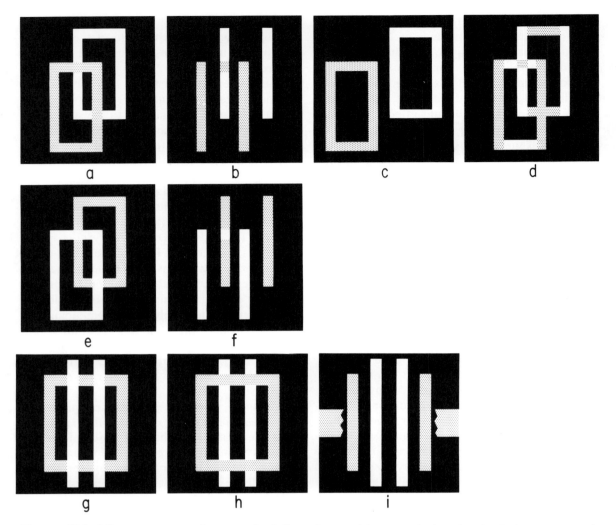

FIGURE 23.3. Nine patterns used to test the influence of perceived figure/ground and depth relations within an inducing pattern on phantom visibility. The interposition cues designating the dark gray parts as ground to the white parts in patterns (e) and (g) reduced phantom visibility.

Matthews, & Berbaum, 1974; Smith & Over, 1977). These and other data suggest that the mechanisms responsible for illusory contours may overlap substantially with mechanisms involved in the normal detection of brightness gradients (Grossberg & Mingolla, 1985; Shapley & Gordon, 1985; Weisstein, 1970; Weisstein & Maguire, 1978). Phantom contours have also been found to interact with real contours in selective adaptation. Weisstein, Maguire, and Berbaum (1977) found that exposure to moving visual phantoms gave rise to an appropriate motion aftereffect in the retinal region where phantoms had been seen. Analogous results have been obtained with illusory contours (Smith & Over, 1979). Maguire (1978) demonstrated the converse. Exposure to real contours in motion led to subsequent direction-selective increases in the latency of the appearance of the phantom illusion. Direction-selective adaptation of the illusion was evident even when the retinal area adapted was restricted to the region corresponding to the occluding surface where no actual contours are in motion. These results parallel masking results with illusory contours and indicate a substantial overlap between mechanisms that produce illusory contours and those that process real contours and surfaces.

A similar point is made in a recent study (Brown, 1985). Orientation sensitivity for briefly flashed line segments was tested in regions on the occluding surface where phantoms were seen as compared with physically identical regions where no phantoms were visible. Sensitivity was greater within the phantom regions, paralleling results that show that orientation sensitivity is superior in those regions of an ambiguous figure (Rubin's faces/vase figure) that are currently perceived as figure (Wong & Weisstein, 1982). No directly analogous study has yet been performed with illusory contours. Coren and Theodor (1977), however, did demonstrate that the illusory brightness changes associated with the two sides of an illusory edge affected luminance thresholds for light spots on either side of the edge.

Subjective contours have also been found to reduce both reaction time and error rate for dot localization in the same way as real contours (Pomerantz, Goldberg, Golden, & Tetewsky, 1981).

These results with phantom and illusory contours are quite compatible with neural models that attribute illusory contours to computation by complex cells in V1 or V2 (Grossberg & Mingolla, 1985; von der Heydt, Peterhans, & Baumgarten, 1984). Recent demonstrations indicate that the mechanism responsible for illusory contours is sensitive to the amount but not the direction of contrast of inducing contours in the figure (Prazdny, 1983; Shapley & Gordon, 1985). An analogous demonstration can be produced with phantom-inducing displays. The inducing figure is shown in Figure 23.4.

The top and bottom of the inducing pattern in the typical phantom display are phase shifted so that dark and bright bars on top and bottom are 180° out of phase. Phantom contours are clearly seen in the central region when the figure is observed in a dimly illuminated room.

The large number of common properties between phantom and the Kanizsa type illusory

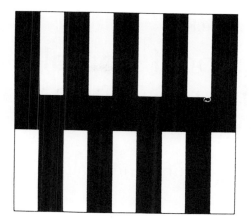

FIGURE 23.4. Display to illustrate that direction of stimulus contrast is not critical to phantom appearance.

contours suggests that they are each manifestations of spatially limited contour completion mechanisms sensitive to the magnitude, but not the direction, of stimulus contrast. These contour-generating mechanisms interact with mechanisms of brightness assimilation to define apparent brightness of surfaces in the figure (Grossberg & Mingolla, 1985). These mechanisms appear closely related to mechanisms that detect real contours, as illusory and real contours interact in a number of experimental situations.

The unique properties of phantom contours, such as the dependence under some conditions upon display motion, appear due to their production by configurations that are atypical of the set of patterns known to produce illusory contours. Figural cues in these displays are relatively weak. Thus, the displays are more sensitive to relative lightness, common motion, cues about the relative spatial position of surfaces, and other surface-defining information. Further exploration of the way different sources of surface-defining information interact to strengthen and weaken illusory contours should do much to advance our knowledge of visual perception.

CHAPTER 24

Amodal Completion and Illusory Figures: An Information-Processing Analysis

Nicola Bruno and Walter Gerbino

An illusory figure is an occluding figure. In all compelling instances, perception of the illusion occurs together with amodal completion of the inducing elements. However, it is presently uncertain whether or not this relation should be interpreted causally. The purpose of this chapter is to look at completion from an information-processing point of view. A better understanding of the completion process might help clarify its role in the perception of illusory figures and give us some insight into how these illusions are produced within the visual system.

The Co-occurrence of Completion and Illusory Figures

Is phenomenal completion necessary for the perception of illusory figures? This general question can be rephrased in two ways. We may ask whether it is possible to observe examples of illusory figures in the absence of phenomenal completion. The answer is generally no. Only a few demonstrations question this general conclusion (Kennedy, 1978a), but whether the effects discussed in these demonstrations relate to standard illusory surfaces is dubious (Minguzzi, 1983; Parks, 1984). A separate question is whether incompleteness in the inducing elements is necessary for the phenomenon to occur. Kanizsa (1955a) gave a positive answer, arguing that four crosses, being complete, "stable and regular" elements, do not produce illusory figures. Opposing Kanizsa, however, are reports of illusory figures with geometrically regular inducers, like squares and triangles (Sambin, 1974a), and even with the

crosses of Kanizsa's demonstration (Day & Kasperczyk, 1983a).

However, if these latter observations seem to rule out geometrical incompleteness as a necessary factor, they do not exclude phenomenal completion. First, it is not clear whether the geometrically regular inducers remain phenomenally regular, once the illusion is perceived. To the contrary, some have observed that they tend to continue amodally behind the illusory occluder (Minguzzi, 1982). Second, completion does not always occur in the direction of regularization (Kanizsa, 1975b); therefore, it might well occur with regular inducers. Thus, completion of the inducing elements seems to be present in all instances of illusory figures. Figural incompleteness, on the other hand, might be related to particularly effective illusory effects, as suggested by the fact that incomplete inducers yield more salient instances of the phenomenon (Day & Kasperczyk, 1983a).

Two Hypotheses on Completion and Illusory Figures

The systematic co-occurrence of completion and illusory figures deserves an explanation. How does the completion process relate to the production of the illusion? Two contrasting views can be found in the literature. According to one (Kanizsa, 1955a, 1974, 1976), illusory surfaces are a by-product of the tendency to complete certain structures. Through completion, incomplete inducers can be transformed into stable, more regular figures. To reach this preferred organization, however, the visual system must provide an occluder; thus the illusory surface is formed, despite the absence of local stimulus information to specify it.

In contrast with Kanizsa, Gregory (1972) and later Rock and Anson (1979) proposed that illusory figures are produced by reasoning-like, problem-solving processes. Some low-probability feature of the inducers—the presence of "gaps" for Gregory, figural incompleteness, alignment and perceptual set for Rock and Anson—activate a search for a solution capable of accounting for or explaining such a feature. Thus, the system postulates—hypothesizes—the occluding figure, and this is what is perceived.

In their treatment of the stimulus factors associated with illusory figures, the two accounts overlap. Perception of an illusory figure is predicted in the presence of figural incompleteness, and the illusion allows for completion of the incomplete elements. The two accounts differ, however, in the actual mechanism proposed to be responsible for completion. According to Kanizsa, the transformation of the homogeneous field into an illusory figure is due to spontaneous, preattentional processing guided by organizational forces; for Gregory and Rock, on the other hand, the process is better described in terms of more cognitive, reasoning-like mechanisms. The difference might be regarded as purely terminological, that

is, dependent on one's choice of a metaphor for perceptual processing. What is certainly true, however, is that little is known about the completion process, and even less about completion with illusory figures. The study we present here is a first attempt to address this issue.

An Information-Processing Analysis

To investigate how completion behind an illusory surface is achieved, we adopted the experimental paradigm developed by Gerbino and Salmaso (1985). Observers performed a same–different matching task on stimuli involving forms that were physically and phenomenally complete (here referred to as *complete* forms), forms that were physically incomplete but phenomenally completing behind either line-drawn or illusory occluders (*completed* forms), and forms both physically and phenomenally incomplete (*truncated* forms).

All comparisons are described in Figure 24.1. Target stimuli and comparison patterns were presented in succession at the center of a computer-controlled screen (exposure = 333 msec; ISI = 350 msec). The target was always presented first. Observers were asked to compare complete targets (diamonds or hexagons) with

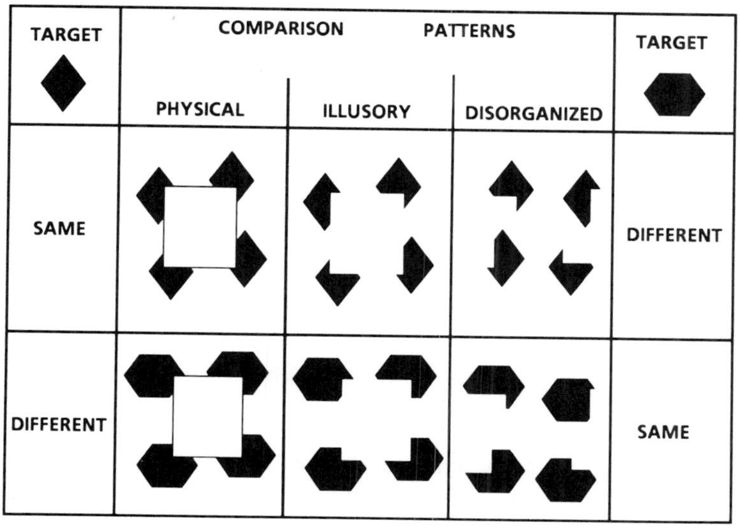

FIGURE 24.1. Twelve possible matches resulted from the combination of two targets (diamond, hexagon) with six comparison patterns. All stimuli had 333 msec exposure. The ISI was 350 msec.

comparison patterns made out of physically identical forms. As Figure 24.1 shows, however, these varied in their phenomenal appearance: In the *physical* and *illusory* conditions, they looked like complete shapes partly occluded by a line drawing or an illusory rectangle, in the *disorganized* condition, like truncated shapes. The main dependent variable was reaction time; error rates were computed as well, but since they were generally negligible they will not be discussed. Viewers were instructed to judge sameness on the basis of category. Thus, a comparison between a complete rectangle and a truncated rectangle was a positive match, regardless of the phenomenal dissimilarity between the two forms.

Considerable evidence in the literature shows that illusory surfaces tend to be functionally similar to equivalent luminance gradient figures. For instance, illusory figures have been shown to act like their "objective" counterparts in producing geometrical illusions (Gregory, 1972; Meyer & Garges, 1979; Pastore, 1971), and various figural aftereffects (Smith & Over, 1976, 1979), in stroboscopic motion (Ramachandran, 1985b; Sigman & Rock, 1974; von Grünau, 1979), and in facilitating performance in information-processing tasks (Pomerantz, Goldberg, Golder, & Tetewsky, 1981). Can this equivalence be extended to completion effects? If so, we should expect same matches in the illusory and physical conditions to be roughly equivalent. If, on the other hand, completion behind an illusory surface requires more cognitive, attention-demanding processes than completion behind a physical occluder, we should predict that same matches in the illusory condition will require more time. And finally, if completion depends upon categorizing a truncated form as a modification of a complete prototype, then same matches in the illusory condition should be equivalent to those in the disorganized condition.

The results are summarized in Figure 24.2. The mean reaction times were 624 msec ± 15 in the physical condition, 646 msec ± 14.5 in the illusory condition, and 689 msec ± 17 in the disorganized condition. Thus, same matches in the disorganized condition require more time ($p < .05$), suggesting that completion behind illusory surfaces occurs at a more primitive level than categorization. As indicated by a compari-

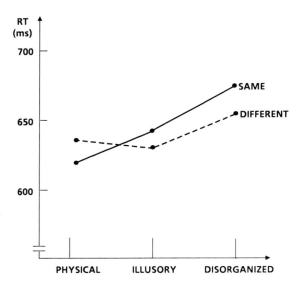

FIGURE 24.2. Average latencies in the study. Same matches are equivalent in the physical and in the illusory conditions. In the disorganized condition, however, the matches were slower ($p < .05$). The result suggests that completion behind illusory figures is different than categorization and can be achieved as fast as completion behind a physical occluder.

son of mean latencies in the illusory and physical conditions, on the other hand, completion behind an illusory figure does not require longer processing than its luminance gradient counterpart. Different matches, finally, were statistically equivalent in all conditions.

Final Considerations

Two indications emerge from our data. The first concerns the level of the completion process. Gerbino and Salmaso (1985) have recently suggested that completion could be considered as an instance of transformation within the visual code (Posner, 1978). Our result agrees well with this suggestion and with Kanizsa's notion of an automatic, early completion. Furthermore, since the illusory occluder must be already available for the inducers to complete behind it, the outcome of the experiment also suggests that illusory figures themselves are produced early in visual processing, possibly at the level of the *boundary completion* process hypothesized by Grossberg and Mingolla (1985a). The second indication concerns the role of attention. Research by Pritchard and Warm (1983) suggests that illusory figures involve a greater attentional load than physical ones. Insofar as our data point to an early, preattentional availability of the illusory occluder, they provide no evidence for the claim. Since the question of the role of attention was not addressed directly by our study, however, this latter conclusion needs further support.

Finally, to the question of whether the completion process is better described in terms of spontaneous organization or perceptual problem solving, our present data do not speak. Inferentialistic explanations evoke mechanisms that are different in nature than the automatic process suggested by our data. As Cutting (1986) pointed out, however, inference comes in two kinds: inductive and deductive. If perceptual processes are inductive, then they must involve top-down components from memory and cognition and operate on a probabilistic basis. Our data seem to suggest completion is not a process of this kind. If, on the other hand, perceptual processes are deductive, then all premises come from stimulus information and design features of the system, and inference proceeds automatically like a mathematical proof. In this latter sense, we believe, inference is as spontaneous as organization. Which description better captures the essence of the completion process is therefore a question for further investigation.

Acknowledgments. The authors thank James Cutting, Michael Kelly, and Robert Millard, for reviewing earlier drafts of this manuscript.

CHAPTER 25

Illusory Contours, Texture Segregation, and a Configural Inferiority Effect

Glenn E. Meyer and David Fish

Components of objects seem better or faster perceived in their object context than when standing alone. Such phenomena are now referred to as *object superiority* or *configural superiority* effects (Weisstein & Harris, 1974; Pomerantz, Sager, & Stoever, 1977). We attempted to explore the intersection of the configural superiority effect, illusory contours, and texture segregation with the hope of giving us some insights into these phenomena.

First, a brief look at the major camps of illusory-contour theories. The first regards the illusory contour as a passive output of a "deceived" neurophysiology. The inducing elements are thought to activate various types of cell receptive fields or Fourier systems to produce an edge even though the edge is physically incomplete. The production of the tilt, motion and color-contingent aftereffects, Poggendorf illusion, stroboscopic motion and visual masking with illusory contour stimuli (Meyer & Garges, 1979; Smith & Over, 1975, 1976, 1979; von Grünau, 1979; Weisstein, Matthews, & Berbaum, 1974), along with spatial-frequency based analyses of illusory contours (Ginsburg, chap. 13) are supportive of this viewpoint. These findings suggest that illusory contours and surfaces are equivalent to, although perhaps weaker than, real edges and objects and would produce effects similar to real edges due to the commonality of mechanism.

The second set of theories, while not denying the role of neural mechanisms in most cases, propose that higher-order processes are the major factors in illusory-contour formation. The cognitive process is usually a variant of depth stratification, interposition, or an attention-based problem-solving strategy of perceptual interpretation (Kanizsa, 1976; Meyer & Senecal, 1983; Rock & Anson, 1979). Data which support this point of view usually find a nonequivalency between an illusory contour and a real contour in some perceptual task like contour disappearance (Halpern & Warm, 1981), the rod–frame task (Streibel, Barnes, Julness, & Ebenholz, 1980) and orientation discrimination (Pomerantz, Goldberg, Golder, & Tetewsky, 1981), and some optical illusions (Meyer, 1986). Typically, the illusory contour does not produce the effect found with the real contour even though the illusory edge is perceptually very powerful. Support also comes from research demonstrating that illusory edges can be made to disappear by perceptual reorganization of reversible figures (Meyer & Phillips, 1980), are subject to processing capacity demands (Pritchard & Warm, 1983), are more visible if a depth stratification is present (Meyer & Senecal, 1983), and show learning and attentional effects (Rock & Anson, 1979). Such findings are not totally explanable by passive responding of the known array of the visual system neurons. Again, this is not to deny the neuronal process but to say there is more than just that. Many of the chapters in this volume hold this position.

There are also various points of view regarding the object and configural superiority effects. Candidates for the crucial process are three-dimensionality, connectedness, structural relevance, line masking, fixation point detail, and perceptual discriminability/redundancy relationships (Enns and Prinzmetal, 1984). These arguments are not usually couched in neurophysiological terms.

Given the differing viewpoints, it would be of interest to see if illusory edges could be used to produce a configural or object superiority effect. Neuronally based theories might be expected to predict object superiority effects from illusory edges if they regard the illusory edge as a consequence of normal edge processing or even a necessary and useful part of vision. The effects might be weaker but in the same direction.

A cognitive approach to illusory contours gives rise to various predictions which depend on your rationale for the configural and object effects. If the object effects are rather late-occurring processes and the illusory contour is an early construction, as in Gerbino and Kanizsa (chap. 27, this volume), one might expect to find an illusory-configural enhancement. If the configural effect is due to relatively early perceptual processing as suggested by Pomerantz (1981) and illusory contours take a fair amount of time to construct, they may not aid in element detection. It is also possible that an illusory-contour context might interfere with element detection. Other types of configurations do slow processing and degrade accuracy (Banks & Prinzmetal, 1976). One could speculate that the attentional capacity necessary for an active illusory-contour process could also be a resource drain. Analyses such as Kennedy's (chap. 28, this volume) suggest that certain illusory surfaces would be ineffective as subjects are quite aware of their unreality despite the surfaces' visibility.

To test these possibilities, we chose in Experiments 1 and 2 to replicate a configural superiority effect reported by Pomerantz et al. (1977) and Pomerantz (1981). Pomerantz found that a discrimination between 45° and 135° lines was aided by an L context that formed triangle or arrow elements (see Figs. 25.1 & 25.2). The same elements may aid in texture segregation (Julesz, 1981b). The L-shaped element is easily replaced by an illusory contour L and various control Ls (see Figs. 25.1 & 25.2). Experiment 3 tested whether illusory contours aid in the detection of elements which actually contribute to the illusory contour. Experiment 4 and 5 used

texture segregation to explore the results of Experiments 1, 2, and 3.

Experiment 1

Method

The stimuli consisted of four lines in a horizontal array. Three lines were oriented at 135° and one at 45°. The latter was used as the target and it could be placed in any of the four positions within six contexts (Fig. 25.1).

Figures 25.1A–C were used as controls. Figure 25.1F is the condition with no context. Figure 25.1E is a variant of the Pomerantz et al. (1977) figure which did produce faster detections of the 45° line as compared to the no context condition. Figure 25.1D is an illusory-contour version.

Procedure

A trial was started by the presentation of the fixation point for 500 msec. The target array was then presented for 200 msec and the blank field returned. Subjects had to press a button corresponding to the position of the 45° line. Instructions emphasized speed and accuracy equally.

Results

Mean reaction times and errors were computed for each type of stimulus context and position in the stimulus array. The context main effect was significant for the mean correct reaction times and error rates ($p < .001$). Conditions 25.1A–D (hollow dots, solid dots, empty contours, and illusory contours) did not significantly differ from each other but did differ from the faster arrow/triangle (E) and line alone (F) arrays. The latter (E and F) did not differ from each other. Error rate was highly correlated with mean correct reaction time ($r = .98$, $p < .001$).

Discussion

There are several important points to be made. First, we did not find a significant advantage for the arrows/triangles context as Pomerantz et al.

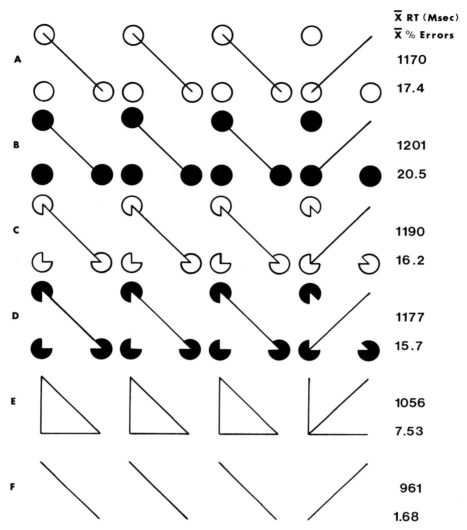

$\overline{X}$ RT (Msec)

$\overline{X}$ % Errors

A   1170   17.4

B   1201   20.5

C   1190   16.2

D   1177   15.7

E   1056   7.53

F   961   1.68

FIGURE 25.1. Examples of stimulus displays used in Experiment 1. Target is the 45° line which was presented in all four positions. Adjacent to the display is the mean reaction time and error rate for that stimulus. Context display types: A. Hollow-dot. B. Solid-dot. C. Hollow contour. D. Illusory contour. E. Triangle and arrow. F. lines alone or no context. The 135° and 45° lines were 0.75° of visual angle in length and 0.02° wide. The targets in (A)–(D) would be contained in a square subtending 5.5° by 5.5°; (E) and (F) would fit in a 5.05° square.

Four-hundred-eighty slides were presented (80 for each stimulus, 20 for each position). Fifteen subjects were tested.

(1977) did with similar elements. However, Weisstein and Harris (1974) did not originally find their object context to be better than a "lines alone" condition. Their objects were better than their controls. While later experiments did demonstrate actual advantages for object conditions (Williams & Weisstein, 1981, Pomerantz et al., 1977; Pomerantz, 1981), our results are not atypical in this regard.

The most interesting finding is that the illusory-contour conditions are significantly slower and more error prone than the lines alone and arrow/triangle conditions. In fact, this context is as bad as the other control conditions. The presence of the illusory context did not aid and, if anything, seemed to be a hinderance. Examining our reaction times and error rates, we find that they are close to those reported by

Pomerantz (1981; Pomerantz et al. 1977). Also, the increase in errors with reaction time seems to rule out a speed–accuracy tradeoff slowing the illusory contours (Pachella, 1974).

Pomerantz (1981) suggests two factors which may be operative in his task. The first is the production of an emergent feature by the addition of the context. In this case, the feature may be closure as the context makes some lines into triangles. This type of feature may be rapidly and automatically processed. Such features may also be processed by "closed channels" such that the component lines which determine closure are not available for use until after or at the same time as the closure feature is available. If our illusory contexts generate such a cue, it seems to take longer to use than when it occurs in real lines, or perhaps something masks this cue (see our Experiment 4).

Pomerantz's second factor is that the actual four target lines in his display can form a gestalt which may interfere with target detection. His lines were arranged in a square (see Fig. 25.2). In the no-context or lines-alone condition, the lines might group in such a manner that the supposedly different target line is seen as part of an organized figure and not different. A matching line is seen as not part of the figure and said to be different. This can be seen in Figure 25.2B. The left lower 135° line, the right lower 45° line, and the upper right 135° line can be viewed as an empty box. Thus, incorrectly, the upper left 135° line is picked as different—even though it matches the two other 135° lines. This does not happen in the arrow/triangle context (Fig. 25.2A) where the closure cue predominates. Perhaps, our horizontal array did not contain this interfering factor. This would explain why the lines alone were not inferior to the triangle/ angle context. Of course, this implies that closure was not very powerful in our situation. There is also the possibility that the horizontal array interacted with the subjective contour to eliminate the benefits of closure or produced a grouping not conducive to detecting the line. Experiment 2 was run to test if arranging the elements in a square matrix would replicate Pomerantz's context superiority effect and, perhaps, aid the subjective contours. One might expect the latter if the illusory-closure cue would make target detection "immune" to devouring, incorrect gestalts.

Experiment 2

The figures were similar to those in Experiment 1 except that they were now arranged in a square. However, only the lines alone, arrows/ triangles, and illusory-contour contexts were used to see if the latter were still inferior to the first two contexts.

Results

The means for reaction times and error rate are presented in Figure 25.2. Each of the stimuli differed from each other ($p < .05$). Again, errors and time were highly correlated ($r = .97$, $p < .05$).

Discussion

Experiment 2 replicated the findings of Pomerantz et al. (1977). Importantly, the illusory-contour condition was still inferior to the triangle/arrow and even poorer than the now second-place line-alone context. A brief bit of introspection when examining Figure 25.2 indicates that the pacmanoid components seem to mask the closure cues and box structure which Pomerantz (1981) feels are important to the configural-superiority effects. We will return to this in Experiments 3, 4, and 5.

Experiment 3

In our first two experiments, one might object that the target line was not really part of the illusory context. After all, the illusory triangle produces a "whiter than white" figure and the target line is black. The target, therefore, might not be part of an analysis based on the closure of a lighter triangle. Experiment 3, therefore, tried to directly test whether a sense of closure in an illusory-contour figure could aid in a reaction time task. If closure is an emergent feature, we might find that the production of an illusory contour which is "closed" would aid in detecting an element which is necessary for the "closed" illusory contour to be visible.

The task was to detect the position of a dot which had the appearance of a "pacperson moving south," as one of the subjects so aptly

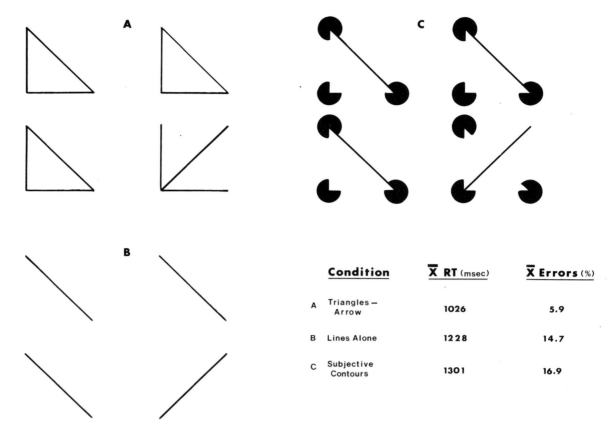

	Condition	$\overline{X}$ RT (msec)	$\overline{X}$ Errors (%)
A	Triangles — Arrow	1026	5.9
B	Lines Alone	1228	14.7
C	Subjective Contours	1301	16.9

FIGURE 25.2. Examples of stimulus displays used in Experiment 2. Target is the 45° line which was presented in all four positions. In the lower right corner are the mean reaction times and error rates for the stimuli. Display types: A. Triangles and arrows. B. Lines alone. C. Illusory contours. Ten subjects were tested.

put it. As seen in Figure 25.3, all stimuli had a top row of four dots. The subjects had to find the one with the cutout. In Figure 25.3A, the cutout leads to the production of an illusory triangle while the solid dots do not. Figure 25.3D is a dots-alone array. Figure 25.3B was to test if the alignment of the edges of the "pac-people" was an aid to detection even if the illusory contour was not present. Figure 25.3C represents a hollow dots-alone condition to control for the amount of black area present in the array.

Method

The subjects were now instructed to detect the cutout dot of the top row.

Results

The mean reaction times and error rates are presented in Figure 25.3. The dots-alone conditions did not significantly differ from each other but were faster and less prone to error than the context conditions ($p < .001$).

The hollow-contour and illusory-contour conditions did not differ significantly. Errors were again highly correlated with reaction time ($r = .99$, $df = 2$, $p < .005$).

Discussion

Obviously, the illusory contour continues to be a less than helpful part of the situation. It seems that if closure is produced by the subjective

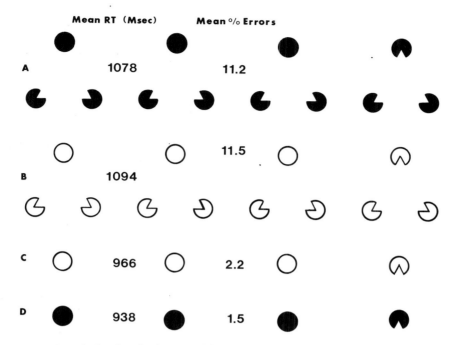

FIGURE 25.3. Examples of stimulus displays used in Experiment 3. The target is the "pacman facing south" in the upper row of four elements in (A) and (B) or in the row of four when presented alone as in (C) and (D). The target appeared in all four positions. Mean reaction times and error rates are presented in the first two positions. Display types: A. Illusory contours. B. Hollow contours. C. Hollow dots. D. Solid dots. Each dot was 0.22° in diameter and located on the apices of an equilateral triangle with 0.6° sides. The four target dots of the top row were equally spaced over 3.2°. Fifteen subjects were tested.

contour, it does not aid in detecting the target. One could conceptualize the task, when faced with the array in Figure 25.3A, as locating the illusory triangle. However, subjects, when questioned, said they explicitly tried to ignore the context as it distracted them! If closure aids in the Pomerantz arrow/triangle vs. line alone task, it does not help if the closure cue is "illusory." In all of our experiments, the illusory-contour conditions were equivalent to controls.

Several reasons are possible for the failure of the illusory contour to produce a configural superiority effect. There is evidence that illusory contours take time to form and are not immediately available for at least 100 msec or perhaps longer (see Petry & Gannon, chap. 21, this volume; Rock & Anson, 1979; Von Grünau, 1979; Gellatly, 1980). Thus, in our task, the illusory contour might not "be there" to aid in line detection. While this is an attractive explanation, it does not predict that the illusory-contour conditions would be worse than the line-alone con-

ditions. If the contour isn't there, why not just use the targets themselves? Obviously, this was not done as the illusory contours were slower than lines alone. In all the control conditions, there seemed to be significant interference.

It has also been stated that the formation of illusory contours might be involved in a capacity-driven process (Pritchard & Warm, 1983). Perhaps the production of the contour would drain resources from target detection and slow it down. This would be congruent with the increase in errors, which suggests an interference with the detection process. One could also suggest that the subjects are waiting for the subjective context "to come in," as in a horserace, and hold in abeyance the processing of the target. At this point, feeling a need to respond, they may choose on the basis of an incomplete or faulty target analysis. This would also increase times and errors (Pachella, 1974). Delay of response might occur if the subject is forced to wait for a sense of closure due to the subjective contour activating Pomerantz's closed channel, although this seems rather stretched to us.

We find the attentional hypothesis to be the more appealing of the two but neither is satisfactory. Recall that in all three experiments, the illusory contours were equally as bad as the control conditions which did not produce any contours! This suggests that the problem lies not in the illusory-contour formation process but in some other aspect of these contexts.

Texture Segregation: Experiments 4 and 5

In our first three experiments, it seems that the illusory-contour conditions were producing some sort of interference. Looking at our stimuli, we were impressed at the perceptual regularity or texturelike quality that the contour-inducing elements gave to the display. Perhaps this quality interfered with target detection.

There has been a current resurgence in interest in texture segregation, as this ability may be related to preattentive visual processing and the definition of basic visual features (Julesz, 1980, 1981a, 1981b; Julesz & Bergen, 1983; Treisman & Gelade, 1980). The basic task is to see if an area of a stimulus stands out easily (or without the need for focal attention) from the rest of the stimulus.

Since texture detection seems such a powerful and early process, we felt it might be interfering with our task. One might consider detection of the target line in Experiments 1 and 2 and the pacman in Experiment 3 as similar to a texture task. Julesz (1981a, 1981b) has demonstrated texture segregation with an arrow and triangle texture. At one point, Julesz (1981b) felt the crucial cue to be closure, in agreement with Pomerantz (1981), but now he suggests the important difference is the number of line terminators, with the arrow having more than the triangle (Julesz, 1981a; Julesz & Bergen, 1983).

In our task, could texture interfere? Kimchi and Palmer's (1982) report suggests we have enough elements for our patterns to take on a textural quality. Work by Fox (1978) has demonstrated interference effects in texture segregation. In his Figure 6 (p. 30), an orientation-

based texture is eliminated by surrounding the elements with a circle. Fox's Figure 9 (pp. 44–45) shows that an orientation-based texture can be masked by a superimposed texture of dots which are in close proximity to the texture's elements. Similarly, Callaghan, Lasaga, and Garner (1986) report that variations in hue can disrupt an orientation-based texture segregation. In our task, could the presence of the illusory contours' inducing elements and the other contexts be interfering?

In Experiment 4 we searched for a configural superiority effect in a texture segregation task based on 45° vs. 135° lines but with different contexts, some of which used Fox (1978) "camouflage" and some of which tested whether or not illusory contours by themselves would produce textural segregation. Our task was to have subjects rate the strength of the apparent texture or of the "pop out" effect (Beck, 1983).

It would be interesting if given time for illusory contours to develop, these contours would aid in the perceptual strength of a texture segregation. Something more complicated might be involved than a simple preattentive process if an illusion which seems to need focal attention (Meyer & Phillips, 1980; Pritchard & Warm, 1983; Rock & Anson, 1979) aided in texture segregation. Beck (1983) has reported that illusory-contour lines will enhance in texture segregation if they form a higher-order structure of lines across the texture. However, we are testing if discrete illusory-contour elements will segregate. These discrete elements should have a sense of closure as compared to the surrounding elements and perhaps a hint of depth segregation if the illusory-contour triangles are seen in front of the inducing elements.

Experiment 4

Five textures were developed to test for a configural superiority effect using illusory contours and to test for camouflage of one texture by another. The textures are presented in Figure 25.4.

The patterns were composed of a 2 by 2 element central patch containing 135° lines, surrounded by elements with 45° lines. Each pattern differed in the other components of the

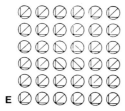

FIGURE 25.4. Texture stimuli used in Experiment 4: A. Hollow contours. B. Orientation. C. Arrow and triangle. D. Illusory contour. E. Arrow and triangle surrounded by circles. Each texture was presented to each subject on a separate sheet, with order randomized. Size of individual elements at average viewing distances was similar to that of the elements in the tachistoscopically presented displays in Experiments 1–3. Sixty subjects were tested. Subjects were pretrained on several textures that differed in clarity.

elements. Figure 25.4C was a texture segregation based on arrows and triangles, while 25.4B was composed of lines alone. These represented the basic elements of the original configuration superiority effects. Figure 25.4D was an illusory-contour version. Figure 25.4E used Fox's (1978) technique of surrounding circles to see if this would mask the texture segregation of arrows vs. triangles. Figure 25.4A (hollow contours) had edges similar to Figure 25.4D (illusory contours), but produced no apparent illusory triangles.

Results

The mean ratings are presented in Figure 25.5. There was a significant effect of texture type ($p < .001$). It was found that the lines-alone texture and triangle/arrows did not differ significantly from each other but did from the illusory contour and hollow contour. These latter two were not significantly different from each other. However, the first four textures rated significantly higher than the last camouflaged texture.

Discussion

We have found that a texture segregation based on differences in orientation basically is "hurt" by contexts. Again, the illusory contour did not help. Given a free viewing situation with a non-timed response, subjects should have had enough time to construct the illusory contour such that the subjective triangle could aid in texture discrimination.

The results of the experiment suggest that the closure generated by an illusory contour did not act as a visual primitive and aid in the texture discrimination. Also, if the illusory contours gave an impression of depth stratification, it was not helpful, even though with other textures, depth is a powerful cue.

The next question is why is there so much interference in these textures. As seen in Figure 25.5, the powerful triangles and arrows texture was much weakened by surrounding the elements with circles, essentially replicating Fox (1978). The illusory contours and hollow contours were also not as strong.

The reason probably lies in the processes involved in a texture segregation. It is clear that extra elements or uncorrelated stimulus variation can disturb the ease of texture segregation (Fox, 1979; Callaghan et al., 1986). One can look at our possible causes of interference from several perspectives. First, the elements of the patterns which are not lines or arrows/triangles form a constant and homogeneous texture over the entire stimulus. One clearly sees a texture of circles, dots, or contour elements. The texture of lines or triangles/arrows has to be separated from this "solid" or undifferentiated texture. This may be hard to do and masks our target texture segregation. Second, surrounding each line or triangle/arrow element with a cir-

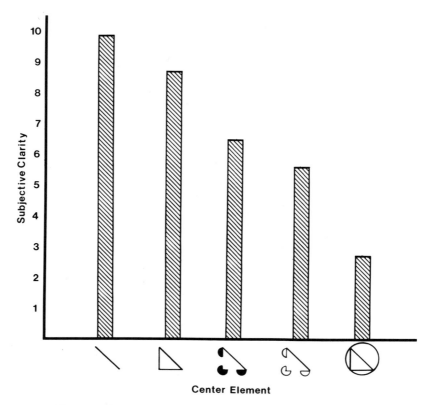

FIGURE 25.5. Mean ratings for the textures in Figure 25.4.

cle, dot, or contour pattern reduces the perceived difference between these elements. Enns and Prinzmetal (1984) feel such differences underlie the contextual superiority effects. Thus, if the strong appearance of the dots, circles, and inducing contours makes elements more similar, this would reduce the texture segregation. The illusory-contour condition may produce a triangle which might have aided in segregation by increasing perceived differences, but the inducing elements simultaneously could have reduced these differences. In the reaction time experiments, the dots and inducing contours increase similarity and destroy and context effect. The illusory triangle may not have had the time to form and could not aid in discrimination. Closure seemed not to be a powerful factor. It is possible that if it was used as a clue, it was masked by the surrounding elements. The circles surrounding the arrows/triangle texture were also devastating. The circles have their own sense of closure which may dilute the distinctiveness of the arrows closure. If the hypothetical closed chan-

nels of closure signal that closure exists across the whole texture, it may hard to pick out an added patch in the middle.

Experiment 5

The rationale of this experiment is similar to that of Experiment 3, which found the presence of an illusory contour did not aid in the detection of an element necessary for the perception of a closed illusory triangle. It would seem that closure did not help, nor did the presence of an illusory object. Perhaps this was due to there not being enough time for the illusory contour to form. If there was, closure and objectness might have aided.

There is another possibility based on target distinctiveness. In Experiment 3, the illusory-contour and hollow-target arrays have two out of three identical elements (see Fig. 25.3). The dot-alone targets have no common elements. Distinctiveness would predict the latter's better reaction times.

In this experiment, we attempted to test whether closure and its resultant objectness were more important than distinctiveness. Four textures were used (see Figure 25.6). The center of each was a four-element texture composed of various right triangles. The surround has no triangles. Figure 25.6D presents the clearest case. Four solid black triangles are surrounded by elements made of three solid dots at the apices of a similar but invisible triangle. Figure 25.6B represents an illusory contour version of the same. Figure 25.6C is a hollow-contour control. Figure 25.6A is the crucial test as it contains the illusory-contour center and surrounding elements made of the pacmen rotated so as to not form any illusory contours in the surround (any of which are seen take a long time to see and are extremely fragile). Obviously, we wanted to see if the illusory texture (25.6B) would be effective. It contains orientation differences and the presence of an illusory contour. The latter would add distinctiveness due to presence of the illusory triangle and also

would add closure as a clue. Also, the illusory contours might add brightness differences and a depth stratification. Both of these are potent cues for a texture segregation (Julesz & Bergen, 1983). The hollow contours control for the presence of the orientation differences between the center of the texture and the outside. Figure 25.6A is an important test as it contains the illusory contour's objects, depth, brightness, and closure. However, it may not be as distinct since the elements of the illusory contour out contain orientations similar to the center elements and are scattered around the outside. With a similar display, Rock & Anson (1979) found that a single illusory triangle was quite difficult to detect. It did not "pop out." If distinctiveness rather than an immediate appreciation of closure is important, we would predict that Figure 25.6A would be a poor texture.

Method

Testing was similar to Experiment 4.

Results

The means of the ratings were as follows:

Figure 25.6A—illusory contours surrounded by pacmen = 1.92.
Figure 25.6B—illusory contours surrounded by dots = 5.57.
Figure 25.6C—hollow contours surrounded by hollow dots = 4.24.
Figure 25.6D—triangles surrounded by dots = 8.04.

All means were significantly different from each other ($p < .01$).

It is no surprise that the solid triangle texture (Fig. 25.6D) had the highest clarity rating. The illusory-contour texture was next, although much lower in textural segregation. The question is whether the closure of the illusory contour had a major role or was it some other property of this display. Both the illusory-contour display and the hollow-contour display contained the same orientation information but the former was rated as stronger. However, closure does not seem to be the crucial factor in light of the very low rating of Figure 25.6A. The center elements still contained the closure cue, if such is really generated by an illusory contour, but

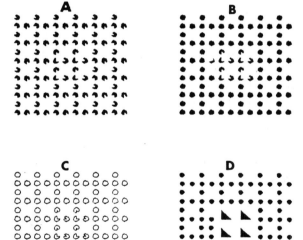

FIGURE 25.6. Textures used in Experiment 5. All have a center patch of four elements which differ from the surrounding ones. Display types: A. Illusory contours surrounded by pacman elements rotated so as to not produce a subjective triangle. B. Illusory contour surrounded by dots. C. Hollow contours surrounded by hollow dots. D. Solid triangles surrounded by solid dots. Forty-nine subjects were tested.

the similarity of the surrounding rotated pacmen destroyed texture segregation. This finding agrees with that of Rock and Anson (1979) that similar distractors make it quite difficult to appreciate the illusory contour. The closure is thus not preattentively apparent. We conclude that closure per se is not the factor operating in the illusory-contour texture. It seems more likely that if the illusory contour forms, its presence makes the center items more discriminable, and it is this factor that mediates the texture segregation. Enns (1986) found closure was a usable cue only if it was easily discriminable in a pattern.

General Discussion and Summary

The purpose of our study was to look for an equivalency between illusory contexts and real ones in the configural superiority effect. We did not find it. Instead, our reaction time and error measures found illusory-contour contexts to be hindrances. This led us to suspect an interference from the illusory-contour inducing elements. We investigated this with the texture segregation tasks and found some support for this idea. The numerous dotlike pacmen interfered with detecting the discrepant elements. Experiment 5 seemed to demonstrate that element discriminability is more important, in accord with Enns and Prinzmetal (1984). The idea of closure as a closed, preattentive, and early available channel was not strongly supported by our data. Perhaps, amodal completion of elements is accomplished quickly, as suggested by Brono and Gerbino (chap. 24, this volume) but the illusory contour seems to be available later (see Petry & Gannon, chap. 21). Our reaction times in a task requiring the analysis of the contour were significantly slower than Bruno and Gerbino's.

We did not find the illusory contour to be equivalent to the real contour. Theories which postulate such an equivalence need to take into account the differential times involved in processing both real and illusory surfaces and objects. If the construction of the illusory contour is thought to take place in the same neural loci as real-contour evaluation, there should be some rationale for the differences in temporal processing. The illusory contour was not an aid in reaction tasks or texture discrimination. Also, we found that texture segregation is not as easy and automatic as some suggest. Discriminability seems such an important factor (Enns, 1986) that our use of it to diagnose visual primitives must be used cautiously. Interference is certainly possible (Callaghan et al., 1986; Fox, 1979). We did not find that the depth, closure, brightness, or objectness induced by an illusory contour (Experiment 5) could act against the interfering context. These results also suggest that object superiority effects may not be a unique class of phenomena but must be considered in the light of texture segregation effects and the influences of similarity. The illusory contour seems important inasmuch as it is an objectlike construct but with temporal properties that enable us to probe some of the predictions made by theories of these processes.

SECTION VI
Illusory-Contour Appearance

Section VI, the final section, is concerned with the appearance of illusory contours in laboratory and applied settings.

Chapter 26, by Coren, Porac, and Theodor, discusses the role of perceptual and cognitive set in the appearance of illusory contours.

In Chapter 27, Gerbino and Kanizsa argue against a cognitive constructionist model of illusory contours and in favor of a perceptual organization product view. They present new and counterintuitive examples of illusory contours based on assimilation and amodal completion.

In Chapter 28, Kennedy describes a series of experiments on the apparent illusory quality of subjective contours and stimulus conditions under which this bicamerality exists. The results are discussed in terms of possible physiological and perceptual mechanisms.

Chapter 29, by Gellatly and Bishop, describes changes in perception of illusory contours through training procedures analagous to skill acquisition. They compare the process to reading and discuss theoretical implications.

In Chapter 30, Gillam discusses the role of perceptual grouping and illusory-contour salience. She points out that illusory contours are frequently seen under conditions of poor rather than good perceptual grouping.

Chapter 31, the final chapter in the book, by Nicholas Wade, extends illusory contours into the realm of cognition, art, and appearance. Wade describes and depicts illustrations he calls *allusory* contours, since the images invoked depend on and interrelate cognitive and perceptual processes.

CHAPTER 26

Set and Subjective Contour

Stanley Coren, Clare Porac, and Leonard H. Theodor

The perception of contours usually results from the presence of sharp local gradients in luminance or wavelength. This volume is, as you know, oriented toward an understanding of the set of stimulus arrays in which lines or edges appear to the observer despite the absence of such physical stimulus variations. These illusory demarcations have been called *subjective contours,* to distinguish them from *objective contours,* which are percepts associated with measurable physical modulations in the stimulus.

As is typical of most instances of perceptual illusion, many different hypotheses have been offered to explain the existence of subjective contours. Also, analogous to the study of visual illusions is the fact that all of these theories may be classified under two general rubrics: the first subsumes a number of *structural* or *physiological* mechanisms, while the second includes *cognitive mechanisms* or *judgmental strategy* mechanisms.

Physiological Theories

In the more physiologically oriented set of theories we find a number of processes suggested. For example, since most subjectively contoured figures also show systematic brightness effects, the same mechanisms which account for brightness contrast have been invoked to explain findings by Brigner and Gallagher (1974), Coren and Theodor (1977), Day and Jory (1978, 1980), Frisby and Clatsworthy (1975), and Jory and Day (1979). Other investigators have suggested that subjective contours

arise from the interactions among the receptive fields of orientation-specific cortical cells (e.g., Jung; 1973; Jung & Spillman, 1970; Kennedy, 1979; Smith & Over, 1975, 1979), or that they are due to Fourier analysis processes in the visual system (Becker & Knopp, 1978; Ginsburg, 1975). As a class, though, these structural theories have not fared as well as might be hoped. Thus, there are difficulties with brightness contrast explanations since objectively contoured figures which ought to maximize brightness contrast do not produce similar effects (Coren & Theodor, 1975). Furthermore, several investigators have presented subjective figures in the absence of subjective brightness differences (Parks, 1980a; Spillman & Redies, 1981; Ware, 1980). Edge detector interactions seem unlikely since blurring often improves the strength of these effects (Spillman, 1975). The Fourier analysis argument has been weakened by the fact that in some figures subjective contours can be observed which do not correspond with the theoretically relevant low spatial frequency component (Parks & Pendergrass, 1982).

Cognitive Theories

The class of cognitive or judgmental theories which have been offered in juxtaposition to the physiologically based processes also form a rather varied group. For example, Kanizsa (1974, 1976) suggests that illusory contours arise because of the operation of a principle analogous to the Gestalt Law of Closure. Other theorists view the perception of the subjectively contoured figure as some form of problem solving or unconscious inference. Accordingly, the figure is "derived" or "abstracted" from inferences provided by the partial figural cues present in the stimulus arrays, in much the same manner that meaningful configurations are extracted from incomplete outline drawings or cartoons (Bradley & Dumais, 1975; Gregory, 1972; Kennedy, 1976a,b; Piggins, 1975; Rock & Anson, 1979).

A rather specific cognitive theory has been suggested by Coren (1972). He noted that most subjective-contour inducing figures contain implicit depth cues. Thus, Figure 26.1a contains implicit interposition cues, consistent with a white square interposed in front of four black circles (with its corners resting on them), and also interposed in front of the set of intersecting black lines. He also presented a number of other configurations in which depth cues could be used to produce subjective contours, such as 26.1b, which forms a horizontal subjective edge through the use of texture gradients, or 26.1c, where shadowing is used to create the subjective contours outlining the word FEET. According to Coren's hypothesis, the subjective contours emerge when the observer perceptually reorganizes the configuration according to these cues. The resultant three-dimensional percept is simpler, in measurable information content, than the actual two-dimensional array. While some support for this theoretical position comes from informal observations that subjec-

tive contours are almost invariably accompanied by the impression of segregation of the array into several levels of depth, data from more formal research also tends to support this theory. Some indirect measures, based upon placing targets on or beside illusory figures have shown that size constancy can be triggered by the apparent depth in subjective contour arrays (Coren, 1972; Porac, 1978). Other investigators directly manipulated the depth cues in a stereoscopic paradigm. When the subjective-contour arrays were presented in a stereoscope, in the presence of binocular disparity cues which were in opposition to the implicit depth cues in the pattern, the subjective contours tended to disappear, as would be expected if the organization of the array into depth was vital to the etiology of the illusory figure (Gregory & Harris, 1974; Lawson, Cowan, Gibbs, & Whitmore, 1974; Whitmore, Lawson, & Kozora, 1976). A first attempt at a more direct measure of the apparent depth segregation of subjective contour arrays comes from Halpern (1981), who had her subjects reproduce the apparent depth between the illusory figure and its background by marking off a length on a ruled horizontal line. The most direct measures come from Coren and Porac (1983), who used a binocularly seen point of light, adjustable in depth from the observer. This point of light was superimposed upon the subjectively contoured figure or upon the background. The results indicate that in

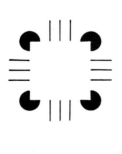
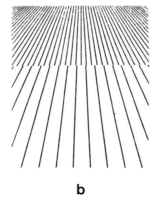
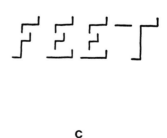

a   b   c

FIGURE 26.1a. A subjective-contour square due to the presence of implicit interposition cues for depth. b. The edge of the apparent cliff is a subjective contour caused by the texture gradient cues, suggesting a shift in apparent depth between the planes (after Coren, 1972). c. The word FEET appearing as subjectively contoured letters caused by the implicit depth cue of shadowing (after Coren, 1972).

those configurations which they measured, whenever there was a subjective contour present, there was also the correspondingly predicted difference in apparent depth.

Perceptual Set and Subjective Contours

In addition to the formal theories suggesting the operation of cognitive mechanisms that we noted above, other lines of evidence have suggested that some well-known perceptual–cognitive processes, such as perceptual set, may also play a role in the appearance of subjective contours. The word *set* is used in a number of different contexts in psychology. Generally speaking it refers to an acquired, often temporary, condition that predisposes an individual toward a particular response or class of responses. A simple example of one form of mental set can be demonstrated by reading the following string of words aloud:

MACBETH, MACARTHUR, MACINTOSH,
MACDILLON, MACCARTHY, MACDOWELL,
MACKENZIE, MACDONALD, MACCLINTOCK,
MACHINES

Now look back at the next to the last word.

Did you succumb to the mental set given by the context and pronounce it Mac Hines? In the absence of the induced set you most certainly would have used the more familiar and common word *machines* (Coren, 1984). Your prior history with the early part of the list induces a set which tends to predispose you to organize each of the inputs into two components (Mac + something). In the perceptual realm, sets to organize the array into objects or arrays varying in depth might induce the perception of subjective contours as well.

Although Coren (1974) noted the possible operation of set in some subjective-contour figures, most of the observations which support this contention are rather anecdotal, or based upon self-evident reasoning. For example, consider again Figure 26.1c, where we see the subjectively contoured word FEET. It is highly unlikely that an individual who is unfamiliar with the English alphabet would see this configuration as anything other than a collection of black lines.

An interesting classroom demonstration can be constructed which demonstrates the operation of perceptual set on the appearance of subjective contours. If a naive group of individuals is shown the configuration depicted in Figure 26.2a and asked to describe what they see, most

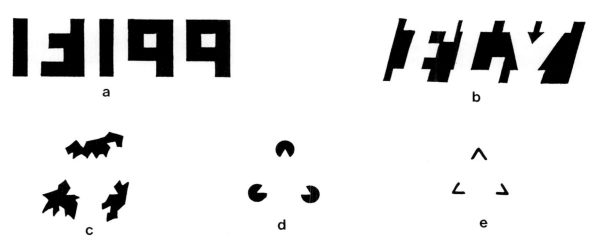

FIGURE 26.2. The configuration in (a) does not usually cause a report of a subjectively contoured word (FILL) unless subjects are first "set" to see subjective letters by a series of subjective-contoured words such as (b), where the word FLY is seen. Similarly, (c) is a figure which subjects seldom spontaneously see as a subjectively contoured triangle unless set to do so by seeing a series of subjectively contoured figures such as (d). In (e), an inverted (point down) subjective triangle may be seen if the set is strong enough.

will give response in which they indicate a string of black figures, namely, a 1 followed by an inverted F, then the numbers 199. If they are next given a series of subjectively contoured letter strings, such as the familiar one shown in Figure 26.2b, which depicts the word FLY, and then they are again given Figure 26.2a to view, they will readily see the subjectively contoured word FILL. Presumably, this shift occurs because they are now *set* to see subjectively contoured letters, which they were not set for initially.

Informal Evidence

There are numerous casual examples of the interaction between perceptual set and the appearance of subjective contours which might be mentioned. Several have already been mentioned in the previous section. One anecdotal example deals with a configuration first presented by Coren (1972), which is depicted as Figure 26.2c. Most naive observers, when shown this configuration in isolation do not see any subjectively contoured figure here, although the angle elements needed to produce a subjective triangle are in fact present. It is interesting to note that, if the observer is first "set" for the perception of subjective contours by viewing a series of configurations such as Figure 26.2d, or those shown later in this chapter as Figures 26.5b or 26.5c, many report seeing the subjective triangle in Figure 26.2c quite spontaneously. In addition, such set may lead to the reporting of subjective figures in arrays which virtually never produce unprompted reports of subjective contours, such as Figure 26.2e. Coren reports that he was quite surprised, upon receiving reviews for his 1972 paper, that one referee noted the perception of an inverted subjective triangle in this configuration. Although he himself had never detected this subjective figure before, when it was pointed out to him by the referee's comments, it did become quite visible. Coren now notes that it is virtually impossible for him to view this array now without seeing the subjectively contoured figure. There is an interesting followup to this tale. At a subjective-contour conference, held at Adelphi University in 1985 (Petry &

Meyer, 1986), Coren told this story and demonstrated a number of similar set effects. His paper was followed shortly thereafter by another paper which used a series of outline figures, all constructed on the same principle as Figure 26.2e as control figures in which no subjective contours were expected to be seen. Unfortunately, since the audience had now been "set" to see subjective contours in such arrays, there was a bit of an undercurrent of conversation during the talk, as one researcher or another nudged his neighbor to point out the now visible configurations, which, of course, were never seen by subjects in the experiment being described since they had not been set to do so.

Most of the existing demonstrations of the effect of perceptual set on the appearance of subjective contours are as informal and anecdotal as those presented above (e.g., Landauer, 1978; Parks, 1984). If the effects are reliable, one would expect them to be demonstrable under laboratory conditions. Therefore, in order to provide some formal experimental measures of the operation of set on the appearance of subjective contours we conducted a pair of experiments, which we will briefly describe below.

Experiment 1: Set and the Shape of Subjective Contours

The first experiment attempted to ascertain whether the shape of subjectively contoured figures could be altered by variations in the observer's viewing set. As a starting point, it was necessary to find some configuration in which the perceived illusory figure was not as unambiguously defined as in the typically used configurations. An example of one such array is seen in the variant of a pattern offered by Ehrenstein (1941), shown in Figure 26.3a. Here observers frequently report the appearance of white circles at the point where the lines should intersect. Such an appearance is not, however, always the case. Occasionally, an observer will report that the shape of the figure at the intersection is a square, rather than a circle. Frequently, however, observers report nothing but a set of broken dashed lines. Usually, when the experimenter points out or suggests the exis-

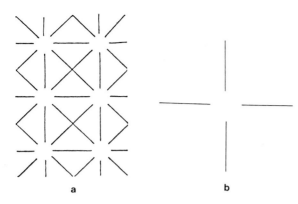

a   b

FIGURE 26.3a. A series of white subjective circles is usually reported in this figure (after Ehrenstein, 1941). b. A minimal configuration for the perception of a subjective contour, in which the seen shape may be either a circle, square, or amorphous light blob, used as the stimulus in the first experiment.

tence of some figures at the intersection, most observers readily reorganize the percept and report the existence of a white, subjectively bounded circle overlapping the intersections of the lines. The fact that many observers require prompting before they report a subjective contour in this configuration is in itself interesting and tends to support the operation of perceptual set in this context. Let us consider the simplest possible inducing configuration for the appearance of a subjective contour which can be extracted from this array. This would be similar to Figure 26.3b. In this configuration we have two alternative perceptual organizations of the array. In the first, we can see four short unitary line elements arranged along the horizontal and vertical axes. In the second we can see two continuous line segments which orthogonally intersect one another, with some white subjectively contoured figure interposed in front of the intersection. If the perceptual organization adopted is the latter, there is not sufficient information in the array to specify the shape of the occluding figure. It could just as well as be a circle, square, diamond, or merely an amorphous blob. Cognitive processing theories of subjective contours would maintain that the specific form of the figure which phenomenally appears to the observer should depend upon particular assumptions which the observer makes in viewing the configuration. Of course,

physiologically based, neural interactive theories should maintain that the shape and phenomenal appearance of the subjectively bounded figure should be independent of the viewing set of the observer.

The stimulus configuration which we used is shown in Figure 26.3b. To induce the various perceptual sets, each stimulus was preceded by a cover sheet containing one of three versions of the following set-inducing instruction:

On the following page you will see a pattern composed of four black lines and a central area. Look at the central area carefully. Many people report seeing a white *figure* in that region. If you see any white figure after studying the figure for a few moments, outline the figure with your pen or pencil. If you can't see the white figure after looking at the pattern for a few moments, check the space provided in the lower right-hand corner of the next page.

The above instruction was designed for the group in which no specific figural set was induced. The other two versions of the instruction sheet differed only in the substitution of a single word. The one occurrence of the word *figure,* which we have italicized in the above instruction (but not in the actual test stimuli), could be replaced with either the word *square* or *circle*. Thus, the observer could either receive a neutral set for a subjective figure at the locus of the intersection of the lines or a specific set for a square or a circle. In addition, a space was provided on the lower right-hand corner of the page, reading, "Check here if you see nothing."

A total of 161 undergraduate volunteers participated in this experiment. Each received only one form of the set instruction and each produced only a single response. Each response was then classified as a circle, a square, amorphous (which included generally "blob" types of figures), or no figure seen. The square category included both outline squares drawn with the bottom line parallel to the edge of the page or squares rotated 45° to form a diamond-like configuration, since no particular orientation of the square had been set in the instructions. The data are presented in Figure 26.4.

Inspection of Figure 26.4 clearly indicates that instructional set interacts with the shape of the subjectively contoured figure seen, and these differences are statistically reliable. It is

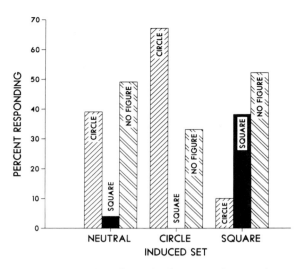

FIGURE 26.4. Data from the first experiment, showing the effect of set on the perception of subjectively contoured figures. Note how the percentages of the seen figures are shifted in the direction of the induced set.

interesting to note that when observers are set merely to see a subjective contour via the neutral instruction, without any specification of what the particular contour is, approximately half (49%) of the observers do not report seeing any figure at all in this minimal array. Of those who do see a subjective figure, the majority of these (39% of the total sample, or 76% of those who see any subjective contour figure at all) report the perception of a circle. When the set is specific for the perception of a circle, the number of reported percepts of a circular subjective contour significantly increases to 67% of the entire sample, thus actually comprising 100% of all those who see any illusory figure in this group, while the proportion of observers reporting no perception of any figure at all is significantly reduced from 49% in the neutral set group, to 33% in this group. On the other hand, when the observer is set for the perception of a square, the number of circle responses is drastically reduced (relative to the neutral set) to only 10% of the sample with a concomitant increase in the number of square responses to 38% of the total sample, or 79% of all the subjects reporting any illusory figure. The increase in the square responses is made even more noticeable, given the fact that this response is minimally present under the neutral set, and totally

absent for the circle set. Thus, it seems clear that if an observer sees a subjective contour in the test stimulus, the subjective contour which he sees is apt to be one which he was set to see. Such a result is consistent with a cognitive processing interpretation of subjective contours; however, it is not particularly in accord with expectations from neural interactive theories which would maintain that the specific pattern seen is predetermined by the nature of the neural or inhibitory interactions.

Experiment 2: An Indirect Measure

While the results of Experiment 1 seem to convincingly associate the apparent shape of a subjective contour with set effects (at least where the subjective shape allows several possibilities), it might be argued that the manipulation is "too strong." Because in the set induction we said, "Many people see a white (figure)," a certain percentage of individuals might respond that they saw the figure, merely on the basis of social or response conformity. Although informal interviews with a subsample of the subjects suggests that they actually did "see" the figure that they were set to see, we felt that a more indirect form of set induction and a more indirect dependent measure would provide a reassuring cross-validation of the results of the above experiment.

An indirect assessment of the effects of set is possible since, as we noted earlier in this chapter, there is both direct and indirect evidence that the appearance of subjective contours is also accompanied by a segregation of the array into depth, with the subjective contour apparently displaced forward, in front of the background (e.g., Coren, 1972; Coren & Porac, 1983; Halpern, 1981; Porac, 1978). We therefore decided to use this depth separation as a dependent variable to measure the effects of set on the emergence of subjective contour, using some techniques for the direct assessment of apparent depth in such arrays which was first introduced by Coren and Porac (1983).

To do this, we first selected a somewhat stronger configuration than the one shown in Figure 26.3b. This array, introduced by Ken-

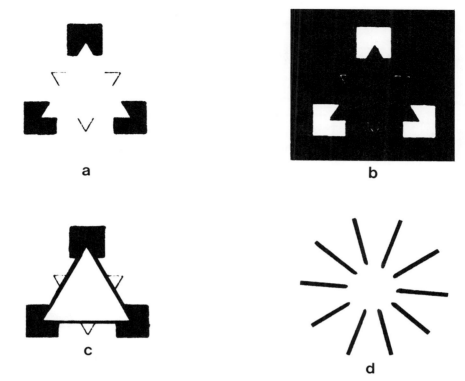

a

b

c

d

FIGURE 26.5a. a and b. Subjective-contour triangles (after Coren, 1972). c. An objective triangle pattern (after Porac, 1976). d. A subjective-contour pattern which may be seen as a circle (after Kennedy, 1978b). All served as stimuli in Experiment 2, and were presented in the order given here.

nedy (1978b), has eight lines (Fig. 26.5d) instead of four, and tends to produce the perception of a white circle interposed on a starburst of lines. However, a sizeable number of observers require prompting to see this.

The apparatus used was similar to that of other investigators attempting to assess apparent depth in parts of configurations (Coren & Festinger, 1967; Gregory, 1966; Kilbride & Leibowitz, 1975) and has been directly used on subjective-contour arrays by Coren and Porac (1983). In essence, the procedure involves the superimposition of a binocularly viewed target on a monocularly viewed stimulus pattern whose depth characteristics one would like to assess. The binocular target, which can be adjusted in apparent depth, can be imaged over any component of the figure. The observer's task is simply to set the adjustable binocular target until it is at the same phenomenal depth as the portion of the stimulus array upon which it is imaged. The actual apparatus used is shown in Figure 26.6a.

Stimuli were prepared as slides and projected upon a rear projection screen. Mounted in front of the screen was a sheet of polarizing material. The image of the adjustable depth spot was reflected to the observer's eyes by means of a half-silvered mirror, through which the polarized monocular stimulus pattern was also visible. A pair of orthogonally oriented Polaroid filters was placed in the viewing port, which allowed the subjective-contour inducing stimuli to be seen by only one eye, while the spot was seen by both eyes. The observer varied the apparent distance of the binocular spot, and the projected distance of the spot provided the measurement of apparent depth directly in millimeters. To determine the apparent difference in depth between the subjectively contoured figure and the background, the spot was imaged on the figure 1° to the inside of the apparent subjective contour (the location marked F in Fig. 26.6b), or to the outside of the subjective contour (the location marked B in Fig. 26.6b) for each figure used.

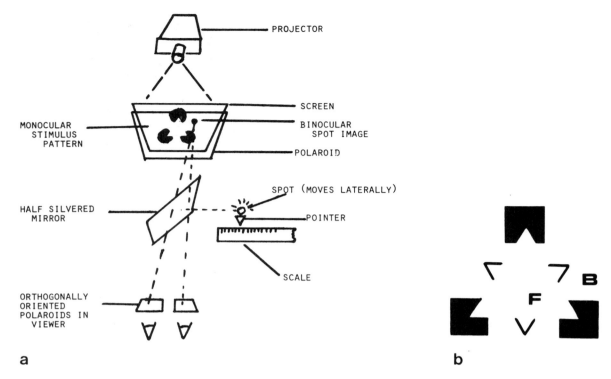

a   **b**

FIGURE 26.6a. The apparatus used to measure the
apparent depth of parts of the subjective-contour figure through superimposition of an adjustable binocular marker on a monocularly seen stimulus. b. The

placement of the test stimuli could either be on the
figure in the locus marked *F* or on the background in
the locus marked *B*.

The set induction was indirectly provided by
context in this study. For the subjects in whom
there was to be no set induced, only the test
figure (Fig. 26.5b) was presented, and measurements of the relative apparent depth of the figure and the background were taken. For the
group in whom set was induced, a real-contour
figure (Figure 26.5a) was first presented, followed by two subjective-contour figures (26.5b
and 26.5c). The subjects made the same depth
judgments on each of these arrays as they
would make for the test figure (Fig. 26.5b). The
prior presentation of subjective-contour figures
should "set" the observer for the perception of
a subjective-contour figure, which should then
manifest itself in the appearance of an apparent
depth segregation between illusory figure and
background. Twenty subjects served in the no-
set condition, and 20 in the set-induction sequence.

First, it is important to assure ourselves that
the technique used is sensitive enough to moni-

tor apparent depth differences. Using this apparatus, we confirmed the findings of Coren and
Porac (1983) in that for both of the subjective-
contour figures (Figs. 26.5b and 26.5c), the illusory contour was seen as closer than the background. These results were statistically
significant, thus replicating Coren and Porac's
(1983) direct measurement of depth segregation
in subjective-contour arrays.

When we turn to the results on Figure 26.5d
as a function of set induction we see that they
are quite straightforward. For the group in
which there was no set induction there is no
significant apparent depth segregation. Informal
interviews with the subjects further supported
the absence of any appearance of an illusory
figure for nearly half of the subjects. For the
group which had the figure presented in the context of other subjective-contour figures and
hence were set for the appearance of subjective
contours, there was a significant difference between the apparent depth of the subjectively

contoured figure and its background. Furthermore, the subjective reports of the observers confirmed that virtually all of this group did have the experience of an illusory figure.

Despite the fact that this study used an indirect measure, it clearly confirms the operation of set upon the perception of subjective contours. This replicates the findings of the previous study, and suggests that cognitive influences play a role in subjective-contour formation.

Cognitive Factors and Subjective-Contour Perception

Let us now look back and assess the relative contribution of cognitive mechanisms to the perception of subjective contours. The two new studies briefly described above seem to produce a pattern of results which confirm the anecdotal and informal observations that perceptual set (a clearly cognitive process) does interact with the appearance of subjective contours. The first experiment utilized a rather explicit set induction and found that the apparent shape of the illusory figure can be influenced by set in an ambiguous subjective-contour inducing array. The second experiment was more subtle, both in set induction and in the dependent variable used. Here, set was induced by presenting an array in the context of other configurations which produce salient subjective contours. The dependent measure was the appearance of segregation of the array into depth, directly measured using the procedures of Coren and Porac (1983). Again, the influence of set manifested itself clearly in the formation of the subjective figure and its secondary perceptual effects.

These results do have theoretical implications about the nature of the processes underlying the perception of subjective contours. A structural or physiological interpretation of subjective contours does not provide the degree of flexibility needed to explain these results. Certainly, no one would reasonably predict that interactions between orientation-specific receptors, lateral inhibitory effects, or the low-frequency components of the Fourier analysis of the patterns would change as a function of the observer's set or expectations. Thus the more structural explanations, which already

seem to have been producing somewhat mixed results as we noted above, seem to be a bit less plausible in light of these data. This is not to say that such physiological factors do not play a role at some level of analysis. Coren and Girgus (1978) have demonstrated that most illusory phenomena have both cognitive *and* physiological contributions which contribute at different levels of visual processing. Rather, this is to suggest that such physiological mechanisms do not play the *primary* causal role in subjective-contour formation.

While these results are quite consistent with cognitive explanations of subjective-contour formation, and difficult to explain in any other terms, they, unfortunately, do not allow us to clearly differentiate among the various theoretical positions. Those who maintain that the achievement of the subjective contour is a form of problem solving or unconscious inference, those who view it as a form of Gestalt closure, and those who feel that subjective contours arise from the reorganization of the configuration on the basis of implicit depth cues can all reasonably accommodate the operation of perceptual set. Set may certainly manifest itself as a predisposition to see objects, to segregate the field into depth planes, or to cognitively close complex arrays into a simpler integrated organization.

At the very least, data such as these demonstrate that the operation of perceptual set in the form of a simple cognitive variable, whose characteristics are influenced by the subject's prior experiences, expectations, and predispositions. Perceptual set may be influenced by either short-term (contextual) or long-term (life history) factors. The fact that such a variable may influence the appearance of subjective contours seems to strengthen the position of all those theorists who ascribe the perception of these illusory figures to higher level cognitive processing.

Acknowledgments. Names of the authors are listed in alphabetical order. This research was supported, in part, by grants from the Natural Sciences and Engineering Research Council of Canada. The authors would like to thank Miriam Blum-Steele and Susan Dixon for their assistance in data collection and manuscript preparation.

CHAPTER 27

Can We See Constructs?

Walter Gerbino and Gaetano Kanizsa

The Place of Illusory Figures in Perceptual Theory

Most empirical evidence about illusory figures was collected in order to show that the phenomenon is better understood within one side of some fashionable dichotomy: as sensory vs. cognitive, peripheral vs. central, or bottom-up vs. top-down. The heuristic value of such a binary mode of thinking is often demonstrated by discoveries of new instances of the phenomenon and by ramifications of research about its determinants.

However, to what extent has this experimental effort contributed to the general understanding of perception? Ultimately, this is the important question. We will argue that illusory figures may be crucial in deciding between basic models of perceptual functioning. Years and years of analytical investigation have shown that illusory figures are less illusory than is perhaps suggested by their name. They are a stable phenomenon, which claims for a meaningful place in perceptual theory.

Preliminarily, let us raise a phenomenological point. Sometimes (for instance, see Pomerantz, Goldberg, Golder, & Tetewsky, 1981) an illusory triangle is described as a way of "depicting" a triangle. The underlying assumption—that illusory figures belong more to pictorial vision than to ordinary seeing—is rather popular, and seems to be supported by some empirical findings (Kennedy, 1979). However, this assumption may rely on a particular kind of stimulus error. Because the effect is generally obtained by pictorial means, one tends to argue that it is peculiar to pictorial vision. The argument is misleading because pictorial vision, properly speaking, involves the double awareness of both a represented object and the means supporting its representation. But any good instance of an illusory figure is not perceived as a depiction (Parks, chap. 8, this volume).

One may legitimately claim that an outline triangle depicts a real triangular surface, because line drawings are a symbolic way of rendering shape; but an "illusory" triangle does not refer to any another triangle. Hence, illusory figures are better described as "real" objects produced by pictorial means than as pictorial effects.

In this sense, they do not stand alone. Other illusions of reality can be obtained under pictorial conditions, for instance, by using linear perspective (Metzger, 1953; Michotte, 1962). Metzger's example, shown in Figure 27.1, which is a modification of an old demonstration by Ladd-Franklin (1887), makes evident the contrast between *represented* and *experienced* three-dimensional space, within the domain of paper-and-ink artefacts. Analogously, the existence of illusory figures makes evident the contrast between a *depicted shape* and a *shaped surface*.

By this fundamental distinction, illusory figures can be qualified as phenomenally real objects. Such an experience of reality is weakly sustained by external constraints, whereas most of the time object perception is strongly sustained by the stimulus. Here is the epistemo-

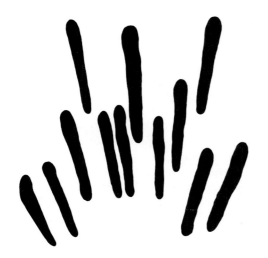

FIGURE 27.1. Metzger's demonstration that pictorial stimuli may generate an illusion of reality. Rods are perceived as standing up when viewed monocularly, from a point near their locus of convergence. (After Metzger, 1953.)

logical relevance of the phenomenon. We are confident that the internal constraints revealed by the study of illusory figures belong to normal functioning of the perceptual system.

The Energetic vs. Informational Dichotomy

In some respect, previously mentioned dichotomies are fundamentally equivalent. All share a common two-factor model where cognitive, central, top-down processes, in one word "the mind," interact with sensory, peripheral, bottom-up processes, in one word "the matter."

It is remarkable that so far illusory figures have been resisting a unilateral explanation, based upon only one side of any of such dichotomies. This is the reason why most students of perception are now admirably tolerant and maintain an eclectic position. But when truth is in the middle, then a dichotomy becomes of little use.

Therefore, for the sake of discussion we will propose another dichotomy, which contrasts energetic vs. informational models. Then we will discuss empirical evidence showing that

what is unique to illusory figures supports only one side of it, the energetic one.

In energetic models, object properties are constrained by laws, i.e., normative principles embodied in natural events, whose teleological interpretation has only a metaphorical value. In informational models, object properties are defined by rules, symbolic devices that control admissible goal-directed operations.

We believe that distinctive features of illusory figures are better understood within an energetic model than within an informational model and that these features constitute typical instances of Gestalt-like properties, i.e., they emerge as a result of spontaneous organizational tendencies acting upon the distribution of forces generated by stimulation. We will stress that they are directly constrained by energy parameters, such as luminance, retinal topography, and retinal size. Obviously, we admit that these constraints can be indirectly represented by rules, corresponding to propositional formulations of natural laws. But this is a different matter, common to all scientific areas.

According to the cognitive view, perceptual processing is the building up of a structural description of the external world, triggered by stimuli, formulated in mentalese, and controlled by parsing rules. While this is nice, it sounds rather abstract. Given their phenomenal character of materiality, why should ordinary percepts not be conceived as "physical" products, constrained by natural laws?

We are suggesting here that illusory figures do not result from visual processing at the semantic level. They may tell us something about the level in which visual units come into existence, a level logically presupposed by the semantic one. In other words, the properties of illusory figures are the product of a noninterpretive, nonfinalistic level, in which the stimulus undergoes a particular lawful transformation.

Retinotopic Constraints on Clarity and Shape

A first evidence for an energetic model comes from the common observation that the clarity of an illusory figure is an inverse function of visual angle (Dumais & Bradley, 1976). Broadly speaking, in order to get a better effect one has to use small displays, or to view oversized displays at a distance. Otherwise, fragments of the illusory figure are visible near the inducers, but they do not reach each other; and beyond a given limit, with large visual angles, only a virtual shape is present, devoid of any modal character. The very existence of an illusory figure depends upon retinal size.

Clearly, arguing that the informational value of the stimulus configuration is affected by retinal size represents an ad hoc hypothesis. One can arbitrarily set the range whereby a given interpolating procedure is applicable, but the choice of any range cannot be easily justified by the claim that within it a given figural hypothesis is more plausible than another.

On the contrary, the influence of visual angle suggests that energetic constraints are present. The illusory figure behaves like an elastic substance under stretching. Despite constant informational plausibility, it lawfully varies in its phenomenal clarity and eventually disappears when an extreme condition is reached.

A direct effect of retinal distance upon shape can be observed in the simple X configuration shown in Figure 27.2. When the pictorial plane is frontal, the central illusory blob has a circular shape; when the picture is slanted, the illusory blob becomes elliptical. Contrary to what one would expect by slanting a physical disk, it is an ellipse having its major axis along the direction of slant (instead of its minor axis). As a conse-

quence of perspective, slanting destroys the central symmetry of line endings. When the picture is slanted around a frontal-horizontal axis, line-endings become projectively nearer along vertical than along horizontal directions, and the blob appears vertically elongated.

If illusory figures were postulated in order to account for occlusions in the outer world, then one should see an X pattern covered by either a constant circular disk or a deformed elliptical disk, corresponding to the projection of a physical disk seen at slant. Because the illusory figure apparently lies upon the slanted surface and looks elongated along the direction of slant, one must conclude that the shape of an illusory figure is not constrained by ratiomorphic constancy mechanisms. The illusory blob emerges, with its specific shape constrained by retinotopic factors, independently from any constructive perceptual hypothesis. Thus, it appears that only after its formation can the illusory blob be interpreted as an occluding surface.

The demonstration above allows us to appreciate how illusory figures continuously change when the whole picture is translated and rotated. But even more impressive results are obtained by manipulating the inducers. Kanizsa (1955a and chap. 4) described these elastic deformations in his original paper, and further work has been done by Bradley and co-workers (Bradley & Lee, 1982; Bradley, 1983).

In this respect, the role of dots is particularly interesting. We have been intrigued for years by the impressive influence of dots on the shape of the figure induced by the so-called Koffka cross (Day & Jory, 1978). By themselves, four dots generate only a virtual square, i.e., a pure shape without a modal surface character. However, when added to the cross configuration (within a well-defined range), they both increase the salience of the illusory figure and continuously modify it in an elegant and lawful manner (see Fig. 27.3).

Depending on the width of the arms of the cross, the central figure can be either a disk or a rounded square. Four symmetrical dots along the diagonals lead to the perception of a perfect square, as well as a whole family of concave squares, depending on the distance of the dots from the center of the figure. The phenomenon is well known, but nobody really understands why dots influence the perception in this way.

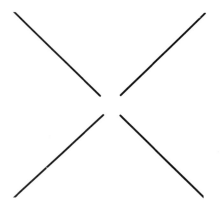

FIGURE 27.2. When the picture plane is frontal, the illusory blob is circular. When the picture plane is slanted, the blob becomes an ellipse with its major axis along the direction of slant.

FIGURE 27.3. The shape of the blob induced by the Koffka cross (on the left) is not well defined. Four dots alone make us perceive simply a virtual square. When the four dots are added to the cross, they define the shape of the blob in a precise manner.

Lines and solid regions—our conventional inducers—can always be interpreted as pieces of information about occlusion; dots cannot, unless they are conceived as very short lines. Do they actually work in this fashion?

Observations with a dynamic display, where subjects could control dot locations by a joy stick, suggest that they do not function as interposition cues. Observers were required to change the illusory shape by moving dots along diagonals, in an interactive computer animation. All observers described the event as one of pushing the contour outwards and braking its contraction inwards. The effect observed during outward motion is particularly compelling. Dots seem to come in contact with a point of the outer border of a rubber sheet, and exert an action on it. Therefore, they are phenomenally located *within* the illusory figure, not outside like conventional inducers, and appear to act as pivots.

This conclusion is supported also by precise static determinations of dot locations necessary to induce a perfectly rectilinear square. When dots are inside the square limits, one sees a perfect square. When dots are outside them, however, one sees a slightly concave square (see Fig. 27.4).

Thus, small elements tend to belong to the illusory figure, instead of being occluded by it. This fact, stressed also by Minguzzi (chap. 7, this volume), indicates that any ratiomorphic interpretation based on occlusion cannot fully explain the specific shape of the illusory figure.

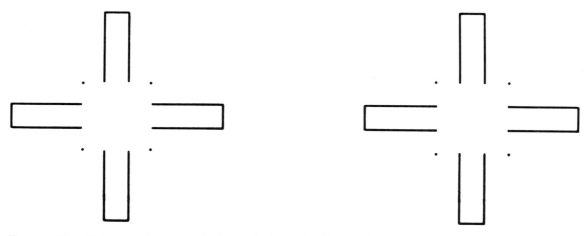

FIGURE 27.4. Dots are phenomenally located within the illusory figure. In fact, one perceives a perfect square when dots are inside the rectilinear corners defined by line endings (left cross), and a square with slightly curved sides when dots are outside them (right cross).

Such a conclusion is supported also by the observation that actually perceived shapes always represent a "minimal outcome," with respect to the infinite number of shapes that could account for a given set of gaps or interruptions—an outcome that, however, is severely limited by retinotopic factors.

The "Meaning" of Color Changes

Color changes observed in illusory figures are difficult to interpret. Several authors (Brigner & Gallagher, 1974; Day & Jory, 1978; Frisby & Clatworthy, 1975; Kennedy, 1979; Sambin 1985) have claimed that processes like assimilation, dissimilation, and contrast are basic to the perception of illusory figures. Despite this claim, some aspects of color changes remain obscure. Most researchers investigated patterns made of black inducers on white paper, and described the illusory figure as higher in brightness, lightness, whiteness, and thingness than the ground. All these attributes seem to go together. When one uses white inducers on black paper, the situation becomes more complex, because the illusory figure is usually described as "blacker but more brilliant." In the achromatic domain, color labeling is a discouraging business.

Hence, we tried to get some useful suggestions from chromatic displays. Beautiful and compelling examples of color changes are obtained in illusory "transparent" figures. Let us consider Figure 27.5. An empiricistic interpretation of transparency has trouble in explaining the central reddish square, because no physical

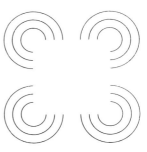

FIGURE 27.6. Line endings produce intensive contrast, but no chromatic induction. See color plate on page xvi.

filter can alter a green background and turn it into red. Therefore, it is difficult to consider this effect to be the product of a perceptual process of color splitting, conceived as the inverse of physical color mixing.

Assimilation, dissimilation, and contrast are better suited to explain the effect. But, do they refer to the qualitative component of color (hue and chroma), or to the intensive component (brightness or lightness)? The reddish square could be the effect of either chromatic assimilation to internal red arcs, or chromatic dissimilation induced by endings of external green arcs; but it could be also the joint effect of both.

Figure 27.6 suggests that green arcs modify the intensity of the central square, but do not exert any antagonistic chromatic induction. The background becomes slightly greenish because of chromatic assimilation, but the central square does not appear reddish (as one should expect on the basis of chromatic contrast or dissimilation).

Briefly, lines produce chromatic assimilation at their sides, and intensive contrast at their endings. This conclusion is supported also by the comparison of Figures 27.7 and 27.8. In both cases the red arcs produce chromatic assimilation within the central illusory square, which appears reddish. But in Figure 27.7 the central square appears dark because the sur-

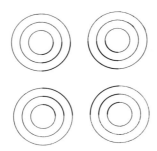

FIGURE 27.5. A reddish square in a greenish surrounding. Contrast or assimilation, or both? (Internal and external sectors are approximately isoluminant.) See color plate on page xvi.

FIGURE 27.7. Chromatic assimilation within the central square. See color plate on page xvi.

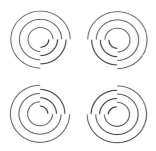

FIGURE 27.8. The central square is brighter than in Figure 27.7 because of intensive contrast, induced by green line endings. See color plate on page xvi.

rounding white area is brightened by red line endings, whereas in Figure 27.8 it appears bright because it undergoes intensive contrast by the green line endings.

The direct comparison of Figures 27.5 and 27.8 is instructive. Conditions for chromatic assimilation are the same in both cases. However, conditions for intensive contrast are absent in Figure 27.5, where there are no line endings. The central square in Figure 27.8 is reddish, but desaturated because of increased brightness.

Figure 27.5 could be considered to be an instance of perceptual transparency. Rather, we believe that it simply results from chromatic assimilation unaltered by brightness contrast, in conditions where the figural structure is preserved. The color change is independent from any attribution of "meaning" to the picture. The assimilated film does not emerge *because* one hypothesizes transparency in the picture and knows that, in reality, transparent media exhibit a film mode of appearance. More simply, physically transparent media—as well as pictorial displays that simulate them—produce optical arrays containing coherent color changes along a border, without abrupt line endings. This co-occurrence of color homogeneity of elements within the same region and absence of line endings sets the conditions for chromatic assimilation without brightness contrast.

We See Products, Not Constructs

Within an informational model, illusory figures are crucial illustrations that the mind is constructive not only at the conceptual level, but also at the perceptual level. According to this approach, perceptual hypotheses acquire the phenomenal character of external reality, when stimuli do not contradict them. In this instance, we see our mental constructions. Hence, the theoretical significance of illusory figures is very broad indeed.

Clearly, illusory figures are very useful in showing that there is more in perception than in the stimulus. However, the relevant point is another question: whether or not empirical evidence supports a constructivistic view. Paradoxically, illusory figures have been used mainly to *verify* the proposition that visual entities are reifications of constructs, although the epistemology behind the informational model is based on falsification. Perceptual hypotheses would be accepted only when they are not falsified by sensory data.

At a close examination, the phenomenology of illusory figures supports the idea that stimuli are transformed according to intrinsic laws of organization; ordinarily but not necessarily, the results of this organization are meaningful and logically plausible.

In addition, the interpretation originally proposed by Kanizsa (1955a and chap. 4) should be evaluated from this point of view. In Kanizsa's explanation, amodal completion of inducers plays a role different from hypothesized occlusion in a cognitive explanation, although they may look similar. A critical feature of an informational account of illusory figures is the following: they are postulated by the visual system, and ultimately perceived owing to the lack of contradictory information, because they represent a logical solution, at the level of phenomenal reality, to a problem posed by gaps and alignments, at the level of proximal stimuli. The explanation based on amodal completion is theoretically different—in the mind of its proponent—because a reasoning-like result would be produced by natural means, i.e., by the intervention of a blind, energy-absorbing process of field segregation. According to this model, a "gap" in an inducer is not an interposition cue, but a locus where the structure of the inducer's form is perturbed. In other words, the formation of contours separating visual regions is not taken for granted. The functional counterpart of a contour is not a landmark, topographically equivalent to the corresponding border in the stimulus pattern. A contour is a unilateral barrier against intrafigural forces that tend towards equilibrium. The local action of each inducer is supported by tensions arising from the distribution of figural forces and is manifested by color dishomogeneities that regularly accompany them. Color contrast and assimilation reveal in which direction the contour is acting as a barrier. The emerging of the whole illusory figure is a cooperative phenomenon, where retinotopic factors are dominant.

Normally, optical information is so rich that it becomes tempting to consider it as the sole determinant of visual experience. Illusory fig-ures—as well as amodal continuation phenomena, so intimately connected to them (Kanizsa & Gerbino, 1982)—constitute an important source of knowledge about vision, because they allow us to explore the constraints imposed by the organism when producing percepts. However, thinking that the nature of these constraints is "mental" must be our very last resource.

Acknowledgments. This work was supported by Consiglio Nazionale delle Ricerche (CNR) Grant no. 81.00049.04.

CHAPTER 28

Lo, Perception Abhors Not a Contradiction

John M. Kennedy

Subjective contours are divisions seen crossing homogeneous regions (see Fig. 28.1a,b). They can resemble lines on paper (that is, lines made of pigment flush with the surface bearing them). They can also look like edges of opaque or semitransparent surfaces (that is, occluding boundaries of surfaces overlapping a background). Further, they can also look like boundaries of shadows (perceptible phenomena flush with the surface bearing them) or like highlights (perceptible phenomena that can appear recessed behind a surface). And they can look like corners (that is, convex and concave dihedral angles, dividing surfaces with different slants). In short, they mimic *all* the main sources of optic structure to which the eye is sensitive, not just occluding edges (Kennedy, 1975).

However, to describe subjective contours as resembling ecological sources of optic structures may be misleading. Indeed, it may be misleading in precisely the same way that describing subjective contours as illusory can be misleading. That which mimics or is illusory is by definition *deceptive* (see Fig. 28.1c,d for a deceptive display, an illusion). In an illusion, the perceiver takes objectively equal things to be unequal. But in contrast with illusions, subjective contours are often described by the perceiver as not deceptive. That is, stating this distinction in an informal way, the naive observer seeing his or her first subjective contour may say, "Oh, I see a line that doesn't exist!"

I have often shown a subjective-contour slide with 30 or 40 lines on it to an audience of freshman students and asked, "Do you all see the line that isn't there?" The students nod their heads, and if asked, point to the line that isn't there.

It is this curious ability of a subjective contour to be seen and to be evidently nonexistent to the naive observer that is the topic of this chapter. I will first establish the fact that subjective contours are *apparently unreal*. Next, the hypothesis that *apparent reality* is a function of contour strength will be rejected. I will then suggest that apparent reality is dependent on a *type* or *height* of processing in the visual system. I will compare the basis for reality judgments of subjective contours to reality judgments of illusions (and, briefly, pictures). And I will note that cognitive contour explanations which rest on the assumption that perception abhors a contradiction cannot handle apparent nonexistence.

Subjective Contours and Disconfirming Evidence Coexist

Most theories totally disregard the capacity of a subjective contour to be seen and to be evidently purely subjective. Directly or indirectly they conform to the notion that subjective contours have the same status for the perceiver as either real contours which exist between two regions of different reflectance on a surface, or two regions of different reflectance one overlapping the other.

Indeed, Coren (1972) in order to remark on the vividness of subjective contours quotes a subject as saying admiringly, "I know it's not real, but how did you do it?" Coren uses the comment to emphasize the figure's strength.

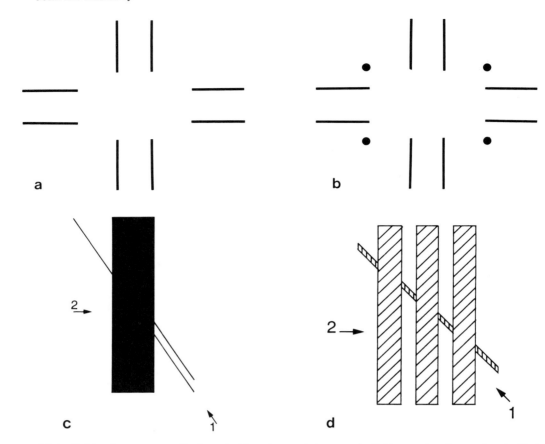

FIGURE 28.1. Subjective-contour displays (a,b) and geometrical illusions (c,d). Subjective contours depend on grouping and connecting the inducing elements. Line elements create black-white contrast effects at their ends, hue assimilation effects alongside, and hue assimilation extensions ahead. Dots aid grouping, so that small dots and large dots can pull the connections, as here, into pincushion shapes whose vertices can be toward the center of the dots, as is evident in the large-dot figure.

But taken at face value, surely an important feature of the comment is that the subject knows the contour is not real! Furthermore, there is not a priori reason to believe that strong contours—real or subjective like these in Figure 28.2—are seen as real and that weak contours are seen as unreal. Some weak contours are perfectly real. And some strong subjective contours are taken to be unreal, Coren's subject reveals.

Some theorists consider subjective contours to be produced by hypothesis-generating procedures in perception. These procedures are said to be active in much of perception. In these theories, since normal perception of real objects and perception of subjective contours are all produced by the same machinery, there is no reason for the perceiver to suspect that some contours are unreal. According to the hypothesis-generating theories, perception is based on the amassing of probabilistic cues. If the cues make a particular source a good bet, the perceptual systems will create a percept of that source. Perceptual information that a source is not present ought to make the percept vanish, a candle flame blown out in a wind of disproof. This line of argument stretches from Berkeley (1604/1922) to Helmholtz (1909/1925) to Gregory (1972), and to Coren (1972), who applied it to subjective contours, and to Rock and Anson (1979), who offer evidence for its application to subjective contours.

One fundamental assumption in all theories that take perception to be logic-like (or hypothesis-testing or inferential) is this: Perception is a dictatorship in which only the voice of the fa-

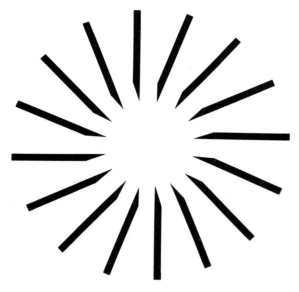

FIGURE 28.2. A strong subjective brightness figure.

vored hypothesis (or conclusion or inference or guess) is heard by the perceiver. The brain may receive incomplete or contradictory information, but it censors the competing petitions and allows only one percept at a time. A thing is or is not. It cannot both be present and be absent. So goes logic, and so therefore goes perception.

What in fact happens when the visual system is given evidence that a subjective contour does not exist? Kennedy (1985) describes just such a test. In a solid frame, two sets of parallel rods were arranged as in Figure 28.3, resembling mismatched wallpaper (Kennedy, 1975). A fine line appears to be joining the tips of the rods,

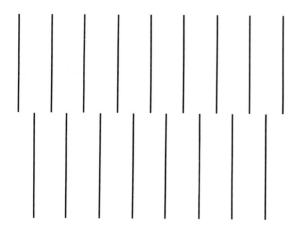

FIGURE 28.3. A subjective edge.

dividing the two sets of parallel rods. Let us call this line the Mind Line (cf. Ware & Kennedy, 1978).

There are two interesting ways to provide perceptual information that the Mind Line does not exist. When a small card is held behind one of the inducing rods of the Mind Line construction and slightly below the Mind Line, a light can be placed so as to cast a shadow of the tip of an inducing rod. Were the Mind Line real it would have a shadow. Alas, only the real rod succeeds in casting a shadow. Like a phantom from the occult, the Mind Line has no shadow. But the perceptual system persists, against the evidence, in maintaining the Mind Line.

Also, when a small mirror is held behind one of the inducing rods in the Mind Line construction, slightly below the Mind Line, and tilted to reflect the tip of the rod, the mirror image reveals the tip but no trace of the Mind Line. The mirror reveals that the Mind Line does not exist. But the perceptual system retains the Mind Line, contravening the perceptual information from the mirror.

In principle, we could in addition use any of several other devices to tell the system that the Mind Line is imaginary. We could magnify one section of the construction through a lens. Or the construction could be tilted so that one part is near and the rest far. The nearby rods are optically too far apart to generate a Mind Line. And we can rotate the construction so that what is near becomes far, and vice versa. When the rods are nearby, only rods are seen. But the Mind Line reappears each time the rods revert from near to far.

In short, the Mind Line is *not* a hypothesis of the perceptual system emerging from a consistent synthesis of all the available perceptual information. The Mind Line can coexist with information that it is unreal.

Impressions of Unreality

The impression that subjective contours are unreal is not vouchsafed only to the intelligentsia. A series of three subjective-contour constructions were shown to children aged 3–4, by Jane Magnan. The constructions were a Mind Line, a wheel figure called Spokes with pointed spokes coming to the center (Fig. 28.4), and a

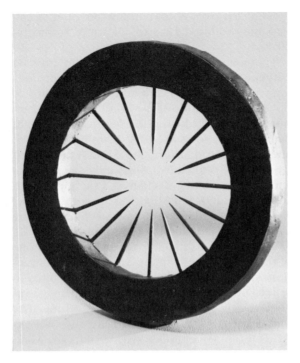

FIGURE 28.4. Spokes construction (by Colin Ware). Children notice the central bright disc and declare it to be insubstantial, made of nothing.

wheel figure called Sunburst, in which the spokes were arranged as in Figure 28.2.

The children were asked what they saw, what they would feel if they put a finger in the region of the subjective contours, and whether anything would be broken if you pushed a finger through the forms. All seven children reported seeing the subjective figures (lines joining the sticks, bright circles). When they were asked about touching the shapes, five said they could not be touched, one's finger would just go through, nothing would be broken, and the like. One 3-year-old said she didn't know about two of the figures but that she could just put a finger through without touching anything for the Sunburst figure. One 3-year-old said the Mind Line could be touched but the other two figures could not.

We have shown five subjective-contour constructions to eight 9-year-old children, adding Misty Strip (Fig. 28.5) and one like Misty Strip except that the inducing rods are in a circle like a cage. Five children reported seeing all five subjective-contour figures. The other three children reported seeing only some of the figures.

All of the five who saw all the figures, when asked what the figures were made of, said they were made of "nothing" or "air." They also said, when asked, that the figures could not be touched or broken by inserting an object.

We have also shown subjective-contour displays—some of them drawings and some of them photographs of constructions—to four groups of adults ($n = 17, 11, 25, 20$) and asked them to pick out any lines or shapes that are unreal. In Figure 28.6 there are a large number of arcs and some lines crossing the arcs. Seventeen adults from the University of Toronto were shown a version of this display in which two arcs (top right) were created by putting cracks in the slide's glass frame, producing an odd, unfamiliar appearance of black lines on the screen each with some light mingled with the black. Fourteen subjects picked only one line in this display as unreal—the subjective contour. Tested again with a group of 11 adults, at Sarah Lawrence College, 9 of the 11 picked only the subjective contour as unreal.

A further group of 25 adults in Toronto were asked about three triangles simultaneously: a "clear" triangle, a "misty" triangle (see Fig.

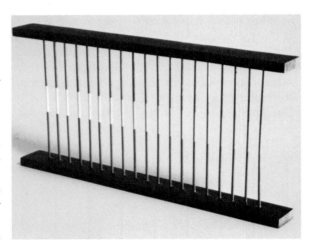

FIGURE 28.5. Misty Strip. The center portion of the rods is painted white, in farther regions, or gray, in nearer regions. Subjects see a Misty Strip join the painted bands. The gradations in the central white strips on each bar cannot readily be reproduced here, but the idea should be clear, and some of the effects should be present for the viewer. Construction by Colin Ware. The color plate of this figure can be found on the color insert on page xv.

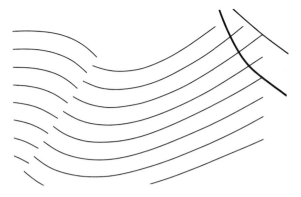

FIGURE 28.6. Drawing of "sheared strata," with two additional arcs at the corner. In a slide presentation the arcs were created by cracks in the glass of the slide, producing an unusual mixture of light and dark along the arc. Subjects generally deemed the contour along the "shear" to be unreal, and the crack-arcs to be real.

28.7), and a Kanizsa triangle. Eighteen of the 25 thought all three of the triangles were unreal.

Another group of 20 adults were asked about a Kanizsa figure (bright center) and a Black Flower or Black-Eyed Susan figure (a darker center subjective-contour figure). See Figure 28.8.

Fifteen subjects saw both the dark and light centers and made reality judgments about both. Eleven said both centers are unreal. Two thought the white center was unreal and the black was real. Two thought both centers were real.

Interestingly, not all the subjective figures were judged unreal. The group of 25 adults judging the three triangles were later asked to judge slides of three constructions shown simultaneously: Mind Line, Spokes, and Misty Strip. Twenty-two out of 24 scorable responses deemed only the Mind Line and the Spokes to be unreal. That is, 22 out of 24 subjects judged the Misty Strip to be real! Why should the Misty Strip be singled out, be different from Spokes and the Mind Line? This is especially remarkable in that the Misty Strip is one of the weaker effects in our displays.

The Sarah Lawrence adults who judged Figure 28.6 were later asked to judge the Misty Strip slide and were asked where the Misty Strip was to be found: in the construction, in the slide by a trick of the photographer, or purely in the eye? Ten reported seeing the subjective figure; while two of these thought the figure was "in the construction," six described it as being in the slide.

If the Misty Strip figure were the only one frequently deemed real, then its perceptual status might be considered complex, or sensitive to sophisticated notions about perceptual displays (see Gibson, 1951, on Rubinian displays and Kennedy, 1974, on Rubin and pictures). However, there is a second display (Fig. 28.9) that often fools subjects into taking subjective effects to be real. It is not a construction and therefore not subject to the complexities in slides of constructions.

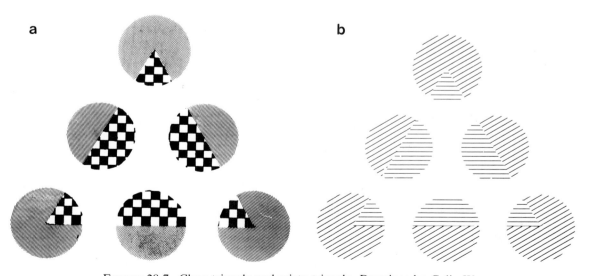

FIGURE 28.7. Clear triangle and misty triangle. Drawings by Colin Ware.

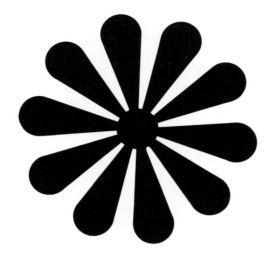

FIGURE 28.8. Black flower.

The 20 Toronto subjects who examined Figure 28.8 were later asked to review 28.9. They were asked what was unreal: the diagonal divisions joining the elbows of the chevrons, the chevrons themselves, and/or the black diagonal bars at the ends of the chevrons? Eighteen reported seeing the diagonal divisions, the white chevrons and the black bars. Seventeen judged the diagonal divisions to be unreal, and no one deemed the black bars to be unreal. Informally, I have noticed that most people are shocked to find the black bars are exactly the same shade as the black regions between the white chev-

rons, and there is no contour between the black bars and these black regions.

Why Are Subjective Contours Apparently Unreal?

For a large number of subjective-contour displays, the subjective figure is deemed to be unreal by naive observers. How is this possible? There are many kinds of explanations, but very few seem genuinely promising.

Explanations Which Fail

1. One explanation would be that subjective contours are always weak. This seems unlikely to be the major factor, since several of the displays are vivid, and some weak displays are judged to have real contours in them. An image's strength does not indicate whether it is real or purely mental.

2. Another possibility is that fixation of subjective contours makes them disappear. This could not work well in the general case, that is, for both real and subjective contours. Any weak star, and the diffuse penumbra of a shadow, disappears when fixated. But fixation followed by disappearance may be a contributory factor at times, alerting the observer to think twice. Further, fixation may be only one of several ways to make subjective contours disappear. One may be able to "set" himself to have subjective contours appear and disappear, rather as he can "set" himself to have figure–ground alternate and to reverse a Necker cube (see Coren et al., chap. 26, this volume).

A fixation–disappearance and "set" explanation is unlikely to apply to children given nondirective questions and to novice observers rapidly picking out an unreal figure from a mass of inducers. It seems more plausible that the contour is seen and is seen to be unreal at the same instant.

3. Another possibility is that subjective contours appear to be different than the inducing contours, and, given the leading question "what is unreal?" the subjective contours are judged to be unreal as a matter of default. This account has difficulty coping with the display involving cracks in a slide, and the odd mixture of light and dark in the slide's projected version

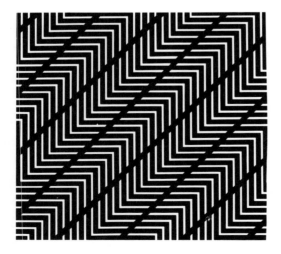

FIGURE 28.9. Version of Zoellner illusion. (After Kanizsa, 1979.)

of the crack. The dominant response to this slide presentation is that only the subjective contour is unreal, and the odd projected version of the crack is deemed real.

4. Another explanation could be that the inducing contours appear in perception first and the subjective contours appear second, even though only a brief period later. Do time differences alone predict reality judgments? Taken literally, the explanation holds that anything noticed later is judged unreal. This account has trouble dealing with displays involving many inducers, not all of which would be noted immediately. Inducers noted later than the first glance are not judged unreal. Further, Bruno and Gerbino (chap. 24, this volume) demonstrate that subjective-contour forms are as fast as many other organizations (but see Petry and Gannon, chap. 21, this volume).

A Proposed Explanation Which May Work

Presumably, two visual systems are operating, one producing subjective contours and one disconfirming them. Could they be at times created by the night vision system (the rods and their connections) while the day vision system contradicts them? Both systems, in this account, operate in the same time frame, rather than in some kind of alternation where the subjective contours are not present for brief spells. This would explain why lowered illumination (emphasizing night vision) strengthens some subjective contours—if this point can be sustained (see the controversy in this volume). It would explain why fixation (emphasizing day vision) weakens or even destroys the contours at times. It would also explain why contrast effects in many subjective contours are based on luminance (a night vision capability) and not on color contrast (a day vision capability). See also Ramachandran (chap. 10, this volume) and Cavanagh (1987), but see Shapley and Gordon (chap. 11, this volume). Note too that this day vision/night vision supposition cannot account for all of the effects related to subjective contours. For example, I find extension contours (Bradley, 1976; Rubin, 1915) are tinged with the color of the inducers (see also Gerbino & Kanizsa, chap. 27, and de Weert & van Kruysbergen, chap. 17, both in this volume, for re-

lated suggestions and demonstrations). Assimilation effects related to subjective contours are also tinged with the color of the inducers. Evidently at times the day vision system contributes to the formation of the contours. Perhaps, then, we could hypothesize that *in those conditions* where it might be that the night vision system is the *only* factor producing subjective contours, it will be easy for the subject to pick out the unreal contour. I offer this day/night comparison simply to illustrate what I mean by two different physiological systems (see Marr, 1982, p. 70). Notice that this evidence could also be used to argue for a contribution from low spatial frequency systems (God help us!), especially if long "microgenesis" times are found to be reliable (see Petry & Gannon, chap. 21, and Ginsburg, chap. 13, this volume).

The day vision/night vision explanation does contain a general principle that I do think should be taken seriously in explaining the apparent unreality of subjective contours. The principle is that there are two systems coexisting. One "contains" the contours, the other does not. This principle can be compared to the "bicameral" principle in picture perception, where apparent depth in the picture coexists with apparent flatness of the elements on the picture surface (Kennedy, 1976a; cf. Parks, chap. 8, this volume).

What possible inducing parameter can vary so that on some occasions strong contours are deemed to be unreal and on some occasions weak contours are deemed to be real?

A dimension of variation that can be somewhat independent of the contour's strength is the angular subtense of the inducers. It is possible that when the inducers are far apart (and only "connected" by a system which has low acuity) the subjective contour is deemed unreal, and when the inducers are close together, the contour is deemed real. Presumably, the contours may appear real when the gaps between inducers subtend small angles, and they may appear unreal when the gaps subtend larger angles. (The binocular subjective contours appearing real may be capable of retinal space rivalry, though some binocular subjective contours are insensitive to rivalry. The ones immune to rivalry may be from wider-gapped inducers, arising high in visual processing.)

In short, subjective contours can be just

that—apparently subjective or unreal to the observers. But they can become apparently real too. This suggests there are criterial visual angles for bringing lower-order visual systems into operation. And higher-order visual systems (operating in most subjective contour displays researched to date) may operate in parallel with other systems in which the contours do not exist. Subjective contours can be nondeceptive, apparently unreal. They can also be deceptive, apparently real. The height-of-processing theory holds that subjective contours—that are apparently unreal—turn into illusory contours—which we cannot tell are unreal—when inducers come close to one another. Subjective contours can become illusory contours.

Comparison with Geometrical Illusions

Just as there have been cognitive theories of subjective contours, stressing hypothesis making by the visual system, so too there have been cognitive theories of geometrical illusions, stressing the application of hypotheses about distance which "scale" the apparent size or direction of components of the illusory figure.

Similarly, just as there have been peripheral theories of subjective-contour formation, stressing contrast and lower-order connections between inducing elements, so too there have been peripheral theories of geometrical illusions, stressing orientation and angle perception of the figure's elements.

Consider analogs between subjective contours and geometrical illusions. If an illusion is caused by peripheral factors, then the observer should not be able to tell what is real and what is not. But, also, adjustment of peripheral factors should both strengthen and dispel the illusion. Further, if the modifications are truly peripheral, subjects should not know which of their changing impressions is the "correct" one.

The reader is invited to examine Figure 28.1c,d from several vantage points. One should be with the illusory figure in the frontal-parallel plane. A second vantage point should

be at a glancing angle, say one aligned with diagonal lines in Figure 28.1c,d. A third should be at another glancing angle, say at right angles to the first glancing angle.

It will be observed that the illusion is present from the normal, frontal-parallel views. It will disappear from one glancing angle (aligned with the diagonals) and will reappear for the second glancing angle.

With Andrew Portal, I have tested Figure 28.1c with 13 subjects, asking them to make judgments of the appearance of the illusory figure from the three vantage points (normal, glancing angle continuing the diagonals, and glancing angle from the side of the figure). Twelve saw the line continuation incorrectly from the normal vantage point, and 12 saw the correct continuation from the glancing angle along the diagonal. Ten had the illusion reinstated from the second glancing angle. But when asked what was the real state of affairs—what was the true continuation of the diagonal lines—their judgments were random. Six were correct, seven incorrect. For Figure 28.1d, 10 subjects judged the display incorrectly from the normal vantage point, all 13 judged the display correctly from the glancing vantage point along the diagonal, and 8 judged incorrectly from the second vantage point. However, when asked what the true state of affairs was, the responses were random: seven judged correctly and six incorrectly.

We have repeated this experiment several times, with the same results. Subjects cannot tell which impression is correct.

Illusions like Figure 28.1 (or the Zoellner illusion, Fig. 28.8) can be made to appear in force, and disappear entirely, by inspecting from various vantage points including extreme glancing angles.

These results with geometrical illusions support the contention that the illusions are peripheral. Adjustments such as viewing from glancing angles affect peripheral factors such as retinal angles. Affecting the peripheral factors creates and destroys the illusion. The illusion is created by peripheral factors, it seems, and in keeping with the peripheral genesis of the illusion, subjects do not know when they are deceived and when they have the correct impression.

Perceptual Effects

It would be conceded by all that observers can learn by indirect or nonperceptual means that the subjective contours and the geometrical illusions are false. Observers could simply be told they are misled. This would not trouble hypothesis-testing theories. The theories could simply hold that perception operates to a degree independently of cognition. It is only perceptual effects that concern the theories. The strength of the present demonstrations is that they undoubtedly use basic perceptual effects: unaided inspection, shadows, and viewing from various angles. Our emphasis here has been on the relation between two contradictory perceptual effects and cognition: between two contradictory perceptual impressions and judgments of reality.

Perception involves impressions of size, shape, color, and brightness. These impressions arise from inducing elements which have their own distinctive powers. Notably, impressions of brightness arise from luminance differences, from contrast effects at the ends of inducers, and from assimilation effects (Fig. 28.10) at the sides of inducers and ahead of inducers as extension contours. These form the basis for subjective contours, which depend on connections made between inducers by grouping mechanisms. The results are impressions of divisions, which are strong when contrast and assimilation effects differ on either side of the divisions. These impressions can coexist with other impressions which contradict them. Cog-

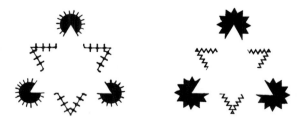

FIGURE 28.10. These figures suggest that assimilation, not just contrast, can play a major role in formation of some subjective contours. There are more line endings, or abrupt changes in contour direction, outside the subjective figure than bordering the figure. But the figure appears bright, presumably because the inducing black regions give rise to assimilation. Figures by Colin Ware.

nition enters, like the chair of a debate, not to dispel contradiction but to note contradiction. When all the impressions arise from lower-order mechanisms, no contradictions exist in the visual system and the subject is deceived by illusions (cf. Gibson, 1966, 1979 for an analysis of the normal case). Across time, the perceiver may be given entirely different impressions of an illusory display by adjusting peripheral factors. In this case there is no simultaneous set of perceptual contradictions, and the perceiver may have no sure basis for determining what is true. Then, the perceiver bases his judgments about reality on lower-order impressions, and in the case of subjective contours, if these contradict an impression created higher in the system, he or she is left in no doubt about what is real. What is peripheral appears true.

CHAPTER 29

The Perception of Illusory Contours: A Skills Analysis

Angus Gellatly and Melanie Bishop

Perceptual Processing and Perceptual Skill

In this chapter we set out to argue that an analysis in terms of perceptual skill is required for the perception of both illusory contours and real contours. Although there is already a tradition of studying the perception of real edges as a matter of perceptual skill (Gibson, 1969), this does not appear to have been done previously for illusory contours and shapes. It is expected that adoption of a skills analysis will cause light to be cast on the processes of perceiving both illusory and real contours.

Perception is frequently thought of as a sequence of processing stages. Although the possibility of some degree of feedback or feedforward is generally acknowledged, a popular form of question amongst perceptionists is: At what stage does the X effect arise? What is the locus of the perceptual genesis of X? For example, illusory contours and their associated phenomena, such as illusory shapes and enhanced brightness, tend to be explained either by appeal to physiological mechanisms or to cognitive processes. And these two types of explanation generally imply reference to, respectively, early or late stages in a processing sequence. Hypothetical physiological mechanisms, contrast detectors, or feature detectors, for instance, supposedly respond to patterns of physical energy and give rise to outputs upon which later, cognitive processes can operate. This is held to be the case both for real contours and illusory contours, that physiological stages of processing are followed by cognitive stages of

processing. In our analysis we will retain the notion of a sequence of stages while trying to get away from the physiology/cognition dichotomy. Instead, we will talk about a continuum of perceptual (neural) habits, or procedures, which can be more or less automatic. More automatic habits occur rapidly in response to stimuli, and therefore early in a sequence of processing stages. Less automatic habits are later occurring, and may require effort.

An analogy with reading words will help to clarify the purpose of employing this terminology. Many children learn to read phonically. They first perceive individual letters and letter groups, then sound them out, and finally identify the meaning, or referent, of a word. Recognition of the word in terms of its meaning is at a relatively late stage in the sequence of processes. With practice, however, the children may become skilled readers, able to identify a word holistically without first recognizing individual letters or deriving the sound of the word (see, e.g., Sloboda, 1986). Word recognition migrates to an earlier stage of processing.

Now reading is about as cognitive a skill as one could hope to think of, yet there would seem to be little point in asking if reading—or a component of it like word recognition—ought to be explained physiologically or cognitively. Many interesting questions can be asked about reading but this does not seem to be one of them. Clearly reading, or word recognition, is dependent on processes that are both physiological and cognitive, not one or the other. Nor is reading an exceptional skill in this respect. One would not be likely to ask of walking either whether it should be explained physiologically or cognitively. The purpose of talking about illusory-contour perception in terms of more or less automatic neural habits is, then, that it allows us to get away from the physiology/cognition dichotomy and to assimilate perception to skills in general. The advantage of this is that a great deal is already known about the analysis of motor and cognitive skills.

If the kind of approach we are advocating can be a fruitful one, then two things should follow immediately. First, it should be possible to point both to examples of illusory contours derived from highly practiced procedures that occur early in processing and also to examples where the procedures are far from automatic and occur later in processing. Second, it should be possible to demonstrate an effect of practice on the locus of some such procedures, and therefore on the apparent locus of perceptual genesis of the associated contours. The remainder of this chapter is an attempt to fulfill these two requirements, albeit in a fairly provisional manner.

Early Genesis of Contours

An example of illusory contours with an early locus of genesis can be seen in the simplified Kanizsa triangle of Figure 29.1. Gellatly (1980) studied the perceptual genesis of the triangle using Werner's (1935) technique of ring masking. Very brief exposures of Figure 29.1 were alternated with 100-msec presentations of Figure 29.2, the three rings of which coincided with the circular contours of the inducing disks in Figure 29.1. With suitable exposure durations subjects reported a pulsing white triangle

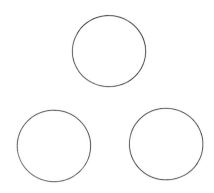

FIGURE 29.2. Masking stimulus with complete disks.

slightly behind the rings, but they did not report any phenomenal awareness of the inducing disks. Masked by the rings, the inducing disks themselves were subliminal. Yet they were still able to induce perception of the triangle. This indicates that the triangle must have been generated at an even earlier stage of processing than the stage at which ring masking occurred. It also shows that once the triangle was posited by the visual system it could withstand deletion of the disks on which that positing originally depended.

A further interesting finding was that when Figure 29.3 replaced Figure 29.2 as mask, perception of the triangle was greatly inhibited. Even when the exposure duration of Figure 29.1 was increased to the point where the disks surpassed threshold, the triangle still did not appear. A several hundred msec exposure of Figure 29.1 was required before the triangle ceased to be masked by the following Figure 29.3. It seems that just as the inducing disks

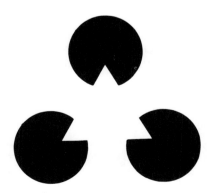

FIGURE 29.1. Inducing disks and illusory triangle.

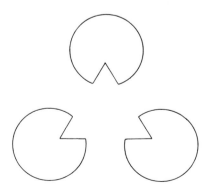

FIGURE 29.3. Masking stimulus with sectored disks.

could be registered and then subsequently deleted when masked by Figure 29.2, so also the triangle could be posited at an early stage but then deleted as a consequence of the arrival of Figure 29.3. Presumably the posited triangle was not deleted when followed by Figure 29.2 because the visual system still needed to make sense of the (unmasked) edges that are seen as the apices of the triangle. (However such contours are not sufficient on their own for genesis of the triangle, since Figure 29.3 does not substitute for Figure 29.1 under any conditions of presentation.) By contrast, when Figure 29.3 follows Figure 29.1 the triangle can be deleted because perception of Figure 29.3 alone can account for the presence of those same edges.

Rock and Anson (1979) reported other evidence that the Kanizsa triangle has an early locus of genesis but that, if rapidly followed by inconsistent information, it can be deleted before conscious representation. Also, Remole et al. (1985) found that flicker halos could be obtained near the edges of a Kanizsa-style rectangle just as they can near to real contours. Since flicker halos are thought to themselves arise early in perceptual processing this again indicates early genesis of illusory contours. It shows that the automatic procedures responsible for the representation of both real and illusory contours in these cases have similar sensitivity to flicker.

Late Genesis of Contours

There is little problem, then, in finding examples of illusory contours that are generated early in processing. How about examples of the second kind, that depend on unpracticed procedures occurring relatively late in processing? A possibility that suggests itself here is the generation of contours and shapes as a result of apparent motion. For if perception of a shape can be induced by the alternation of two stimulus displays this would imply relatively late generation, since the two displays must themselves have been processed before a shape can be posited.

Anstis (1970) reported an effect of this kind for random-dot stereograms, but it is of interest to know if similar results can be obtained with stimulus patterns more typical of those used to produce monocularly visible illusory contours

(Parks, 1984). A problem with Anstis's effect is that the apparent square perceived with the stereograms was no longer visible when alternation of the two displays ceased. The square never became visible in a single stereogram. That means that its locus of generation must have remained late on in the processing sequence; a necessary consequence of the use of stereograms. Our aim is to demonstrate not only that apparent motion can lead to the generation of an illusory shape, but that with practice the locus of genesis of the shape can migrate forwards.

We have now carried out an experiment which demonstrates such an effect, and which at the same time throws light on a proposal of Kanizsa's. According to Kanizsa (1976), a necessary condition for the perception of illusory contours is the presence of incomplete figural elements that induce the perception. If alternation of two figures that contain no obviously incomplete elements (Figures 29.4a and 29.4b) can lead to generation of an illusory shape, then Kanizsa's proposal will require at least some modification.

In our experiment, two groups of 18 subjects each were individually asked to look into a tachistoscope in which Figure 29.4a was visible. The subjects were asked to describe what they saw. All of them reported a number of black shapes aligned on a white background, but none mentioned perceiving a central white rectangle. The subjects were then shown a copy of Figure 29.1, and the illusory nature of the triangle was pointed out to them. They were then asked to look again at the figure in the tachistoscope and to say if they could see any illusory contours contained within it. At this juncture only one subject, from the experimental group, reported the presence of a white rectangle with enhanced brightness. All the other subjects claimed that there was no change in their perceptions.

For subjects in the experimental group the tachistoscope was then set to display Figures 29.4a and 29.4b in alternating 600-msec exposures. The subjects were once again asked to describe what they saw. These reports varied considerably; some subjects had an immediate perception of a white rectangle sliding from side to side and covering and uncovering the black elements at the ends of the figures; others required some degree of prompting before the

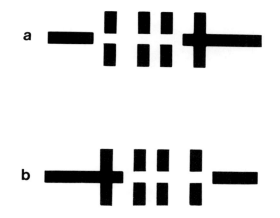

FIGURE 29.4a and b. Stimuli for the perceptual learning of illusory contours.

rectangle appeared. In some of these cases, the only prompting necessary was a request to try to see the changing figure as a whole, rather than in terms of its elements, but in other cases it was necessary to ask the subject to try to see a white rectangle moving from side to side. Eventually, however, all subjects in the experimental group agreed to perceiving a rectangle with illusory contours and enhanced brightness.

As a last stage in the experiment these subjects were then asked to look again at one of the two figures statically displayed. All of them reported that a rectangle was still visible, although only one of them had previously reported perceiving a rectangle under these conditions. Subjects also saw the figure again seven days after the experiment, and 12 of the 18 once more reported the phenomenal presence of the rectangle.

Subjects in the control group never saw the two figures in alternation. They continued to examine Figure 29.4a while being prompted to try to see an illusory white rectangle at its center. They were also exposed to Figure 29.4b to try to help them understand how a rectangle might be contained within the figures, but only two of the subjects were able to report perception of any rectangle. On viewing Figure 29.4a seven days later, again only these two subjects reported the rectangle.

The difference in the number of reports of a rectangle from subjects in the two groups is a marked one. The experimenter's demand that subjects perceive a rectangle was not effective except when alternating presentations of the two figures was introduced to facilitate perception of a rectangle in apparent motion. It seems that for these naive subjects the illusory rectangle can be generated only at a relatively late stage of processing. It is part of a possible interpretation of the figure, or of the two figures in alternation, that may require an effort of will. This is a reminder that perception really can involve nonautomatic as well as automatic processes. The fact that the experimental subjects became more able to perceive the rectangle in a static figure after viewing the two figures in alternation demonstrates how an interpretation—or set of neural habits—can become more available with practice. In the course of the experiment, certain procedures became more automatic for these subjects.

Effort, Automaticity, and Perceptual Skill

The above findings are consistent with an earlier demonstration that binocularly generated illusory contours can, with practice, come to be seen in a monocularly viewed figure (Gellatly, 1982). They also serve to recall some of the lessons of Gestalt psychology. For the naive subject to perceive Figure 29.5 as depicting a cow may well require an initial effort of will. Yet once a meaningful interpretation has been achieved, it is then difficult to get rid of. The cow comes to appear with a clarity and an immediacy comparable to those of the triangle in figure 29.1. And while the same degree of clarity cannot be claimed for the rectangle of Figures 29.4a and 29.4b even after prolonged exposure to alternation, an increase in availability has been demonstrated. In all cases it appears that with practice procedures of interpretation—what we have dubbed neural habits—become more automatic and migrate to an earlier stage of processing. As with any skill, what was at first acquired only laboriously grows easier. Once the appropriate neural connections have been made they can achieve a considerable autonomy from the subject's will.

With respect to Kanizsa's hypothesis about the necessity of incomplete elements for inducing illusory shapes, the present investigation

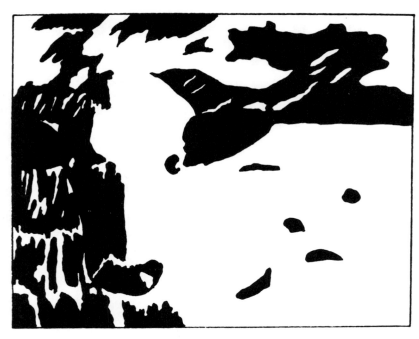

FIGURE 29.5. The hidden cow. An example of perceptual learning. (After Dallenbach, 1951.)

suggests that the notion of what constitutes an incomplete figural element is not a simple one. The elements of Figures 29.4a and 29.4b appear to be complete unless a partially occluding rectangle is assumed, but if that assumption is made then they are incomplete. Incompleteness can be defined only with reference to the set of the perceiver. The completeness or incompleteness of elements varies with the interpretation given to the overall figure. A change in the definition of completeness occurred for the subjects of this study once they had been induced to see a white rectangle in apparent motion, the fresh interpretation being transferred back to the static configurations also. A similar view of the nature of the incompleteness of elements was also reached by Rock and Anson (1979).

The above are not new lessons in psychology but they appear to have sometimes been forgotten in the debate over the proper explanation of illusory contours and shapes. In part this may be because attention has, understandably, focused on relatively easily perceived shapes like the triangle in Figure 29.1. For many—though not all—people, the triangle cannot be perceptually excluded except by concentrating on a

small area of the figure rather than on the stimulus as a whole. Perception of the triangle seems to be determined by highly practiced and automatic procedures of interpretation. These are most likely the procedures that yield figure/ground segregation and overall figural organization. They can be assumed to instantiate Gestalt principles such as similarity and proximity and, important for Figure 29.1, good continuation, as well as rules for local and global consistency. It is the difficulty of *not* seeing the triangle which attests to the high level of automaticity obtained by these procedures. On the other hand, other illusory figures lack the immediacy of the triangle and may become perceptible only as a result of procedures that have to be set up—with effort—during prolonged viewing.

Our point is that, rather than talking of physiological mechanisms versus cognitive constructions, it may be helpful to think of automatic and less automatic procedures for interpretation. Experience and practice may be assumed to shift any one procedure, or set of procedures, along this continuum, as is the case for any other skill. An illusory shape will have an immediacy for a subject in proportion to the automaticity of the neural habits which yield that interpretation of the stimulus configuration in which it is contained. Where subjects do not have the appropriate neural habits available, it may be necessary to stimulate acquisition of the habits by starting with relatively simple applications of them. For the case of the rectangle the simple application is with the alternating figures, because these are more readily given an interpretation that includes the rectangle than is either figure alone. For the cow in Figure 29.5 the appropriate habits are more easily acquired if part of the missing outline is supplied. This method of teaching new skills by starting from simple tasks and then, once the basics are mastered, moving on to those requiring more finely tuned procedures is common in the field of motor performance. Yet whether new motor skills have a physiological or a cognitive basis is not a question that it is usually helpful to ask. In its reliance on more or less automated habits, perception of both real and illusory contours can be seen to resemble other skills. This fact was emphasized long ago in Gestalt studies of perceptual learning. For the present, not a great deal can be added to the description the Gestaltists gave of these habits, but Rock and Anson (1979) have listed some of the cues that may evoke them in the case of illusory contours.

CHAPTER 30

Perceptual Grouping and Subjective Contours

Barbara Gillam

The appearance of subjective contours is so compelling that they are often treated as phenomena with little connection to other aspects of form perception, although the chapters by Day, Rock, Kellman and Loukides, and Mingolla and Grossberg in the present volume do deal with this connection in various ways. In this chapter an attempt is made to examine the relationship between the presence of perceptual grouping and the tendency to see subjective contours. Interestingly, there can be an inverse relationship under certain conditions.

We have argued (Gillam & Grant, 1984) that the occurrence of subjective contours of the occluding type depends on a readiness to treat discrete lines in a figure as connected. This is not a circular statement, since such a readiness can be demonstrated independently of subjective contours or amodal completion. If they are presented under conditions of ambiguous rotary motion in depth, collinear lines and parallel lines will demonstrate a strong tendency to be assigned a common resolution, as shown by the fact that they reverse together (Gillam, 1972; Gillam & Grant, 1984). In the case of collinear lines we maintain that this nonindependence will be manifested as a response to the gap separating the lines as a case of occlusion, rather than a separation into two objects, if there is minimal stimulus support. All that is required in this regard seems to be a minimal depiction of an occluding shape coincident with the gaps in the collinear lines. Take for example the well-known incomplete triangle shown in Figure 30.1. On the basis of our previous work on perceptual unity, we know that there is a strong tendency to respond to the collinear lines of a

figure such as this as connected. The addition of the three dots elicits perception of an occluding triangle linking the edges of the gaps in the incomplete triangle so that the fragments of the latter are amodally completed. On this view, amodal completion and subjective contours are two components of a single perceptual response, which can be regarded as a refinement of an underlying, independently established, perceptual structure.

In this chapter I shall show that this view of subjective contours is true only to a very limited extent. To a surprising degree, whether or not subjective contours appear depends very little on the perceptual unity of those contours which appear to be occluded *by* the subjective contours. Furthermore, the appearance of subjective contours along a set of line terminations is strongest for lines which have the *least* tendency to group.

First I shall consider the stimulus situation in which the grouping of collinear fragments does contribute to the perception of subjective contours in the gap separating them.

Perceptual "Wholes" and Subjective Contours

In the research referred to above (Gillam & Grant, 1984) we were able to distinguish operationally between two varieties of grouping which turn out to have different roles in the formation of subjective contours. The strongest form of grouping, found for collinear lines with small gaps relative to line length, we called *unit formation*. This means that the discrete lines

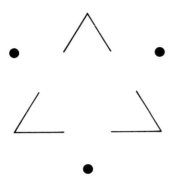

FIGURE 30.1. The subjective triangle joining the dots apparently depends on the presence of collinear line segments.

form an emergent unit, not only reversing together but appearing to be at all times rigidly connected. The parts are no longer available for separate responses. A looser form of connection, occurring with larger gaps, we called *aggregation*. This term means that although the discrete lines are responded to as a unit for some purposes, such as the resolution of ambiguous rotary motion in depth, they may be responded to independently for other purposes, for example appearing to be in a nonrigid relationship to each other. They show a lack of complete independence but do not form a unit. In the former case, when collinear lines are close enough to each other to form units or perceptual wholes, the gaps alone support perception of occlusion if arranged in sequence as in Figure 30.2, with subjective contours delineating the edges in the gaps. This occurs without any additional stimulus support. The discrete components are treated perceptually as parts of the same object, thus supporting an occlusion resolution for the gaps.

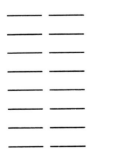

FIGURE 30.2. Subjective contours readily appear across a series of small gaps.

The type of subjective contour shown in Figure 30.2 may illustrate the situation discussed by John Kennedy[1] in Chapter 28 in this volume, in which subjects cannot discriminate subjective from real contours. In his Figure 28.9, collinearity of the interrupted lines is the only support for the contours, which are more compelling than ours because of the density of the inducing lines.

When Collinearity Is Not Enough—Subjective Contours Delineating Large Areas

When the separation of two collinear lines is relatively large, the lines have much less tendency to form a unit (Gillam & Grant, 1984). They will be aggregated for some responses (treated as members of a common class for which the same resolution is appropriate). Clearly their collinearity is perceptually available. However, under conditions in which collinear lines are not close enough to form a perceptual whole on the basis of their proximity alone, more contextual support would probably be necessary in order for the gap to be seen as an occlusion rather than a separation. This does seem to be the case. If the gaps of Figure 30.2 are enlarged (as in Fig. 30.3) the tendency to see subjective contours diminishes. Collinearity alone is not enough in this case, and it is necessary to look to other stimulus properties to elicit perception of an occluding surface with subjective contours and amodal completion of the collinear lines. Four stimulus properties are described below which do enhance the effect of

[1] The effectiveness of the subjective black bands in the Kennedy figure depends on the perceived collinearity of the white bands, which renders the white bands an effectively continuous background across the entire area with the black bands as figures. However, if the figure is tilted so that the black bands are oriented vertically instead of obliquely, the white Vs lose their apparent collinearity because of the Poggendorff illusion. Their loss of continuity tends to make them become figures and the black then becomes ground. The tendency to see subjective contours along the interruptions in the white markedly reduces. This observation supports Rock's point about the importance of figure/ground organization in the formation of subjective contours.

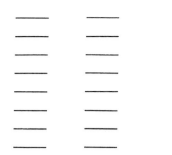

FIGURE 30.3. For large gaps, subjective contours are much weaker than in Figure 30.2. The lines are the same in length and separation.

occlusion and subjective contours in this type of figure.

Shape Depiction

In Figure 30.1 the critical feature necessary to produce the appearance of amodal completion and subjective contours was the depiction of a figure consistent with the edges of the gaps in the collinear fragments. Figure 30.4 gives another example for which the addition of a few dots depicting a diamond results in perception of an occluding diamond-shaped surface filling

the gaps in the collinear lines. Neither dots nor lines alone are sufficient. Note that although the shape is clearly suggested by the dots alone, the presence of the line terminations along its outline makes it appear palpable.

Closure

Closure is often considered irrelevant to the formation of subjective contours, with Figure 30.1 (minus dots) given as an example of its ineffectiveness. Subjective contours do not form to complete the triangle. It would be odd, however, if collinear lines were automatically joined by subjective contours, since parts of a single line are far more likely to be obscured by something overlaying the line than for any other reason. An automatic filling-in process would result in the appearance of lines as if by magic in regions physically hidden. Subjective contours completing collinear lines do occur, as in Kanizsa's classic figure of the incomplete circles (Chap. 4, Fig. 4.11), but only where there is stimulus support for a response to such lines as occluding edges. In the more general case, gaps in lines exist because of occlusion by another figure. If subjective contours occur it is not to join up collinear lines but collinear terminations. This is obvious in Figures 30.1 and 30.2. It is in this context that closure plays a role in the formation of subjective contours. Figure 30.5 shows that collinear terminations are more likely to elicit perception of subjective contours delineating an occluding surface, if seeing such a surface would allow closure of a set of figures, in this case rectangles.

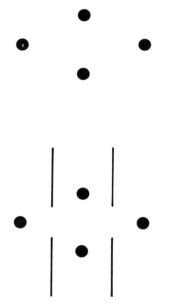

FIGURE 30.4. A diamond shape is suggested by dots alone, but is seen only when collinear lines terminate on its implicit outline.

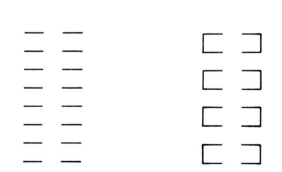

FIGURE 30.5. Subjective contours are stronger when the presence of a perceived occluding surface results in closure of rectangles.

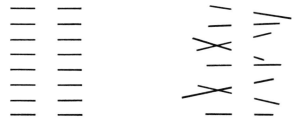

FIGURE 30.6. Subjective contours are stronger when the lines interrupted by collinear gaps are unrelated otherwise.

Poor Organization

Lines which are of random lengths and orientations are more likely to be processed independently of each other than a set of regular lines (Gillam 1976). It is rather surprising, then, to find that subjective contours and perception of occlusion in response to collinear terminations in a set of lines are more salient when the lines are irregular (see Fig. 30.6) than when they are regular in length, separation, and orientation, and hence strongly grouped. This might seem paradoxical. However, a tendency to give more weight in the contour process to orderly terminations of *irregular* arrangements would be ecologically correct, if it is assumed that subjective contours arise as part of the perception of occluding surfaces. Regular terminations of unconnected contours are far more likely to indicate a boundary of an overlaying object than are the collinear terminations of a regular object. The latter could arise simply as part of the object's regularity.

Orientation and Shape of the Gap in Relation to the Lines

Figure 30.7 shows that if the shape formed by the gap is not orthogonal to the terminating lines or is outlined by curved terminations when the lines are straight, a subjective contour is more easily seen. This suggests that stimulus properties consistent with the interruption to the contours arising from an unrelated object, i.e., one with no regular relationship to the lines, are most likely to be seen as an overlay, with accompanying subjective contours.

The Importance of Amodal Completion

So far, it has been assumed that the factors we have isolated and illustrated in Figures 30.4 to 30.7 only work because line collinearity across the gaps allows for amodal completion, given other stimulus support. However, to what degree do the perception of occlusion and subjective contours actually depend on the possibility of amodal completion? Surprisingly, if Figures 30.4 to 30.7 are drawn with the same terminations but without collinearity across the gap, the effect seems very much the same. (See Fig. 30.8.) Subjective contours are still quite apparent although, of course, whether as apparent as with collinear lines is a matter for future experiment.

The lack of importance of collinearity raises the possibility that a *single* row of terminations may be sufficient for the appearance of subjective contours. Single versions are shown for Figures 30.4 to 30.7. (See Fig. 30.9.) Subjective contours are weaker here. The advantage of the double terminations might arise from the fact that they outline an extended occluding surface which single terminations do not. The possibility of amodal completion across the surface does not seem important. However, a similar strengthening of subjective contours occurs when terminations abut each other. (See Fig. 30.10.)

There are some conditions in which single terminations seem to be very effective. This is

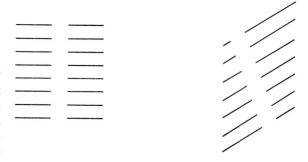

FIGURE 30.7. Subjective contours are stronger when the orientation of the gap sequence is unrelated to the principal axes of the lines in which the gaps occur.

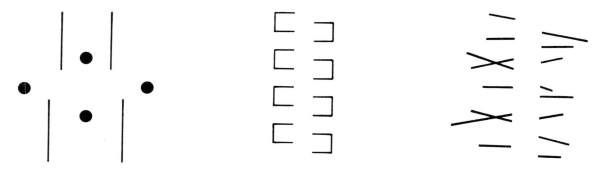

FIGURE 30.8. Showing that collinearity across the gaps is not essential for creating the effects shown in Figures 30.4, 30.5, and 30.6.

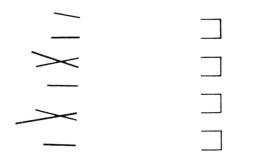

FIGURE 30.9. Showing that a single set of line terminations creates only a weak tendency to form subjective contours relative to a double set.

obvious from Park's zebra figure (chap. 8, Fig. 8.4) and from my Figure 30.11. Here the terminations form curved lines, consistent with the terminations lying on a self-occluding contour. The fact that subjective contours arise so readily under these conditions reinforces the prevalent view that they represent a process of delineating a surface to separate it perceptually from its background.

Conclusions

In the literature there is a convention of drawing subjective contour-inducing figures with lines that are collinear across the region de-

signed to appear occluding. This convention is based on the implicit assumption that the connection between the lines will enhance the appearance of occlusion and hence subjective contours. This assumption does not appear to be warranted. Grouping of lines across a gap (collinearity grouping) seems to be important only if the gap size relative to the line length is very small.

Similarity grouping plays a negative role, in that the more similar a set of lines are and therefore the stronger their tendency to appear as a unit, the less likely it is that their collinear terminations will elicit subjective contours. Order among disorder is particularly powerful.

Although I have argued a somewhat ecological case, that subjective contours arise when stimulus features associated with occlusion are present, it does not seem useful to presume that the process is cognitive, in the sense of thoughtlike or evaluative. It is more parsimonious to argue that stimulus properties, including relative ones, determine the percept directly. The perception of contour in this case results presumably from learned or evolved responses to certain stimulus arrangements which have a high probability of arising from occlusion of one surface by another.

A theory based on the effect of line termina-

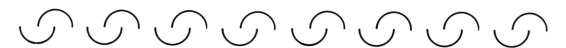

FIGURE 30.10. Double terminations with no gaps also form a powerful subjective contour.

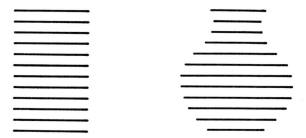

FIGURE 30.11. Subjective contours are more powerful for curved terminations, suggesting a self-occluding contour.

tions will not do unless it incorporates relative properties of the lines terminated, properties such as length, orientation, and separation.

It is unlikely that the processes giving rise to subjective contours have arisen solely for dealing with the situations in which we like to dem-onstrate them: situations in which there is no contrast demarcating the boundary of an over-laying object. A single overlaying object in the environment can be bounded by a great variety of contrasts, some negative and some positive, and it may well be the case that the processes which give rise to subjective contours have de-veloped to give boundary contours a constant appearance as single physical entities despite the vicissitudes of their contrast status. Their perceptual quality depends on information about object relations. The existence of subjec-tive contours shows, as Day (Chap. 5) has pointed out, that perception of a contour is based upon a variety of sources of information. Subjective contours can be thought of as mani-festations of a process of contour constancy. Subjective contours do not reveal a process of filling in gaps, so much as a contour process insensitive to gaps.

CHAPTER 31

Allusory Contours*

Nicholas Wade

This visual epilogue is presented in the hope that the illustrations will both entertain and pose a few puzzles about the nature of illusory contours. Most of the issues raised by the pictures have been addressed earlier in this book, but seeing them in another context might be a suitable way of concluding.

There are at least four levels at which contours can be seen in Figure 31.1: (1) the letters themselves, which are defined physically by the luminance differences; (2) the areas of the incomplete circles, which are defined by the brightness differences averaged within the regions; (3) the patterns within the incomplete circles, which are formed from the differential densities of the typed letters; and (4) the continuities of the sides of the incomplete triangles, for which there is no luminance gradient. The attention of this book is directed principally towards the last type of perceived contour, but we should not lose sight of the problems involved in seeing the others, too.

The illusory figure delineated by the incomplete circles in Figure 31.2 is itself ambiguous: it can be seen either as a vase or as two profiles. Under normal circumstances an incomplete area can signify one object or shape on top of or in front of another, like the triangles in Figure 31.1. According to this principle the profiles would be seen in the central region and parts of the vase at the extremities. Nonetheless, a single figure of either a vase or profiles tends to be seen. In both Figures 31.1 and 31.2 some incompletion or omission—some discontinuity—

is smoothed out by the visual system, so that we see triangles or vase/faces, respectively. However, this does little more than redescribe the phenomenon. There are many incomplete contours that could be completed in these figures, but only certain ones are. Why do we not see illusory contours completing the circles? In other words, why do we see so few illusory contours when there are so many potential completions possible? Could it be the case that if a perceptual completion is to be made then it will be the simplest one? But how is simplicity to be defined? Even here the thorny issue of figure/ground segregation has to be faced. Perhaps this will be made more apparent with Figure 31.3. The form of the Sydney Opera House is defined by omissions from concentric arcs in the upper part, and it is made up from arcs in the reflected lower part. The question is: why is the Opera House perceptually completed and not the arcs of the circles? In one sense the potential completions are in competition. This competition is more explicitly obvious in Figure 31.4, where the completions could be made in two ways: is this a Maltese cross or Maltese circles? The competition need not only be between alternative completions, but also between the possible depth planes in which the illusory contours are seen to lie in this impossible figure (Fig. 31.5).

Schumann (1900) showed that completions can occur across vertically separated parts of a circular pattern; in Figure 31.6 (left) they occur along irregular lines. Does the illusory contour between the letters remain when an additional tear is made, as in Figure 31.6 (right)? Are there illusory contours along the vertical tears?

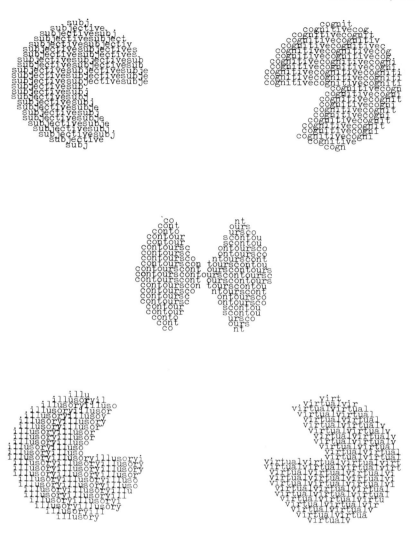

FIGURE 31.1. One phenomenon or many?

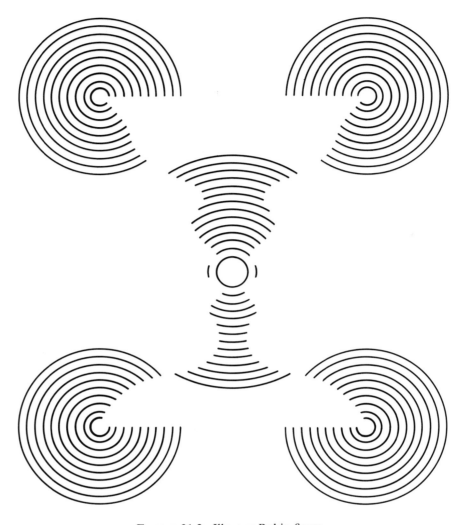

FIGURE 31.2. Illusory Rubin figure.

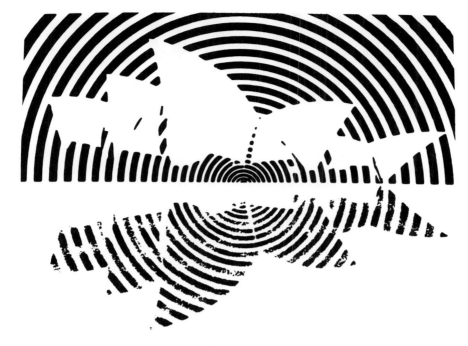

FIGURE 31.3. Op-era house.

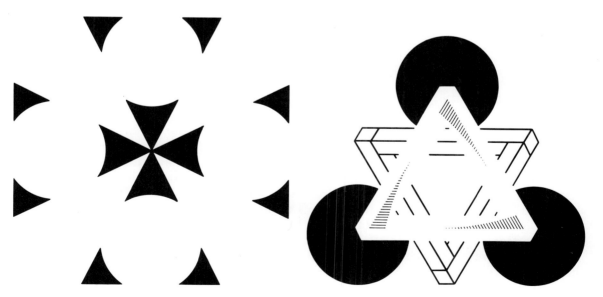

FIGURE 31.4. Competing completions.   FIGURE 31.5. Impossible Kanizsa triangle.

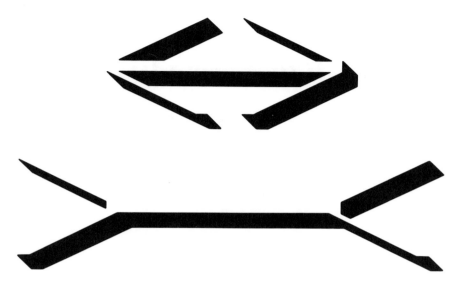

FIGURE 31.6. Torn and Torn Again.

FIGURE 31.7. Depth interpretation of the Müller-Lyer illusion.

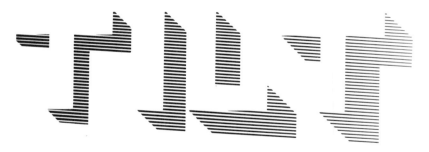

FIGURE 31.8. Inclination.

Shadow effects are often used to create illusory contours, as in Figure 31.7. The dark regions are interpreted as the shadows cast by forms that are in relief with respect to the background. This technique has mostly been used with words: in Figure 31.8 the incomplete shadows of the word appear to be cast on an inclined surface.

Line endings are clearly effective in inducing illusory contours. The contours seen do not meander around the line ends, and they can yield smoothly curved contours like those in Figure

31.9. The same applies to changes in line orientation (Fig. 31.10). Not only does this produce good illusory contours but it also gives an impression of depth. In passing, it is noteworthy that breaking the bilateral symmetry that is almost always present in the Rubin figure tends to favor the visibility of the profiles rather than the vase. It could be the case that the boundary between the orientations is rendered more easily visible because of astigmatic effects. That is, any astigmatism in the viewer's eyes would lead to a difference in the clarity of the contours in

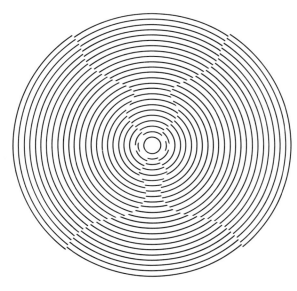

FIGURE 31.9. Mandala.

a portrait of Thomas Young, who first described his own astigmatism at the beginning of the nineteenth century.

Any method of generating perceptual discontinuity provides potential for producing illusory contours. In Figure 31.12 the dark dots formed at the junctions of the white diamond shapes are aligned either concentrically or radially. These are then connected perceptually to give the patterns of illusory circles near the center and radiating lines near the circumference. Similar perceptual completions could be involved in other processes that induce perceptual discontinuities, as Figure 31.13 shows for the familiar Mach bands. There are similar brightness enhancement effects at the extremities of the squashed quadrilaterals in Figure 31.14. The illusory contours, together with the shimmering motion that is seen within the white spaces, add to the impression of waves emanating from the hamburger-like shape in the middle. This partially defined structure is the CN Tower in Toronto.

We now commence with the presentation of allusory rather than illusory contours. An allusory contour is one that hovers near the threshold of vision. It might not be seen initially, but there is always some physical discontinuity,

different orientations, and this could accentuate the perceptual boundary between them. For example, the vertical and horizontal lines in Figure 31.11 create the impression of concentric diamonds that might differ in clarity because of the reader's astigmatism. The figure also carries

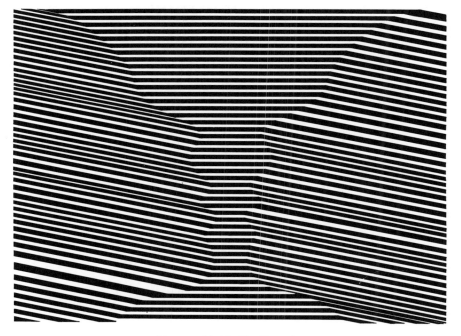

FIGURE 31.10. Profile axis.

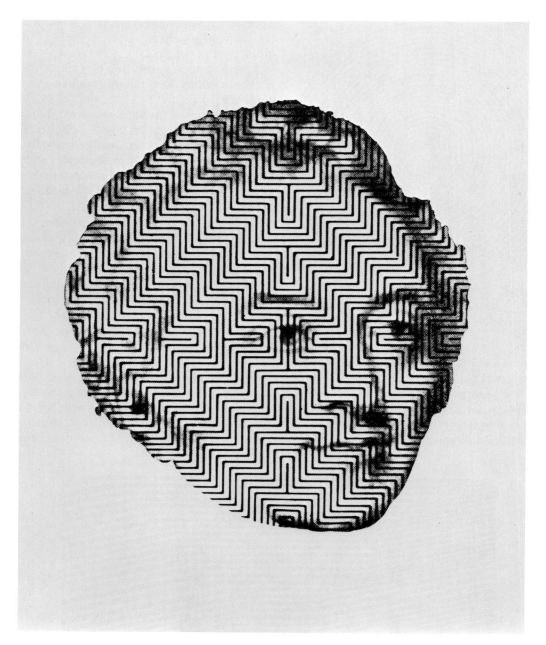

FIGURE 31.11. The astigmatic Thomas Young.

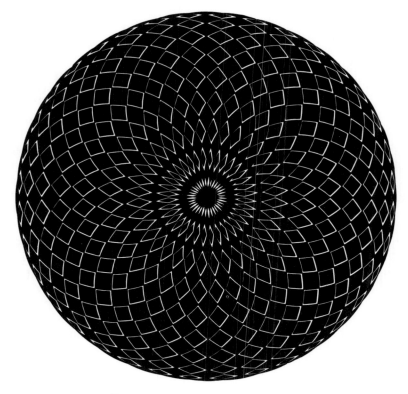

FIGURE 31.12. Good continuations.

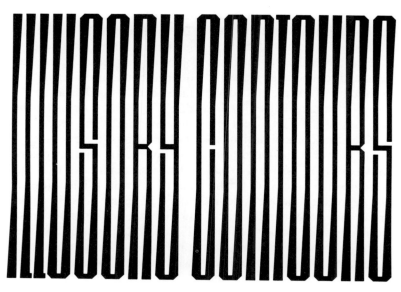

FIGURE 31.13. Border enhancement.

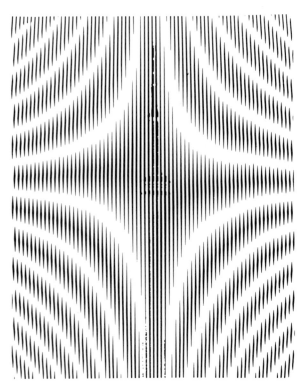

FIGURE 31.14. CN is believing.

shimmering zig-zag forms can appear super-imposed on the pattern (see Wade, 1977, 1982, for a more detailed description of these effects).

The scintillating patterns are less likely to occur when the lines themselves are broken rather than continuous. In Figure 31.17 there are two sets of illusory contours—one describing the concentric circles and the other presenting an allusory portrait of the keynote speaker at the International Conference on Illusory Contours (Petry and Meyer, 1986). They seem to compete for visibility because the circles can be seen when the lines are sharply in focus, whereas the face is more readily apparent when the whole pattern is defocused. The lines themselves do not need to vary very much in thickness in order to set in train the visual processes that lead to the visibility of a face. For example, the slight departures of the tilted lines from straightness in Figure 31.18 defines the portrait of an authority on human visual orientation.

The technique of differential dot size is used in photomechanical printing, and it forms the basis for most of the images we see in newspapers and magazines. With this technique the individual dots vary enormously in size in order to create halftone effects. In Figure 31.19 it might not be possible to discriminate the differences in the sizes of the small dots that make up the larger dots that in turn spell the words *dot matrix*. Again, there is some process of brightness averaging that defines the circular regions of the dots as darker than the background areas. The question to be asked for this and the remaining illustrations is whether we see isolated blobs or a coherent figure that has perceptually defined boundaries. Again, complex forms like faces can be hidden in such regular arrays of dots (Fig. 31.20). Actually, the portrait is not in the dots, but in the spaces between them—the darker regions have smaller white dots so it is the inverse of photomechanical reproduction. The dots do not have to be geometrically regular to provide a basis for such allusory contours. Irregular dots (in color, of course) were used by the Neo-impressionists to create forms. Figure 31.21 pays due homage to the founder of that style—Georges Seurat. For the readers with suitably poor eyesight Seurat's signature (in light dots) might be visible at the bottom left of the picture!

however slight, that will define the incomplete parts of the figure alluded to.

In all the examples that follow the allusory figures might not be visible without some degree of image degradation. This can be achieved by viewing the pictures from afar, by defocusing the image, or by moving it in such a way that the dominant contours become blurred. For example, in Figure 31.15 the words *illusory* and *contours* are repeated throughout in a clearly defined typescript, but the words are embedded in the two parts again—this time defined by differences in the densities of the component letters. In Figure 31.16 the thickness of horizontal lines varies in such a way that the words *illusory contours* can occasionally be seen. When they are visible there is some process of brightness averaging that segregates the areas defining the letters from the more regular background. There are many more illusory effects that can be seen in this figure, even when it is sharply in focus, and some of them are colored: after looking at the pattern for some time the lines become wavy rather than straight, and

```
LUSORYILLUSORYILLUSORYILLUSORYILLUSORYILLUSORYILLUSORYILLUSORYILLUSORYILLUSORYILLUSORYILLUSORYIL
USORYILLUSORYILLUSORYILLUSORYILLUSORYILLUSORYILLUSORYILLUSORYILLUSORYILLUSORYILLUSORYILLUSORYIL
SORYILLUSORYILLUSORYILLUSORYILLUSORYILLUSORYILLUSORYILLUSORYILLUSORYILLUSORYILLUSORYILLUSORYILL
ORYILLUSORYILLUSORYILLUSORYILLUSORYILLUSORYILLUSORYILLUSORYILLUSORYILLUSORYILLUSORYILLUSORYILLU
RYILLUSORYILLUSORYILLUSORYILLUSORYILLUSORYILLUSORYILLUSORYILLUSORYILLUSORYILLUSORYILLUSORYILLUS
YILLUSORYILLUSORYILLUSORYILLUSORYILLUSORYILLUSORYILLUSORYILLUSORYILLUSORYILLUSORYILLUSORYILLUSO
ILLUSORYILLUSORYILLUSORYILLUSORYILLUSORYILLUSORYILLUSORYILLUSORYILLUSORYILLUSORYILLUSORYILLUSOR
LLUSORYILLUSORYILLUSORYILLUSORYILLUSORYILLUSORYILLUSORYILLUSORYILLUSORYILLUSORYILLUSORYILLUSORY
LUSORYILLUSORYILLUSORYILLUSORYILLUSORYILLUSORYILLUSORYILLUSORYILLUSORYILLUSORYILLUSORYILLUSORYI
USORYILLUSORYILLUSORYILLUSORYILLUSORYILLUSORYILLUSORYILLUSORYILLUSORYILLUSORYILLUSORYILLUSORYIL
SORYILLUSORYILLUSORYILLUSORYILLUSORYILLUSORYILLUSORYILLUSORYILLUSORYILLUSORYILLUSORYILLUSORYILL
ORYILLUSORYILLUSORYILLUSORYILLUSORYILLUSORYILLUSORYILLUSORYILLUSORYILLUSORYILLUSORYILLUSORYILLU
RYILLUSORYILLUSORYILLUSORYILLUSORYILLUSORYILLUSORYILLUSORYILLUSORYILLUSORYILLUSORYILLUSORYILLUS
YILLUSORYILLUSORYILLUSORYILLUSORYILLUSORYILLUSORYILLUSORYILLUSORYILLUSORYILLUSORYILLUSORYILLUSO
ILLUSORYILLUSORYILLUSORYILLUSORYILLUSORYILLUSORYILLUSORYILLUSORYILLUSORYILLUSORYILLUSORYILLUSOR
LLUSORYILLUSORYILLUSORYILLUSORYILLUSORYILLUSORYILLUSORYILLUSORYILLUSORYILLUSORYILLUSORYILLUSORY
LUSORYILLUSORYILLUSORYILLUSORYILLUSORYILLUSORYILLUSORYILLUSORYILLUSORYILLUSORYILLUSORYILLUSORYI
USORYILLUSORYILLUSORYILLUSORYILLUSORYILLUSORYILLUSORYILLUSORYILLUSORYILLUSORYILLUSORYILLUSORYIL
SORYILLUSORYILLUSORYILLUSORYILLUSORYILLUSORYILLUSORYILLUSORYILLUSORYILLUSORYILLUSORYILLUSORYILL
ORYILLUSORYILLUSORYILLUSORYILLUSORYILLUSORYILLUSORYILLUSORYILLUSORYILLUSORYILLUSORYILLUSORYILLU
RYILLUSORYILLUSORYILLUSORYILLUSORYILLUSORYILLUSORYILLUSORYILLUSORYILLUSORYILLUSORYILLUSORYILLUS
YILLUSORYILLUSORYILLUSORYILLUSORYILLUSORYILLUSORYILLUSORYILLUSORYILLUSORYILLUSORYILLUSORYILLUSO
ILLUSORYILLUSORYILLUSORYILLUSORYILLUSORYILLUSORYILLUSORYILLUSORYILLUSORYILLUSORYILLUSORYILLUSOR
LLUSORYILLUSORYILLUSORYILLUSORYILLUSORYILLUSORYILLUSORYILLUSORYILLUSORYILLUSORYILLUSORYILLUSORY
LUSORYILLUSORYILLUSORYILLUSORYILLUSORYILLUSORYILLUSORYILLUSORYILLUSORYILLUSORYILLUSORYILLUSORYI
USORYILLUSORYILLUSORYILLUSORYILLUSORYILLUSORYILLUSORYILLUSORYILLUSORYILLUSORYILLUSORYILLUSORYIL
SORYILLUSORYILLUSORYILLUSORYILLUSORYILLUSORYILLUSORYILLUSORYILLUSORYILLUSORYILLUSORYILLUSORYILL
ORYILLUSORYILLUSORYILLUSORYILLUSORYILLUSORYILLUSORYILLUSORYILLUSORYILLUSORYILLUSORYILLUSORYILLU
RYILLUSORYILLUSORYILLUSORYILLUSORY
```

```
                                    ...CONTOURSCONTOURSCONTOURSCONTOURSCONTOURSCONT
URSCONTOURSCONTOURSCONTOURSCONTOURSCONTOURSCONTOURSCONTOURSCONTOURSCONTOURSCONTOURSCONTOURSCONTO
RSCONTOURSCONTOURSCONTOURSCONTOURSCONTOURSCONTOURSCONTOURSCONTOURSCONTOURSCONTOURSCONTOURSCONTOU
SCONTOURSCONTOURSCONTOURSCONTOURSCONTOURSCONTOURSCONTOURSCONTOURSCONTOURSCONTOURSCONTOURSCONTOUR
CONTOURSCONTOURSCONTOURSCONTOURSCONTOURSCONTOURSCONTOURSCONTOURSCONTOURSCONTOURSCONTOURSCONTOURS
ONTOURSCONTOURSCONTOURSCONTOURSCONTOURSCONTOURSCONTOURSCONTOURSCONTOURSCONTOURSCONTOURSCONTOURSC
NTOURSCONTOURSCONTOURSCONTOURSCONTOURSCONTOURSCONTOURSCONTOURSCONTOURSCONTOURSCONTOURSCONTOURSCO
TOURSCONTOURSCONTOURSCONTOURSCONTOURSCONTOURSCONTOURSCONTOURSCONTOURSCONTOURSCONTOURSCONTOURSCON
OURSCONTOURSCONTOURSCONTOURSCONTOURSCONTOURSCONTOURSCONTOURSCONTOURSCONTOURSCONTOURSCONTOURSCONT
URSCONTOURSCONTOURSCONTOURSCONTOURSCONTOURSCONTOURSCONTOURSCONTOURSCONTOURSCONTOURSCONTOURSCONTO
RSCONTOURSCONTOURSCONTOURSCONTOURSCONTOURSCONTOURSCONTOURSCONTOURSCONTOURSCONTOURSCONTOURSCONTOU
SCONTOURSCONTOURSCONTOURSCONTOURSCONTOURSCONTOURSCONTOURSCONTOURSCONTOURSCONTOURSCONTOURSCONTOUR
CONTOURSCONTOURSCONTOURSCONTOURSCONTOURSCONTOURSCONTOURSCONTOURSCONTOURSCONTOURSCONTOURSCONTOURS
ONTOURSCONTOURSCONTOURSCONTOURSCONTOURSCONTOURSCONTOURSCONTOURSCONTOURSCONTOURSCONTOURSCONTOURSC
NTOURSCONTOURSCONTOURSCONTOURSCONTOURSCONTOURSCONTOURSCONTOURSCONTOURSCONTOURSCONTOURSCONTOURSCO
TOURSCONTOURSCONTOURSCONTOURSCONTOURSCONTOURSCONTOURSCONTOURSCONTOURSCONTOURSCONTOURSCONTOURSCON
OURSCONTOURSCONTOURSCONTOURSCONTOURSCONTOURSCONTOURSCONTOURSCONTOURSCONTOURSCONTOURSCONTOURSCONT
URSCONTOURSCONTOURSCONTOURSCONTOURSCONTOURSCONTOURSCONTOURSCONTOURSCONTOURSCONTOURSCONTOURSCONTO
RSCONTOURSCONTOURSCONTOURSCONTOURSCONTOURSCONTOURSCONTOURSCONTOURSCONTOURSCONTOURSCONTOURSCONTOU
SCONTOURSCONTOURSCONTOURSCONTOURSCONTOURSCONTOURSCONTOURSCONTOURSCONTOURSCONTOURSCONTOURSCONTOUR
CONTOURSCONTOURSCONTOURSCONTOURSCONTOURSCONTOURSCONTOURSCONTOURSCONTOURSCONTOURSCONTOURSCONTOURS
ONTOURSCONTOURSCONTOURSCONTOURSCONTOURSCONTOURSCONTOURSCONTOURSCONTOURSCONTOURSCONTOURSCONTOURSC
NTOURSCONTOURSCONTOURSCONTOURSCONTOURSCONTOURSCONTOURSCONTOURSCONTOURSCONTOURSCONTOURSCONTOURSCON
TOURSCONTOURSCONTOURSCONTOURSCONTOURSCONTOURSCONTOURSCONTOURSCONTOURSCONTOURSCONTOURSCONTOURSCON
OURSCONTOURSCONTOURSCONTOURSCONTOURSCONTOURSCONTOURSCONTOURSCONTOURSCONTOURSCONTOURSCONTOURSCONT
URSCONTOURSCONTOURSCONTOURSCONTOURSCONTOURSCONTOURSCONTOURSCONTOURSCONTOURSCONTOURSCONTOURSCONTO
RSCONTOURSCONTOURSCONTOURSCONTOURSCONTOURSCONTOURSCONTOURSCONTOURSCONTOURSCONTOURSCONTOURSCONTOU
SCONTOURSCONTOURSCONTOURSCONTOURSCONTOURSCONTOURSCONTOURSCONTOURSCONTOURSCONTOURSCONTOURSCONTOUR
```

FIGURE 31.15. Illusory contours.

FIGURE 31.16. Allusory illusory contours.

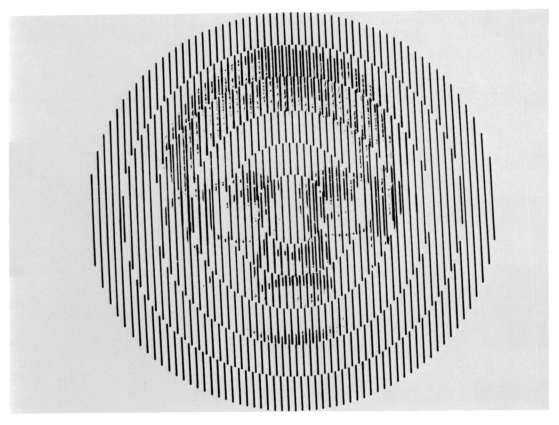

FIGURE 31.17. Day focused.

FIGURE 31.18. Human facial orientation (Ian Howard).

Pattern regularities that occur in nature can also be employed to embed images. In Figure 31.22 the striated configurations of the ocular dominance regions in the visual cortex are employed to carry the portraits of Hubel and Wiesel. Two portraits are also hidden in Figure 31.23. The design itself is made up from the intersections of vertical and radiating lines, with their attendant interference fringes. On the right side is a positive portrait of the artist Ludwig Wilding, whereas a negative portrait is on the left. In common with photographic images generally, the positive image is easier to recognise than the negative. Minimal information is provided for the facial features in Figure 31.24, but when the slight discontinuities defining the eye, nose, and mouth are detected then the profile can be seen.

Musical scores or written text provide powerful aids to visual allusion because focused vision is required to read them and this can render the embedded image harder to discern (see Wade, 1985, for further examples). Figure 31.25 is an allusory celebration of Bach's tercentenary, whereas Figure 31.26 contains text from an even older source. Here we see Ben Jonson's

FIGURE 31.19. Dot matrices.

FIGURE 31.20. Chris scene.

FIGURE 31.21. Pointillism.

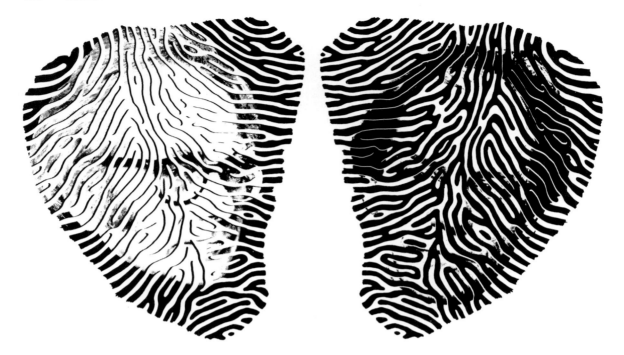

FIGURE 31.22. Feature detectives.

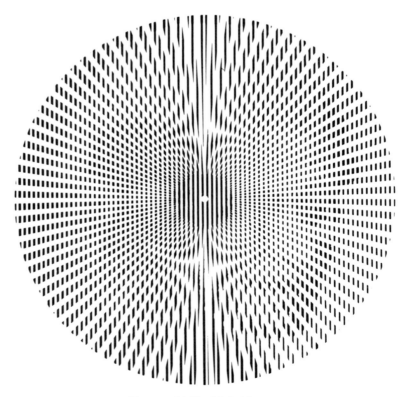

FIGURE 31.23. Moiré images.

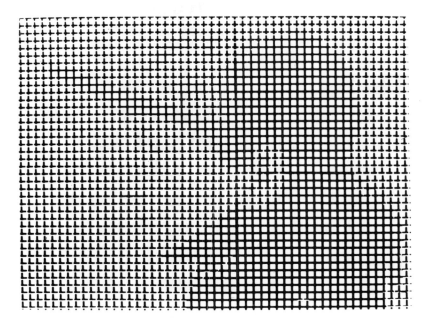

FIGURE 31.24. Jockey.

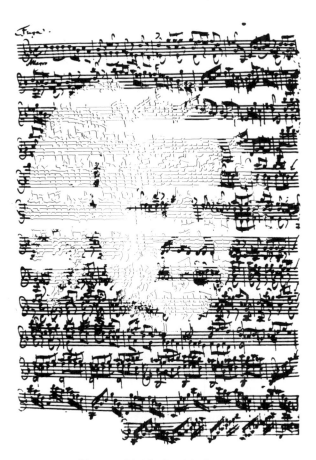

FIGURE 31.25. Bach's fugue.

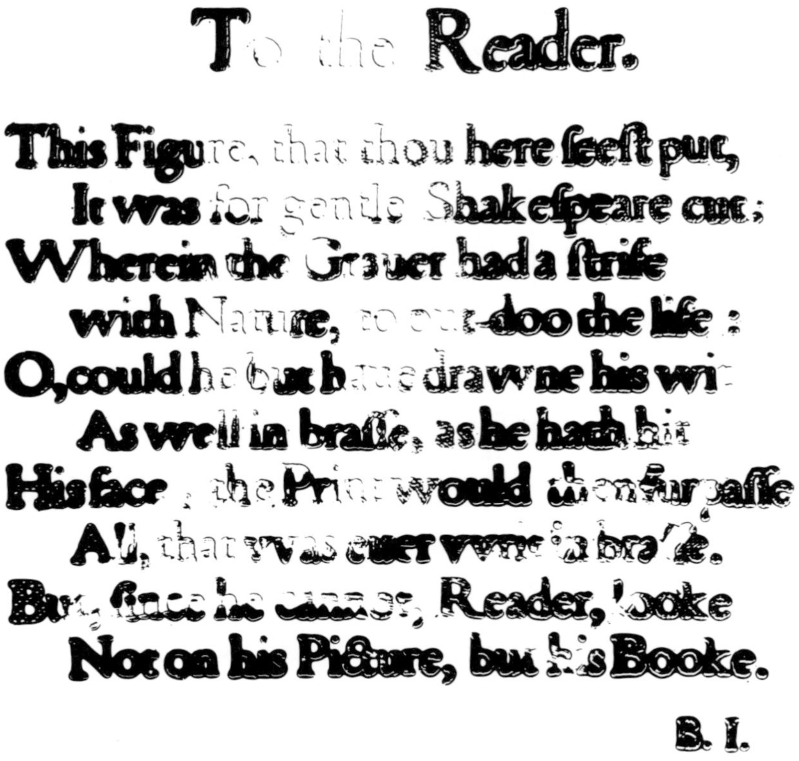

To the Reader.

This Figure, that thou here seeſt put,
It was for gentle Shakeſpeare cut;
Wherein the Grauer had a ſtrife
with Nature, to out-doo the life :
O, could he but haue drawne his wit
As well in braſſe, as he hath hit
His face ; the Print would then ſurpaſſe
All, that was euer writ in braſſe.
But, ſince he cannot, Reader, looke
Not on his Picture, but his Booke.

B. I.

FIGURE 31.26. Droeschout's Shakespeare.

preface to the First Folio edition of Shakespeare's plays. Jonson is writing about the portrait of Shakespeare, drawn by Martin Droeschout, that is on the opposite, title page of that edition. You, too, can see the portrait by suitably defocusing the text. When reading the text you are fulfilling Jonson's request because in the process of reading, the portrait cannot be seen, and when you see the face the text is illegible. Not all of us share Jonson's or Shakespeare's facility with words, and so we need to consult one of those books which provide lists of word alternatives. The cross-referenced system compiled by that student of vision, Peter Mark Roget (Fig. 31.27), is perhaps the best known. One of the words not in his compilation is *quale,* although this was used by the eminent psychologist William James. In Figure 31.28 we see a quale, or vague form, of James in text that is taken from his *Principles of Psychology.*

Do we need an allusory visual system to account for allusory contours? Perhaps not, because Figure 31.29 provides a representation of the visual system as we presently understand it.

Rays of light enter the eye through a small aperture and then strike the retina. Within the retina there are three neural levels consisting of the receptors, bipolar cells, and retinal ganglion cells—all of which have lateral connections via the horizontal and amacrine cells (could these be the site for the Hermann-Hering grid effects?). The axons from the ganglion cells travel to the visual cortex, undergoing partial decussation so that the nasal and temporal hemiretinae project to opposite hemispheres; however there is some bilateral projection along the vertical midline. At the level of the visual cortex there is an organization in terms of vertical columns, within which are six horizontal layers (could these be the site for illusory contours?). We should not overlook the fact that we have two eyes and there is a large degree of binocular overlap of the monocular visual fields, in which there is binocular brightness enhancement. It would have to be admitted that, while this representation of the eye and brain is certainly not illusory, it might reasonably be said to be allusory.

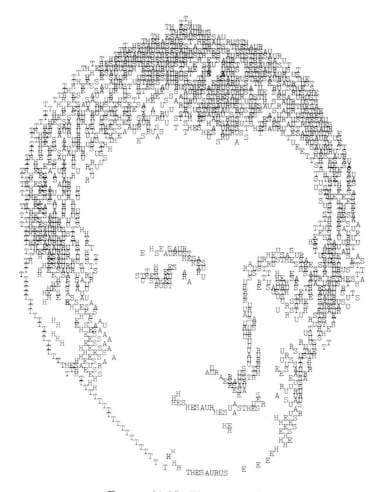

FIGURE 31.27. Thesaurus of Roget.

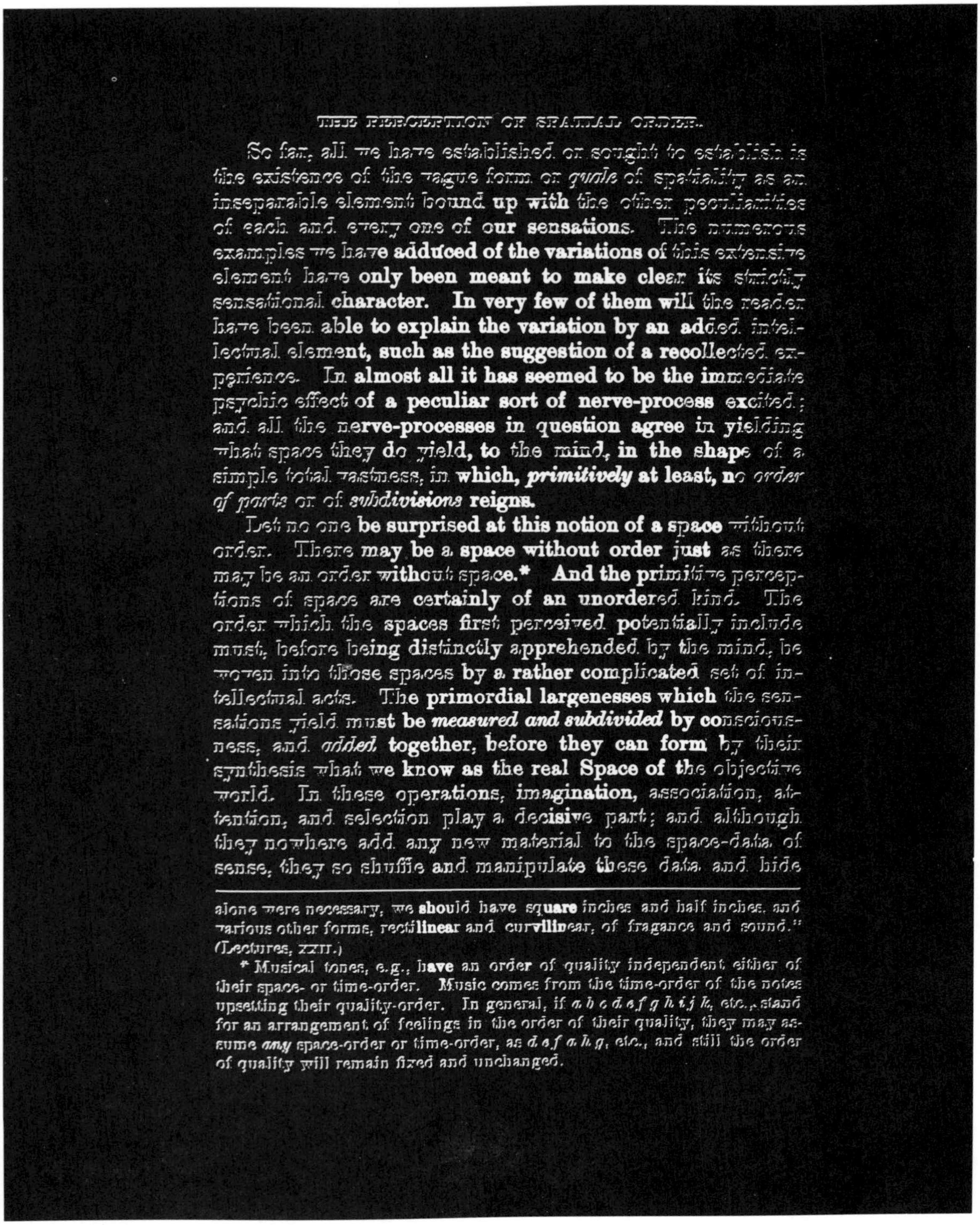

THE PERCEPTION OF SPATIAL ORDER.

So far, all we have established, or sought to establish, is the existence of the vague form or *quale* of spatiality as an inseparable element bound up with the other peculiarities of each and every one of our sensations. The numerous examples we have adduced of the variations of this extensive element have only been meant to make clear its strictly sensational character. In very few of them will the reader have been able to explain the variation by an added intellectual element, such as the suggestion of a recollected experience. In almost all it has seemed to be the immediate psychic effect of a peculiar sort of nerve-process excited; and all the nerve-processes in question agree in yielding what space they do yield, to the mind, in the shape of a simple total vastness, in which, *primitively* at least, no *order of parts* or of *subdivisions* reigns.

Let no one be surprised at this notion of a space without order. There may be a space without order just as there may be an order without space.* And the primitive perceptions of space are certainly of an unordered kind. The order which the spaces first perceived potentially include must, before being distinctly apprehended by the mind, be woven into those spaces by a rather complicated set of intellectual acts. The primordial largenesses which the sensations yield must be *measured and subdivided* by consciousness, and *added* together, before they can form by their synthesis what we know as the real Space of the objective world. In these operations, imagination, association, attention, and selection play a decisive part; and although they nowhere add any new material to the space-data of sense, they so shuffle and manipulate these data and hide

---

alone were necessary, we should have square inches and half inches, and various other forms, rectilinear and curvilinear, of fragance and sound." (Lectures, XIII.)

* Musical tones, e.g., have an order of quality independent either of their space- or time-order. Music comes from the time-order of the notes upsetting their quality-order. In general, if *a b c d e f g h i j k*, etc., stand for an arrangement of feelings in the order of their quality, they may assume *any* space-order or time-order, as *d e f a h g*, etc., and still the order of quality will remain fixed and unchanged.

FIGURE 31.28. Quale of William James.

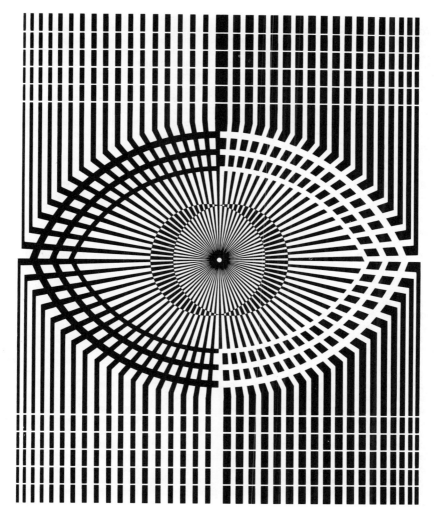

FIGURE 31.29. Eye and brain.

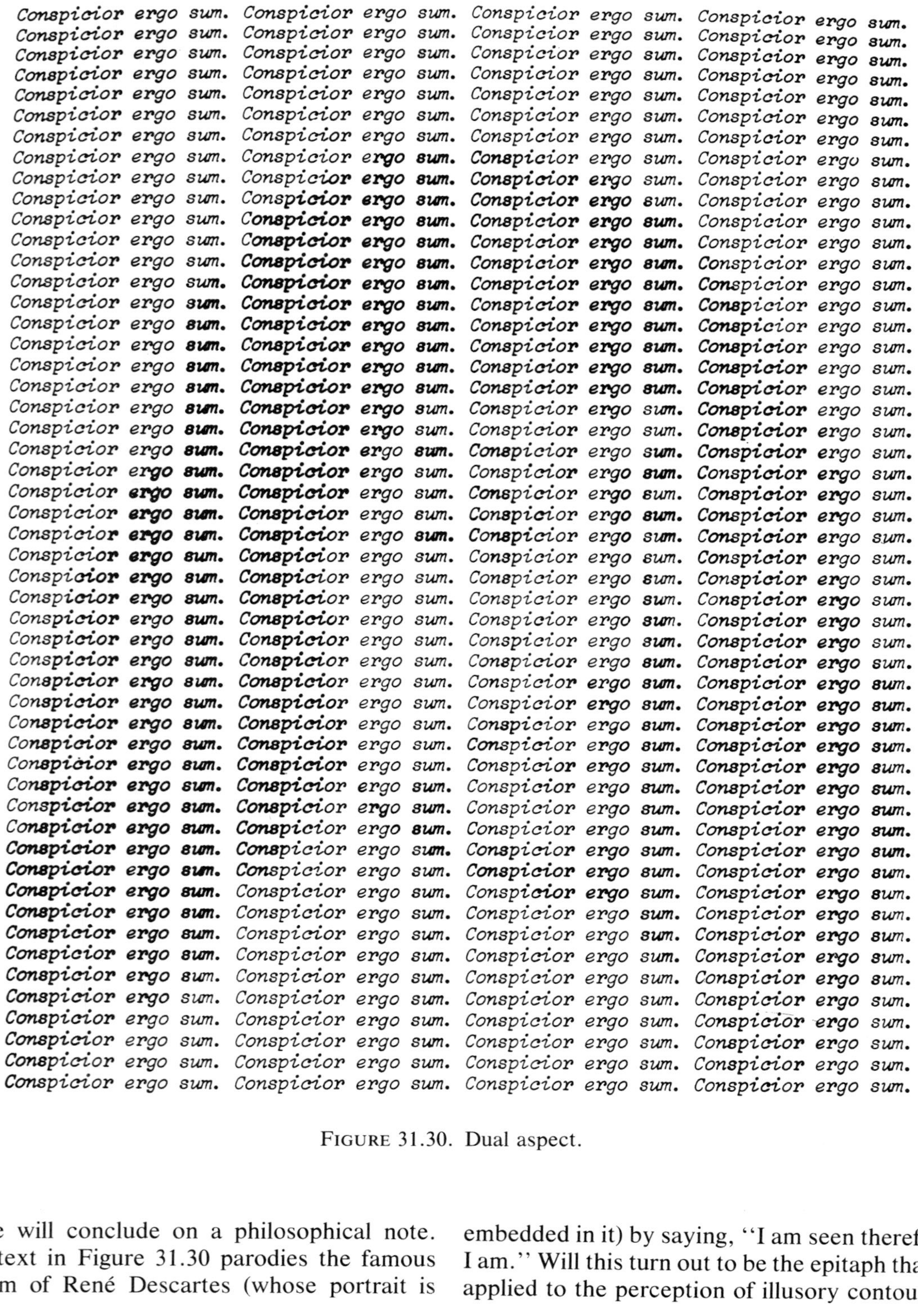

Conspicior ergo sum. repeated across the figure forming a portrait.

FIGURE 31.30. Dual aspect.

We will conclude on a philosophical note. The text in Figure 31.30 parodies the famous dictum of René Descartes (whose portrait is embedded in it) by saying, "I am seen therefore I am." Will this turn out to be the epitaph that is applied to the perception of illusory contours?

References

Abravanel, E. (1982). Perceiving subjective contours during early childhood. *Journal of Experimental Child Psychology, 33,* 280–287.

Albers, J. (1975). *Interaction of color.* New Haven: Yale University Press.

Andersen, G. J., & Braunstein, M. L. (1983). Dynamic occlusion in the perception of rotation in depth. *Perception and Psychophysics, 34,* 356–362.

Anstis, A. M. (1970). Phi movements as a subtraction process. *Vision Research, 10,* 1411–1430.

Arnheim, R. (1974). *Art and visual perception.* Berkeley: University of California Press.

Arnheim, R. (1986). The two faces of gestalt psychology. *American Psychologist, 41,* 820–824.

Bachman, T. (1978). Cognitive contours: Overview and a preliminary theory. *Problems of Communication and Perception, Transactions of the State University of Tartuensis: Studies in Psychology, 7(474),* 31–60.

Banks, W. P., & Prinzmetal, W. (1976). Configurational effects in visual information processing. *Perception & Psychophysics, 19,* 361–367.

Barbur, J. L. (1981). Subthreshold addition of real and apparent motion. *Vision Research, 21,* 557–564.

Barlow, H. B. (1981). Critical limiting factors in the design of the eyes and visual cortex. *Proceedings of the Royal Society of London, B 212,* 1–34.

Barlow, H. B., Blakemore, C. B., & Pettigrew, J. D. (1967). The neural mechanism of binocular depth discrimination. *Journal of Physiology, 193,* 327–342.

Bartley, S. H. (1941). *Vision, a study of its basis.* New York: Van Nostrand.

Beck, J. (1966). Effect of orientation and shape similarity on perceptual grouping. *Perception and Psychophysics, 1,* 300–302.

Beck, J. (1978). Additive and sutractive color mixture in color transparency. *Perception and Psychophysics, 23,* 265–267.

Beck, J. (1983). Textural segmentation, second-order statistics, and textural elements. *Biological Cybernetics, 48,* 125–130.

Beck, J., Prazdny, K., & Ivry, R. (1984). The perception of transparency with achromatic colors. *Perception and Psychophysics, 35,* 408–422.

Beck, J., Prazdny, K., & Rosenfeld, A. (1983). A theory of textural segmentation. In J. Beck, B. Hope, & A. Rosenfeld (Eds.), *Human and machine vision.* New York: Academic Press.

Becker, M. F., & Knopp, J. (1978). Processing of visual illusions in the frequency and spatial domains. *Perception and Psychophysics, 23,* 521–526.

Bejor, G. (1947). La totalizzazione percettiva in campo rotante. In *Contributi dell'Istituto di Psicologia dell'Università di Padova.* Padova.

Benary, W. (1924). Beobachtung zu einem Experiment uber Helligkeitskontrat. *Psychologisch Forschung, 5,* 131–142. (Reprinted in W. Ellis, *A source book of Gestalt psychology,* Selection 8. The Humanities Press, 1950).

Berkeley, G. (1922). *A new theory of vision* (Everyman's Library Edition). New York: Dutton. (Original work published 1604).

Bertenthal, B. I., Campos, J. J., & Haith, M. M. (1980). Development of visual organization: The perception of subjective contours. *Child Development, 51,* 1072–1080.

Berry, W. T., Johson, A. F., & Jaspert, W. P. (1962). *The encyclopedia of type faces.* New York: Pitman Publishing Company.

Blomfield, S. (1973). Implicit features and stereoscopy. *Nature: New Biology, 245,* 147.

Bobak, P., Reichert, B., Petry, S., & Schneck, M. (1979, April). *A comparison of brightness and sensitivity changes with blurred and sharp-edged stimuli of varying durations.* Paper presented at the spring meeting of the Association for Research in Vision and Ophthalmology (ARVO), Sarasota, FL.

Bourassa, C. M. (1986). Models for sensation and perception: A selective history. *Human Neurobiology, 5,* 23–36.

Bowen, R. W., & Pokorny, J. (1978). Target edge sharpness and temporal brightness enhancement. *Vision Research, 18,* 1691–1695.

Boynton, R. B., Hayhoe, M., & MacLeod, D. I. A. (1977). The gap effect: Chromatic and achromatic visual discrimination as affected by field separation. *Optica Acta, 24,* 159–77.

Braddick, O. J. (1974). A short-range process in apparent motion. *Vision Research, 14,* 519–527.

Bradley, D. R. (1976). Personal communication. Cited in Kennedy, J. M. (1976). Sun figure: An illusory diffuse contour resulting from an arrangement of dots. *Perception, 5,* 479–481.

Bradley, D. R. (1982). Binocular rivalry of real vs. subjective contours. *Perception and Psychophysics, 32,* 85–87.

Bradley, D. R. (1983). Nuove osservazioni sui margini soggettive. *Giornale Italiano di Psicologia, X,* 329–358 (available in translation).

Bradley, D. R., & Dumais, S. T. (1975). Ambiguous cognitive contours. *Nature, 257,* 582–584.

Bradley, D. R., & Dumais, S. T. (1984). The effects of illumination level and retinal size on the depth stratification of subjective-contour figures. *Perception, 13,* 155–164.

Bradley, D. R., Dumais, S. T., & Petry, H. M. (1976). Reply to Cavonius. *Nature, 261,* 77–78.

Bradley, D. R., & Hirsch, R. G. (1987). Cognitive style and subjective contours. Unpublished manuscript.

Bradley, D. R., & Lee, K. (1982). Animated subjective contours. *Perception and Psychophysics, 32,* 393–395.

Bradley, D. R., & Mates, S. M. (1985). Perceptual organization and apparent brightness in subjective-contour figures. *Perception, 14,* 645–653.

Bradley, D. R., & Pennella, M. A. (1987). The effects of eye movements on the apparent strength of subjective contours. Unpublished manuscript.

Bradley, D. R., & Petry, H. M. (1977). Organizational determinants of subjective contour: The subjective Necker cube. *American Journal of Psychology, 90,* 253–262.

Bradley, D. R., & Wood, L. C. (1987). The effects of rotation on the apparent shape of real and subjective contours. Unpublished manuscript.

Brady, M., & Grimson, W. E. (1981). *The perception of subjective surfaces.* MIT AI Memo No. 666.

Brandeis, D. U., Lehmann, D., & Mueller, R. U.

(1985). Late EP negativity and perception of Kanisza triangle. *Biological Psychiatry, 20,* 192–193.

Braunstein, M. L. (1962). Depth perception in rotating dot patterns: Effects of numerosity and perspective. *Journal of Experimental Psychology, 64,* 415–420.

Braunstein, M. L. (1966). Sensitivity of the observer to transformations of the visual field. *Journal of Experimental Psychology, 72,* 683–689.

Braunstein, M. L. (1976). *Depth perception through motion.* New York: Academic Press.

Braunstein, M. L. (1983). Perception of rotation in depth: The psychophysical evidence. In *AMC SIGGRAPH and SIGART interdisciplinary workshops on motion: Representation and perception* (pp. 119–124). New York: The Association for Computing Machinery.

Breitmeyer, B. G. (1980). Unmasking visual masking: A look at the "why" behind the veil of the "how." *Psychological Review, 87,* 52–69.

Brigner, W. L., & Gallagher, M. B. (1974). Subjective contour: Apparent depth or simultaneous brightness contrast? *Perception and Motor Skills, 38,* 1047–1053.

Brown, J. M. (1985). *Phantom contour completion: A figure/ground approach.* Unpublished doctoral dissertation, State University of New York at Buffalo.

Brown, J. M., & Weisstein, N. (1985a). Flickering phantoms: A figure/ground approach. *Proceedings and Abstracts of the Annual Meeting of the Eastern Psychological Society, 57,* 38.

Brown, J. M. & Weisstein, N. (1985b). *Visual phantoms enhance target visibility: An illustration of the power of figural organization.* Manuscript submitted for publication.

Brown, J. M., & Weisstein, N. (1986). Depth information within phantom inducing regions can influence phantom visibility. *Proceedings and Abstracts of the Annual Meeting of the Eastern Psychological Association, 57,* 63.

Brunswik, E. (1935). *Experimentelle psychologie in demonstrationen.* Wien: J. Springer.

Brussell, E. M., Stober, S. R., & Bodinger, D. M. (1977). Sensory information and subjective contour. *American Journal of Psychology, 90*(1), 145–156.

Burkhardt, D. A. (1966). Brightness and the increment threshold. *Journal of the Optical Society of America, 56,* 979–981.

Buzzati, P. (1974). *La percezione visiva di figure presentate in condizioni di variazione di illuminazione (effetto Liebmann)* [Visual perception of figures presented with varying light conditions (Liebmann effect)]. Tesi di Laurea. Istituto di Psicologia, Università di Padova.

Caelli, T., Flanagan, P., & Green, S. (1982). On the limits of perceptual complementarity in the kinetic depth effect. *Perception and Psychophysics, 31*, 437–445.

Callaghan, T. C., Lasaga, M. L., & Garner, W. R. (1986). Visual texture segregation based on orientation and hue. *Perception & Psychophysics, 39*, 46.

Cavanagh, P. (1985, November). *Subjective contours signaled by luminance, vetoed by motion or depth*. Paper presented at the meeting of the Psychonomic Society, Boston, MA.

Cavanagh, P. (1987). Reconstructing the third dimension: Interactions between color, texture, motion, binocular disparity and shape. In *Computer vision, graphics and image processing*. New York: Academic Press, pp. 171–195.

Cavanagh, P., Boeglin, J., & Favreau, O. (1985). Perception of motion in equiluminous kinematograms. *Perception, 14*, 151–162.

Cavanagh, P., Tyler, C. W., & Favreau, O. E. (1983). Perceived velocity of moving chromatic gratings. *Journal of the Optical Society of America, 73*, 893–899.

Cheathan, P. G. (1952). Visual latency as a function of stimulus brightness and contour shape. *Journal of Experimental Psychology, 43*, 369–380.

Cohen, M. A., & Grossberg, S. (1984). Neural dynamics of brightness perception: Features, boundaries, diffusion, and resonance. *Perception and Psychophysics, 36*, 428–456.

Coren, S. (1969). Brightness contrast as a function of figure-ground relations. *Journal of Experimental Psychology, 80*, 517–524.

Coren, S. (1972). Subjective contour and apparent depth. *Psychological Review, 79*, 359–367.

Coren, S. (1974). Reply to Banks and Coffin. *Psychological Review, 81*, 266.

Coren, S. (1984). Set. In R. J. Corsini (Ed.), *The encyclopedia of psychology* (Vol. 3, pp. 296–298). New York: Wiley.

Coren, S., & Festinger, L. (1967). An alternate view of the "Gibson normalization effect." *Perception and Psychophysics, 2*, 621–626.

Coren, S., & Girgus, J. S. (1978). *Seeing is deceiving: The psychology of visual illusions*. Hillsdale, NJ: Lawrence Erlbaum Associates.

Coren, S. C., & Komoda, M. K. (1973). The effect of cues to illumination on apparent brightness. *American Journal of Psychology, 86*, 345–349.

Coren, S., & Porac, C. (1983). Subjective contours and apparent depth: A direct test. *Perception and Psychophysics, 33*, 197–200.

Coren, S., & Theodor, L. H. (1975). Subjective contour: The inadequacy of brightness contrast as an explanation. *Bulletin of the Psychonomic Society, 6*, 87–89.

Coren, S., & Theodor, L. H. (1977). Neural interactions and subjective contours. *Perception, 6*, 107–111.

Cornsweet, T. N. (1962). The staircase-method in psychophysics. *American Journal of Psychology, 75*, 485–491.

Cornsweet, T. N. (1970). *Visual Perception*. New York: Academic Press.

Cornsweet, T. N., & Teller, D. Y. (1965). Relation of increment thresholds to brightness and luminance. *Journal of the Optical Society of America, 55*, 1303–1308.

Craik, K. J. W., & Zangwill, O. L. (1939). Observations relating to the threshold of a small figure within the contour of a closed-line figure. *British Journal of Psychology, 30*, 139–150.

Crassini, B., & Broerse, J. (1983). *Making ambiguous figures unambiguous: The influence of real and induced colours on perceptual alternation*. Paper presented at the Tenth Experimental Psychology Conference, Hobart College, Geneva, NY.

Cutting, J. E. (1986). *Perception with an eye for motion*. Cambridge, MA: MIT Press.

Dawson, M. E., Schell, A. M., Beers, J. R., & Kelly, A. (1982). Allocation of cognitive processing capacity during human autonomic classical conditioning. *Journal of Experimental Psychology: General, 11*, 273–295.

Day, R. H. (1983). Neon color spreading, partially delineated borders, and the formation of illusory contours. *Perception and Psychophysics, 34*, 488–490.

Day, R. H. (1986). Enhancement of edges by contrast, depth and figure: The origin of illusory contours. In J. D. Pettigrew, K. J. Sanderson, & W. R. Levick (Eds.), *Visual neurosciences*. Cambridge: Cambridge University Press.

Day, R. H., & Jory, M. K. (1978). Subjective contours, visual acuity, and line contrast. In J. C. Armington, J. E. Krauskopf, & B. R. Wooten (Eds.), *Visual psychophysics: Its physiological basis*, (pp. 331–340). New York: Academic Press.

Day, R. H., & Jory, M. K. (1980). A note on a second stage in the formation of illusory contours. *Perception and Psychophysics, 27*, 89–91.

Day, R. H., & Kasperczyk, R. T. (1983a). Amodal completion as a basis for illusory contours. *Perception and Psychophysics, 33*, 355–364.

Day, R. H., & Kasperczyk, R. T. (1983b). Illusory contours in line patterns with apparent depth due to either perspective or overlay. *Perception, 12*, 485–490.

de Weert, C. M. M. (1979). Colour contours and stereopsis. *Vision Research, 19*, 555–564.

de Weert, C. M. M. (1984). Veridical perception: A key to the choice of colors and brightnesses in multicolor displays. In P. Gibson (Ed.), *Mono-

chrome vs. color in electronic displays. Farnborough, RAE, 18. 1–18.8.

DeYoe, E. A., & Van Essen, D. C. (1985). Segregation of efferent connections and receptive field properties in visual area V2 of the Macaque. *Nature, 317,* 58–61.

Donner, J., Lappin, J. S., & Perfetto, G. (1984). Detection of three-dimensional structure in moving optical patterns. *Journal of Experimental Psychology: Human Perception and Performance, 10,* 1–11.

Dumais, S. T., & Bradley, D. R. (1976). The effects of illumination level and retinal size on the apparent strength of subjective contours. *Perception and Psychophysics, 19,* 339–345.

Duncker, K. (1945). On problem solving. *Psychological Monographs, 58,* 1–112.

Ehrenstein, W. (1941). Uber Abwandlungen der L. Hermannschen Helligkeitserscheinung [Modifications of the brightness phenomenon of L. Hermann]. *Zeitschrift für Psychologie, 150,* 83–91.

Ehrenstein, W. (1954). *Probleme der ganzheitpsychologischen Wahrnehmungslehre* (3rd ed.). Leipzig: J. A. Barth.

Enns, J. (1986). Seeing textons in context. *Perception and Psychophysics, 39,* 143–147.

Enns, J. T., & Prinzmetal, W. (1984). The role of redundancy in the object-line effect. *Perception and Psychophysics, 35,* 22–32.

Eriksson, S. E. (1974). A theory of veridical space perception. *Scandinavian Journal of Psychology, 15,* 225–235.

Fehrer, E. & Raab, D. (1962). Reaction time to stimuli masked by metacontrast. *Journal of Experimental Psychology, 63,* 143–147.

Fiorentini, A., & Mazzantini, L. (1966). Neural inhibition in the human fovea: a study of interactions between two line stimuli. *Atti Della Fondazione Giorgio Ronchi, 21,* 738–747.

Fiorentini, A., & Zoli, M. T. (1966). Detection of a target superimposed on a step pattern of illumination. *Atti Della Fondazione Giorgio Ronchi, 21,* 338–356.

Fiorentini, A., & Zoli, M. T. (1967). Detection of a target superimposed to a step pattern of illumination. *Atti Della Fondazione Giorgio Ronchi, 22,* 207–217.

Fox, J. (1978). Continuity, concealment and visual attention. In G. Underwood (Ed.), Strategies of Information Processing (pp. 23–66). New York: Academic Press.

Fox, R. (1981). Stereopsis in animals and human infants: A review of behavioral investigations. In R. N. Aslin, J. R. Alberts, & M. R. Peterson (Eds), *Development of perception, Vol. 2.* New York: Academic Press.

Fox, R., & McDaniel, C. (1982). The perception of biological motion by human infants. *Science, 218,* 486–487.

Frisby, J. P. (1980). *Seeing.* Oxford: Oxford University Press.

Frisby, J. P., & Clatworthy, J. L. (1975). Illusory contours: Curious cases of simultaneous brightness contrast? *Perception, 4,* 349–357.

Fuchs, W. (1967). On transparency. In W. D. Ellis (Ed.), *A source book of Gestalt psychology* (pp. 89–94). New York: Humanities Press. (Original work published 1924)

Galli, A. & Hochheimer, W. (1934). Beobachtungen an Nachzeichnungen mehrdeutiger Feldkonturen. *Zeitschrift für Psychologie, 132.*

Ganz, L. (1975). Temporal factors in visual perception. In Cartarette, E. C. and Friedman, M. P. *Handbook of Perception: Seeing,* Vol. 5, New York: Academic Press, pp. 169–231.

Geldard, F. A. (1972). *The human senses* (2nd ed.). New York: Wiley.

Gellatly, A. R. H. (1980). Perception of an illusory triangle with masked inducing figure. *Perception, 9,* 599–602.

Gellatly, A. R. H. (1982). Perceptual learning of illusory contours and colour. *Perception, 11,* 655–661.

Genter, C. R., & Weisstein, N. (1981). Flickering phantoms: A motion illusion without motion. *Vision Research, 21,* 963–966.

Gerbino, W., & Salmaso, D. (1985). Un analisi processuale del completamento amodale. *Giornale Italiano de Psicologia, 12,* 97–121.

Gibson, E. J. (1969). *Principles of perceptual learning and development.* New York: Appleton Century Crofts.

Gibson, J. J. (1950). *The perception of the visual world.* Boston: Houghton Mifflin.

Gibson, J. J. (1951). What is a form? *Psychological Review, 58,* 403–412.

Gibson, J. J. (1961). Ecological optics. *Vision Research, 1,* 253–262.

Gibson, J. J. (1966). *The senses considered as perceptual systems.* Boston: Houghton Mifflin.

Gibson, J. J. (1979). *The ecological approach to visual perception.* Boston: Houghton Mifflin.

Gibson, J. J., Kaplan, G. A., Reynolds, H. N., & Wheeler, K. (1969). The change from visible to invisible: A study of optical transitions. *Perception and Psychophysics, 5,* 113–116.

Gilchrist, A. (1977). Perceived lightness depends on perceived spatial arrangement. *Science, 195,* 185–187.

Gillam, B. (1972). Perceived common rotary motion of ambiguous stimuli as a criterion of perceptual grouping. *Perception and Psychophysics, 11,* 99–101.

Gillam, B. (1975). New evidence for 'closure' in perception. *Perception and Psychophysics, 17,* 521–524.

Gillam, B. (1976). Grouping of multiple ambiguous contours: Towards an understanding of surface perception. *Perception, 5,* 203–209.

Gillam, B. & Grant, T., Jr. (1982). Aggregation and unit formation in the perception of moving collinear lines. *Perception, 13,* 659–664.

Ginsburg, A. P. (1975). Is the illusory triangle physical or imaginary? *Nature, 257,* 215–220.

Ginsburg, A. P. (1978). *Visual information processing based on spatial filters constrained by biological data* (Doctoral dissertation, University of Cambridge) pp. 78–129. Air Force Applied Medical Research Laboratories Technical Report.

Girgus, J., Rock, I., & Egatz, R. (1977). The effect of knowledge of reversibility on the reversibility of ambiguous figures. *Perception and Psychophysics, 22,* 550–556.

Glass, L., & Switkes, E. (1976). Pattern recognition in humans: Correlations which cannot be perceived. *Perception, 5,* 67–72.

Glynn, A. (1954). Apparent transparency and the tunnel effect. *Quart. Journal of Experimental Psychology, 6,* 3.

Goldberg, D. H., & Pomerantz, J. R. (1982). Models of illusory pausing and sticking. *Journal of Experimental Psychology: Human Perception and Performance, 8,* 547–561.

Goldstein, M. B., & Weintraub, D. J. (1972). The parallel-less Poggendorf: Virtual contours put the illusion down but not out. *Perception and Psychophysics, 11,* 353–355.

Granit, R. (1977). *The Purposive Brain,* The MIT Press, Cambridge, Massachusetts.

Granrud, C. E., Yonas, A., Smith, I. M., Arterburry, M., Glicksman, M., & Sorknes, A. (1984). Infant's sensitivity to accretion and deletion of texture as information for depth at an edge. *Child Development, 55,* 1630–1636.

Greenwald, A. G., Pratkanis, A. R., Leippe, M. R., & Baumgardner, M. H. (1986). Under what conditions does theory obstruct research progress? *Psychological Review, 3,* 216–229.

Gregory, R. L. (1966). *Visual illusion.* In B. Foss (Ed.), *New horizons in psychology.* Baltimore: Penguin Books.

Gregory, R. L. (1970). *The intelligent eye.* London: Wiedenfeld & Nicholson; New York: McGraw-Hill.

Gregory, R. L. (1972). Cognitive contours. *Nature, 238,* 51–52.

Gregory, R. L. (1977). Vision with isoluminant color contrast: 1. A projection technique and observation. *Perception, 6,* 113–119.

Gregory, R. L. (1981). *Mind in science.* London: Weidenfeld & Nicolson.

Gregory, R. L. (1985). *Illusory surfaces as perceptual postulates.* Paper presented at the International Conference on Illusory Contours, Adelphi University, Garden City, NY, November.

Gregory, R. L., & Harris, J. (1974). Illusory contours and stereo depth. *Perception and Psychophysics, 15,* 411–416.

Gregory, R. L., & Heard, P. F. (1979). Border locking and the cafe wall illusion. *Perception, 8,* 365.

Grossberg, S. (1984). Outline of a theory of brightness, color, and form perception. In E. Degreef & J. van Buggenhaut (Eds.), *Trends in mathematical psychology.* Amsterdam: North-Holland.

Grossberg, S., & Mingolla, E. (1985a). Neural dynamics of form perception: Boundary completion, illusory figures, and neon color spreading. *Psychological Review, 92,* 173–211.

Grossberg, S., & Mingolla, E. (1985b). Neural dynamics of perceptual grouping: Textures, boundaries, and emergent segmentations. *Perception and Psychophysics, 38,* 141–171.

Gyoba, J. (1983). Stationary phantoms: A completion effect without motion or flicker. *Vision Research, 22,* 119–134.

Halpern, D. F. (1981). The determinants of illusory-contour perception. *Perception, 10,* 199–213.

Halpern, D. F., & Salzman, B. (1983). The multiple determination of illusory contours: 1. A review. *Perception, 12,* 281–291.

Halpern, D. F., Salzman, B., Harrison, W., & Widaman, K. (1983). The multiple determination of illusory contours: 2. An empirical investigation. *Perception, 12,* 293–303.

Halpern, D. F., & Warm, J. S. (1980). The disappearance of real and subjective contours. *Perception and Psychophysics, 28,* 229–235.

Halpern, D. F., & Warm, J. S. (1984). The disappearance of dichoptically presented real and subjective contours. *Bulletin of the Psychonomic Society, 22,* 433–436.

Hammond, P., & MacKay, D. M. (1977). Differential responsiveness of simple and complex cells in cat striate cortex to visual texture. *Experimental Brain Research, 30,* 275–296.

Hamsher, K. DeS. (1978). Stereopsis and the perception of anomalous contours. *Neuropsychologia, 16,* 453–459.

Harris, C. S., Schwartz, B. J., Patashnik, O., & Lappin, J. S. (1978). Illusory pauses of moving dots. *Bulletin of the Pyschonomic Society, 12,* 257 (abstract).

Harris, J. P., & Gregory, R. L. (1973). Fusion and rivalry of illusory contours. *Perception, 2,* 235–247.

Hartmann, G. W. (1935). *Gestalt psychology: A survey of facts and principles.* New York: Ronald Press.

Hatfield, G., & Epstein, W. (1985). The status of the minimum principle in the theoretical analyis of visual perception. *Psychological Bulletin, 97,* 155–186.

Heider, Moore, G. (1933). New studies in transparency, form and color. *Psychologische Forschung, 17,* 13–55.

Heinemann, E. G. (1955). Simultaneous brightness induction as a function of inducing and test-field luminances. *Journal of Experimental Psychology, 50,* 89–96.

Helmholtz, H. L. F. von (1867). *Handbuch der physiologischen optik.* Leipzig: Voss. English translation: J. P. C. Southall (1924-5), *Helmholtz's treatise on physiological optics.* Opt. Soc. Amer. New York (3 vols.). Reprinted Dover, New York 1962 (3 vols. bound as 2)

Helmholtz, H. (1871). The relation of optics to painting. In R. M. Warren & R. P. Warren (Eds.), (1968), *Helmholtz on perception: Its physiology and development.* (pp. 137–168), New York: Wiley.

Helmholtz, H. (1878). The facts of perception. In R. M. Warren & R. P. Warren (Eds.), (1968), *Helmholtz on perception: Its physiology and development.* (pp. 205–246), Wiley, New York.

Helson, H., & Joy, V. L. (1962). Domains of lightness assimilation and contrast. *Psychologische Beitrage, 6,* 405–415.

Helson, H., & Rohles, F. H., Jr. (1959). A quantitative study of reversal of classical lightness-contrast. *American Journal of Psychology, 72,* 530–538.

Hendrickson, A. E., Hunt, S. P., & Wu, J.-Y. (1981). Immunocytochemical localization of glutamic acid decarboxylase in monkey striate cortex. *Nature, 292,* 605–607.

Hermann, L. (1870). Eine erscheinung des simultanen contrastes. *Pfüger's Archive für die Gesamte Physiologies des Menschen und der Tiere, 3,* 13–15.

Hertz, M. (1929). Das optische Gestaltproblem und der Tierversuch. *Verhandlungen der deutscher zoologische Gesellschaft.* (cited in Metzger 1935)

Higgins, K. E., & Knoblauch, K. (1977). Spatial Broca-Sulzer effect at brief stimulus durations. *Vision Research, 17,* 332–334.

Hochberg, J., & Beck, J. (1954). Apparent spatial arrangement and perceived brightness. *Journal of Experimental Psychology, 47,* 263–266.

Horton, J. C., & Hubel, D. H. (1981). Regular patchy distribution of cytochrome oxidase staining in primary visual cortex of macaque monkey. *Nature, 292,* 762–764.

Hubel, D. H., & Livingstone, M. S. (1985). Complex unoriented cells in a subregion of primate area 18. *Nature, 315,* 325–327.

Hubel, D. H., & Wiesel, T. N. (1962). Receptive fields, binocular interaction and functional architecture in the cat's visual cortex. *Journal of Physiology, 160,* 106.

Hubel, D. H. & Wiesel, T. N. (1970). Cells sensitive to binocular depth in area 18 of the macaque monkey cortex. *Nature, 225,* 41–42.

Hull, C. L. (1952). *A behavior system.* New Haven: Yale University Press.

Jacobi, J. (Ed.). (1951). *Paraclesus.* New York: Pantheon Books.

Jenkins, B., & Ross, J. (1977). McCollough effect depends upon perceived organization. *Perception, 6,* 399–400.

Jerison, H. (1973). *Evolution of brain and intelligence.* New York: Academic Press.

Jerison, H. (1976). Paleoneurology and the evolution of mind. *Scientific American, 234,* 90–101.

Johansson, G. (1970). On theories for visual space perception: A letter to Gibson. *Scandinavian Journal of Psychology, 11,* 67–74.

Johansson, G. (1973). Visual perception of biological motion and a model for its analysis. *Perception and Psychophysics, 14,* 201–211.

Johansson, G. (1974a). Projective transformations as determining visual space perception. In R. B. Macleod & H. L. Pick, Jr. (Eds.), *Perception: Essays in honor of James J. Gibson.* Ithaca, New York: Cornell University Press. 268–275.

Johansson, G. (1974b). Visual perception of rotary motion as transformations of conic sections—A contribution to the theory of visual space perception. *Psychologia, 17,* 226–237.

Johansson, G. (1975). Visual motion perception. *Scientific American, 232,* 76–87.

Jory, M., & Day, R. H. (1979). The relationship between brightness contrast and illusory contours. *Perception, 8,* 3–9.

Julesz, B. (1971). *Foundations of cyclopean perception.* Chicago: University of Chicago Press.

Julesz, B. (1980). Spatial nonlinearities in the instantaneous perception of textures with identical power spectra. *Philosophical Transactions of the Royal Society of London, B., 290,* 83–94.

Julesz, B. (1981a). Textons, the elements of texture perception and their interactions. *Nature, 290,* 91–97.

Julesz, B. (1981b). Figure and ground perception in briefly presented isodipole textures. In M. Kubovy & J. R. Pomerantz (Eds.), *Perceptual Organization,* Hillsdale, New Jersey: Lawerence Erlbaum Associates, Inc. pp. 27–54.

Julesz, B., & Bergen, J. R. (1983). Textons, the fundamental elements in preattentive vision and perception of textures. *The Bell System Technical Journal, 62,* 1619–1645.

Julesz, B., & Chang, J. J. (1976). Interaction between pools of disparity detectors turned to different disparities. *Biological Cybernetics, 22,* 107–119.

Jung, R. (1973). Neurophysiology and perception. In R. Jung (Ed.), *Handbook of sensory physiology,* Vol. 3, Part A (pp. 1–169). New York and Berlin: Springer-Verlag.

Jung, R., & Spillmann, L. (1970). Receptive-field estimation and perceptual integration in human vision. In F. A. Young & D. B. Lindsley (Eds.), *Early experience and visual information processing in perceptual and reading disorders* (pp. 181–197). Washington, D.C.: National Academy of Science.

Kanizsa, G. (1954a). Il gradiente marginale come fattore dell'aspetto fenomenico dei colori. *Archivio di Psicologia Neurologia e Psichiatria, 15,* 3.

Kanizsa, G. (1954b). Linee virtuali e margini fenomenici in assenza di discontinuita di stimolazione *Atti X Convegno Psicologi Italiani.*

Kanizsa, G. (1955a). Margini quasi-percettivi in campi con stimolazione omogenea. *Rivista di Psicologia, 49,* 7–30.

Kanizsa, G. (1955b). Condizioni ed effetti della trasparenza fenomenica. *Rivista di Psicologia, 49,* 31–49.

Kanizsa, G. (1974). Contours without gradients or cognitive contours? *Italian Journal of Psychology, 1,* 93–113.

Kanizsa, G. (1975a). Some new demonstrations of the role of structural factors in brightness contrast. In S. Ertel, L. Kemmler, M. Stadler (Eds.), *Gestaltheorie in der modernen psychologie.* Darmstade: Steinkopff.

Kanizsa, G. (1975b). The role of regularity in perceptual organization. In G. Flores d' Arcais (Ed.), *Studies in Perception: Festschrift for Fabia Metelli.* Milano: Martello Giunti.

Kanizsa, G. (1975c). Amodal completion and phenomenal shrinkage of surfaces in the visual field. *Italian Journal of Psychology, 2,* 187–195.

Kanizsa, G. (1976). Subjective contours. *Scientific American, 235*(4), 48–52.

Kanizsa, G. (1979). *Organization in vision.* New York: Praeger.

Kanizsa, G., & Gerbino, W. (1982). Amodal completion: Seeing or thinking? In J. Beck (Ed.), *Organization and representation in perception.* Hillsdale, NJ: Lawrence Erlbaum Associates.

Kanizsa, G., & Luccio, R. (1986a). Die Doppeldeutigkeiten der Prägnanz. *Gestalt Theory, 8,* 2.

Kanizsa, G., & Luccio, R. (1986b). Prägnanz und ihre Zweideutigkeiten. *Gestalt Theory* (in press).

Katz, S., & Frost, G. (1979). The origins of knowledge in two theories of brain: The cognitive paradox revealed. *Behaviorism, 7,* 35–44.

Kardos, L. (1934). Ding und Schatten. *Zeitschrift für Psychologie, Ergänzung Band, 23.*

Kaufmann-Hayoz, R., Kaufmann, F., & Stucki, M. (1986). Kinetic contours in infants' visual perception. *Child Development, 57,* 292–299.

Kawabata, N. (1984). Perception at the blind spot and similarity grouping. *Perception and Psychophysics, 36,* 151–158.

Kelley, D. (1986). *The evidence of the senses.* Baton Rouge: University of Louisiana Press.

Kellman, P. J., & Cohen, M. H. (1984a). Kinetic subjective contours. *Perception and Psychophysics, 35*(3), 237–244.

Kellman, P. J., & Cohen, M. H. (1984b). *Subjective contours in physically and perceptually homogeneous space.* Unpublished manuscript.

Kellman, P. J., & Spelke, E. S. (1983). Perception of partly occluded objects in infancy. *Cognitive Psychology, 15,* 483–524.

Kennedy, J. M. (1974). *A psychology of picture perception.* San Francisco: Jossey-Bass.

Kennedy, J. M. (1975). Depth at an edge, coplanarity, slant depth, change in direction and change in brightness in the production of subjective contours. *Italian Journal of Psychology, 2,* 107–123.

Kennedy, J. M. (1976a). Sun figure: An illusory diffuse contour resulting from an arrangement of dots. *Perception, 5,* 479–481.

Kennedy, J. M. (1976b). Attention, brightness and the constructive eye. In M. Henle (Ed.), *Vision and Artifact* (pp. 33–48). New York: Springer.

Kennedy, J. M. (1978a). Illusory contours not due to completion. *Perception, 7,* 187–189.

Kennedy, J. M. (1978b). Illusory contours and the ends of lines. *Perception, 7,* 605–607.

Kennedy, J. M. (1979). Subjective contours, contrast, and assimilation. In C. F. Nodine & D. F. Fisher (Eds.), *Perception and pictorial representation.* New York: Praeger, pp. 167–195.

Kennedy, J. M. (1985). It's all done with mirrors: Proof of non-existence. *Perception, 14,* 513–514.

Kennedy, J. M., & Chatterway, L. D. (1975). Subjective contours: Binocular and movement phenomena. *Italian Journal of Psychology, 2,* 333–367.

Kennedy, J. M., & Lee, H. (1976). A figure-density hypothesis and illusory contour brightness. *Perception, 5,* 387–392.

Kennedy, J. M., & Ware, C. (1978). Illusory contours can arise in dot figures. *Perception, 7,* 191–194.

Kilbride, P. L., & Leibowitz, H. W. (1975). Factors affecting the magnitude of the Ponzo illusion among the Baganda. *Perception and Psychophysics, 17,* 543–548.

Kimchi, R., & Palmer, S. E. (1982). Form and texture in hierarchially constructed patterns. *Journal of Experimental Psychology: Human Perception and Performance, 8,* 521–536.

Kitterle, F. L., & Beard, B. L. (1983). Effects of flicker adaptation upon temporal contrast enhancement. *Perception and Psychophysics, 33,* 75–78.

Kitterle, F. L., & Corwin, T. R. (1979). Enhancement of apparent contrast in flashed sinusoidal gratings. *Vision Research, 19,* 33–39.

Klymenko, V. (1984). The spatio-temporal determinants of the motion-induced contour. Unpublished doctoral dissertation, University of Buffalo, NY.

Klymenko, V., & Weisstein, N. (1981). The motion-induced contour. *Perception, 10,* 627–636.

Klymenko, V., & Weisstein, N. (1983). The edge of an event: Invariants of a moving illusory contour. *Perception and Psychophysics, 34,* 140–148.

Klymenko, V., & Weisstein, N. (1984). The razor's edge: A dichotomy between monohedral and dihedral edge perception. *Vision Research, 24,* 995–1002.

Klymenko, V., Weisstein, N., & Ralston, J. V. (in press). Illusory contours, projective transformations and kinetic shape perception. *Acta Psychologia.*

Koffka, K. (1935). *Principles of Gestalt psychology.* New York. Harcourt Brace & Co.

Koffka, K., & Harrower, M. R. (1931). Colour and organization. *Psychologische Forschung, 15,* 145–275.

Köhler, W. (1940). *Dynamics in psychology.* New York: Washington Square Press.

Kondo, H. (1984). *Saké: A drinker's guide.* Tokyo: Kodansha International.

Kontsevich, L. L. (1986). An ambiguous random-dot stereogram which permits continuous change in interpretation. *Vision Research, 26,* 517–519.

Krause, C. L., & Mishler, C. (1985). *Standard catalog of world gold coins.* Iola, WI: Krause Publications.

Krauskopf, J. (1963). Effect of retinal image stabilization on the appearance of heterochromatic targets. *Journal of the Optical Society of America, 53,* 741–744.

Ladd, F. C. (1807). A method for the experimental determination of the horopter. *American Journal of Psychology, 1,* 99–111.

Land, E. H. (1977). The retinex theory of color vision. *Scientific American, 237,* 108–128.

Landauer, A. A. (1978). Subjective states and the perception of subjective contours. In J. P. Sutcliffe (Ed.), *Conceptual analysis and method in psychology: Essays in honor of W. M. O'Neil.* Sydney, Australia: Sydney University Press.

Lappin, J. S., Donner, J. F., & Kottas, B. (1980). Minimal conditions for the visual detection of structure and motion in three dimensions. *Science, 209,* 717–719.

Lawson, R. B., & W. L. Gullick (1967). Stereopsis and anomalous contour. *Vision Research, 7,* 271–297.

Lawson, R. B., Cowan, E., Gibbs, T. D., & Whitmore, C. G. (1974). Stereoscopic enhancement and erasure of subjective contours. *Journal of Experimental Psychology, 103,* 1142–1146.

Leeuwenberg, E. (1981). Metrical aspects of patterns and structural information theory. In M. Kubovy & J. R. Pomerantz (Eds.), *Perceptual organization* (pp. 57–71). Hillsdale, NJ: Lawrence Erlbaum Associates.

Leroi-Gourhan, A. (1967). *Treasures of prehistoric art.* New York: Harry Abrams, Inc.

Liebmann, S. (1927). Über das Verhalten farbiger Formen bei Helligkeitsgleichheit von Figur und Grund. *Psychologische Forschung, 9.*

Lindsay, P. H., & Norman, D. A. (1977). *Human information processing* (2nd ed.). New York: Academic Press.

Livingstone, M. S., & Hubel, D. H. (1982). Thalamic inputs to cytochrome oxidase-rich regions in monkey visual cortex. *Proceedings of the National Academy of Sciences, 79,* 6098–6101.

Livingstone, M. S., & Hubel, D. H. (1984). Anatomy and physiology of a color system in the primate visual cortex. *Journal of Neuroscience, 4,* 309–356.

Lovegrove, W., Martin, F., & Slaghuis, W. (1986). A theoretical and experimental case for a visual deficit in specific reading disability. *Cognitive Neuropsychology, 3* (in press).

Lu, C., & Fender, D. H. (1972). The interaction of colour and luminance in stereoscopic vision. *Investigate Ophthalmology, 11,* 482–489.

Mach, E. (1822). *Die Analyse der Empfindungen.* Jena: Fischer.

Mace, W. (1971). *An investigation of spatial and kinetic information for separation in depth using computer-generated dot patterns.* Unpublished doctoral dissertation, University of Minnesota, Minneapolis.

Macleod, R. B. (1947). The effects of artifical penumbrae on the brightness of included areas. In J. Nuttin (ed.), *Miscellanea A. Michotte.* Louvain: Editions Institut Supérieur de Philosophie.

Maguire, W. (1978). *Contour completion in dynamic visual displays.* Unpublished doctoral dissertation, State University of New York at Buffalo.

Maguire, W., & Blattberg, K. (1986). Effects of contrast of occluder and flicker frequency on displays which produce phantom contours [Abstract]. *Proceedings of the 57th Annual Meeting of the Eastern Psychological Association.*

Maguire, W. M., Meyer, G. E., & Baizer, J. (1980).

The McCollough effect in rhesus monkey. *Investigative Ophthalmology and Visual Science, 19,* 321–324.

Marr, D. (1982). *Vision.* San Francisco: Freeman.

Matthaei, R. (1929). *Das gestaltproblem.* München.

McArthur, D. J. (1982). Computer vision and psychology. *Psychological Bulletin, 92,* 283–309.

McCourt, M. E. (1982). A spatial frequency dependent grating induction effect. *Vision Research, 22,* 119–134.

Metelli, F. (1940). Ricerche sperimentali sulla percezione del movimento. *Rivista di Psicologia, 34.*

Metelli, F. (1974a). The perception of transparency. *Scientific American, 230,* 90–98.

Metelli, F. (1974b). Achromatic color conditions in the perception of transparency. In R. B. MacLeod & H. L. Pick, Jr. (Eds.), *Perception: Essays in honor of James J. Gibson.* Ithaca, NY: Cornell University Press.

Metelli, F. (1982). Some characteristics of gestalt-oriented research in perception. In J. Beck (Ed.), *Organization and representation in perception.* Hillsdale, NJ: Lawrence Erlbaum Associates.

Metelli, F. (1985). Stimulation and perception of transparency. *Psychological Research, 47,* 185–202.

Metzger, W. (1935). Gesetz des Sehens. Frankfurt: Kramer.

Meyer, G. E. (1986). Interactions of subjective contours with the Ponzo, Muller-Lyer and vertical-horizontal illusions. *Bulletin of the Psychonomic Society, 24,* 39–40.

Meyer, G. E., & Chow, Y. M. (1984). *Visual persistence and illusory contours.* Paper presented at the meeting of the Association for Research in Vision and Ophthalmology, Sarasota, FL.

Meyer, G. E., Coleman, A., Dwyer, T., & Lehman, I. (1982). The McCollough effect in children. *Child Development, 53,* 838–840.

Meyer, G. E., Dougherty, T. (1985). The effects of flicker-induced depth on chromatic subjective contours [Abstract]. *Program for the 26th Annual Meeting of the Psychonomic Society,* Boston, 37.

Meyer, G. E., & Garges, C. (1979). Subjective contours and the Poggendorff illusion. *Perception and Psychophysics, 26,* 302–304.

Meyer, G. E., & Phillips, D. (1980). Faces, vases, subjective contours and the McCollough effect. *Perception, 9,* 603–606.

Meyer, G. E., & Senecal, M. (1983). The illusion of transparency and chromatic subjective contours. *Perception and Psychophysics, 34*(1), 56–64.

Micella, F., Pinna, B., & Sambin, M. (1985). *Segregazione di profondità, in figure anomale con differente grado di evidenza* [Depth segregation in a.f. with different strength]. Paper presented at the 4th meeting of Divisione Ricerca di Base in Psicologia, Ravello, Italy.

Michotte, A. (1950). A propos de la permanence phénoménale. *Acta Psychologia, 7.*

Michotte, A. (1954). *La perception de la causalite.* Louvain: Publications Universitaires de Louvain.

Michotte, A. (1962). *Causalité permanence et réalité phénoménales.* Louvain: Publications Universitaires de Louvain.

Michotte, A., Thines, G., & Crabbe, G. (1964). Les complements amodaux des structures perceptives. *Studia Psycologica.* Louvain: Publications Universitaires de Louvain.

Milkman, N., Schick, G., Rossetto, M., Ratliff, F., Shapley, R. & Victor, J. (1980). A two-dimensional computer-controlled visual stimulator. *Behavioral Sciences Methods and Instrumentation, 12,* 283–292.

Minguzzi, G. (1982). *Figure anomale: le modificazioni di chiarezza indoite de fine di linea,* Trieste, Italy: Reports of the Institute of Psychology, University of Trieste.

Minguzzi, G. (1983). La perceziona di superfici anomale, *Ricerche di Psicologia, 26,* 97–118.

Mitchell, D. E. (1969). Qualitative depth localization with diplopic images of dissimilar shape. *Vision Research, 9,* 991–994.

Mitchison, G., & McKee, S. (1985). Interpolation in stereoscopic matching. *Nature, 315,* 402–404.

Mori, G. F., & Ronchi, L. (1960). On the perception of incomplete borders. *Atti della Fondazione Giorgio Ronchi, 15,* 357–368.

Motokawa, K. (1950). Filed retinal induction and optical illusions. *Journal of Neurophysiology, 18,* 413–426.

Mulvanny, P., Macarthur, R., & Sekuler, R. (1982). Thresholds for seeing visual phantoms and moving gratings. *Perception, 11,* 35–46.

Musatti, C. (1937). Forma e movimento. Venezia: *Atti Reale Istituto Veneto di Lettere, Scienze ed Arti, 97.*

Musatti, C. (1953). Ricerche sperimentali sopra la percezione cromatica [Experimental researches on chromatic perception]. *Archivio di Psicologia, Neurologia e Psichiatria, 14,* 541–577.

Mustillo, P., & Fox, R. (1986). The perception of illusory contours in the hypercyclopean domain. *Perception & Psychophysics, 40,* 362–363.

Neuer, R., Liberston, H., & Yoshida, S. (1981). *Ukiyo-E: 250 years of Japanese art.* New York: Mayflower Books.

Nothdurft, H. C. (1985). Discrimination of higher-order textures. *Perception, 14,* 539–543.

Nothdurft, H. C., & Li, C. Y. (1985). Texture discrimination: Representation of orientation and luminance differences in cells of the cat striate cortex. *Vision Research, 25,* 99–113.

Novak, S. (1969). Comparison of increment and decrement thresholds near a light–dark boundary. *Journal of the Optical Society of America, 59,* 1183–1384.

Novak, S., & Sperling, G. (1963). Visual thresholds near a continuously visible or briefly presented light–dark boundary. *Optica Acta, 10,* 187–191.

Ogle, R. N. (1952). On the limits of stereoscopic vision. *Journal of Experimental Psychology, 44,* 253–259.

Orban, G. A. (1984). *Neuronal operations in the visual cortex.* Berlin: Springer-Verlag.

Osgood, C. E. (1953). *Method and theory in experimental psychology.* New York: Oxford University Press.

Pachella, R. G. (1974). The interpretation of reaction time in information processing research. In B. H. Kantowitz (Ed.). *Human information processing: Tutorials in performance and cognition.* Hillsdale, New Jersey: Lawerence Erlbaum Associates, Inc, pp. 41–82.

Parks, T. E. (1979). Subjective figures: Does brightness enhancement depend upon subjective boundary definition? *Perception and Psychophysics, 26,* 418.

Parks, T. E. (1980a). Subjective figures: Some unusual concomitant brightness effects. *Perception, 9,* 239–241.

Parks, T. E. (1980b). Letter to the editor. *Perception, 9,* 723.

Parks, T. E. (1981). Subjective figures: An infrequent, but certainly not unprecedented, effect. *Perception, 10,* 589–590.

Parks, T. E. (1982a). Brightness effects in diffuse and sharp illusory figures of similar configuration. *Perception, 11,* 107–110.

Parks, T. E. (1982b). Illusory contours: On the efficacy of their need for expression. *Perception and Psychophysics, 32,* 286–289.

Parks, T. E. (1982c). Humor. *Perception, 11,* 240.

Parks, T. E. (1984). Illusory figures: A (mostly) atheoretical review. *Psychological Bulletin, 95,* 282–300.

Parks, T. E. (1986). Apparent depth and texture differences in illusory figure patterns: A paradox resolved. *Perception & Psychophysics, 37,* 568–570.

Parks, T. E., & Marks, W. (1983). Sharp-edged vs. diffuse illusory circles: The effects of varying luminance. *Perception and Psychophysics, 33,* 172–176.

Parks, T. E., & Marks, W. (1985). Illusory figures: Individual differences in apparent depth and lightness. *Perception & Psychophysics, 37,* 529–532.

Parks, T. E., & Pendergrass, L. (1982). On the filtered components approach to illusory visual contours. *Perception and Psychophysics, 32,* 491–493.

Parks, T. E., Rock, I., & Anson, R. (1983). Illusory contour lightness: A neglected possibility. *Perception, 12,* 43–47.

Pastore, N. (1971). *Selective history of theories of visual perception, 1650–1950.* New York: Oxford University Press.

Petersik, J. T. (1980). Rotation judgments and depth judgments: Separate of dependent processes. *Perception and Psychophysics, 27,* 588–590.

Petry, S. (1978). Perceptual changes during metacontrast masking. *Vision Research, 18,* 1337–1341.

Petry, S., Grigonis, A., & Reichert, B. (1979). Increase in metacontrast masking following adaptation to flicker. *Perception, 8,* 541–547.

Petry, S., Harbeck, A., Conway, J., & Levey, J. (1983). Stimulus determinants of brightness and distinctness of subjective contours. *Perception & Psychophysics, 34,* 169–174.

Petry, S., Hood, D. C., & Goodkin, F. (1973). Time course of lateral inhibition in the human visual system. *Journal of the Optical Society of America, 63,* 385–386

Petry, S., & Meyer, G. E. (1986). Adelphi International Conference on Illusory Contours: A report on the conference. *Perception and Psychophysics, 39,* pp. 210–222.

Piggins, D. J. (1975). Cognitive space. *Perception, 4,* 337–340.

Poggio, G. F., Motter, B. C., Squatrito, S., & Trotter, V. (1985). Responses of neurons in visual cortex (V1 and V2) of the alert monkey to dynamic random dot stereograms. *Vision Research, 25,* 397–406.

Poggio, G., & Poggio, T. (1984). The analysis of stereopsis. *Annual Review of Neuroscience, 7,* 379–412.

Pomerantz, J. R. (1978). Are complex features derived from simple ones? In E. L. J. Leeuwenberg & H. F. J. M. Buffart (Eds.), *Formal Theories of Visual Perception.* New York: John Wiley & Sons.

Pomerantz, J. R. (1981). Perceptual organization and attention. In M. Kubovy & J. R. Pomerantz (Eds.)., *Perceptual organization.* Hillsdale, NJ: Lawerence Erlbaum Associates, Inc, pp. 141–180.

Pomerantz, J. R., Goldberg, D. M., Golder, P. S., & Tetewsky, S. (1981). Subjective contours can facilitate performance in a reaction-time task. *Perception and Psychophysics, 29,* 605–611.

Pomerantz, J. R., & Kubovy, M. (1981). Perceptual organization: An overview. In M. Kubovy & J. R. Pomerantz (Eds.), *Perceptual organization.* Hillsdale, NJ: Lawrence Erlbaum Associates, Inc.

Pomerantz, J. R., Sager, L. C., & Stoever, R. J. (1977). Perception of wholes and their component parts: Some configurational superiority effects. *Journal of Experimental Psychology: Human Perception and Performance, 3,* 422–435.

Porac, C. (1978). Depth in objective and subjective contour patterns. *Bulletin of the Psychonomic Society, 11,* 103–105.

Posner, M. I. (1978). *Cronometric explorations of the mind.* Hillsdale, NJ: Lawrence Erlbaum Associates.

Prandtl, A. (1927). Uber gleichsinnige Induktion und dei Lichtrerteilung in gitterartigen Mustern. *Zeitschrift für Sinnesphysiologie, 58,* 263–307.

Praturlon, O. (1947). Il fenomeno di quiete apparente nel movimento traslatorio. In *Contributi scientifici dell'Istituto di Psicologia,* Padova.

Prazdny, K. (1983). Illusory contours are not caused by simultaneous brightness contrast. *Perception and Psychophysics, 34,* 403–404.

Prazdny, K. (1985). On the nature of inducing forms generating perception of illusory contours. *Perception and Psychophysics, 37,* 237–242.

Pritchard, W. S., & Warm, J. S. (1983). Attentional processing and the subjective contour illusion. *Journal of Experimental Psychology: General, 112,* 145–175.

Purdy, D. M. (1936). The structure of the visual world: III. The tendency toward simplification of the visual field. *Psychological Review, 43,* 59–82.

Ramachandran, V. S. (1985a). Guest editorial [Special issue on motion perception, V. S. Ramachandran, Ed.]. *Perception, 14,* 97–103.

Ramachandran, V. S. (1985b). Apparent motion of subjective surfaces [Special issue on motion perception, V. S. Ramachandran, Ed.]. *Perception, 14,* 127–134.

Ramachandran, V. S. (1986a). Illusory contours capture stereopsis and apparent motion. *Perception and Psychophysics, 39,* 361–373.

Ramachandran, V. S. (1986b). The utilitarian theory of perception. APA symposium: Theories of perception, September 1986, Washington, D.C.

Ramachandran, V. S., & Anstis, S. M. (1983). Perceptual organization in moving patterns. *Nature, 304,* 529–531.

Ramachandran, V. S., & Anstis, S. M. (1986). Effect of figure-ground segmentation on apparent motion. *Vision Research, 26.*

Ramachandran, V. S., & Cavanagh, P. (1985a). Subjective contours capture stereopsis. *Nature, 317,* 527–530.

Ramachandran, V. S., & Cavanagh, P. (1985b). Motion capture anisotropy in random-dot patterns. *Vision Research, 25.*

Ramachandran, V. S., Clarke, P. G. H., & Whitteridge, D. (1977). Cells selective to binocular depth in the cortex of newborn lambs. *Nature, 268,* 333–335.

Ramachandran, V. S., & Gregory, R. L. (1978). Does colour provide an input to human motion perception. *Nature, 275,* 55–56.

Ramachandran, V. S., & Inada, V. (1985). Spatial phase and frequency in motion capture of random-dot patterns. *Spatial Vision, 1,* 57–67.

Ramachandran, V. S., Rao, V. M., & Vidyasagar, T. R. (1973). The role of contours in stereopsis. *Nature, 242,* 412–414.

Ratliff, F. (1965). *Mach bands: Quantitative studies on neural networks in the retina.* New York: Holden Day.

Redies, C., Crook, J. M., & Creutzfeldt, O. D. (1986). Neuronal responses to borders with and without luminance gradients in cat visual cortex and dorsal lateral geniculate nucleus. *Experimental Brain Research, 61,* 469–481.

Redies, C., & Spillman, L. (1981). The neon color effect in the Ehrenstein illusion. *Perception, 10,* 667–681.

Redies, C., Spillman, L., & Kunz, K. (1984). Colored neon flanks and line gap enhancement. *Vision Research, 24,* 1301–1310.

Remole, A., Ng, A. S. Y., Bothe, L. C., Padfield, P. D., Spafford, M. M., & Szymkis, M. A. (1985). Flicker haloes observed with subjective borders. *Perception, 14,* 31–40.

Restle, F. (1979). Coding theory of the perception of motion configurations. *Psychological Review, 86,* 1–24.

Restle, F. (1981). Coding theory as an integration of Gestalt psychology and information theory. In M. Kubovy & J. R. Pomerantz (Eds.), *Perceptual Organization* (pp. 31–56). Hillsdale, NJ: Lawrence Erlbaum Associates.

Reynolds, R. I. (1976). The microgenetic development of visual illusions. Ph.D. dissertation, Newark: Rutgers University.

Reynolds, R. I. (1981). Perception of an illusory contour as a function of processing time. *Perception, 10,* 107–115.

Richardson, B. L. (1979). The nonequivalence of abrupt and diffuse illusory contours. *Perception, 8,* 589–593.

Rock, I. (1983). *The logic of perception.* Cambridge, MA: Bradford Books/The MIT Press.

Rock, I. (1986). Cognitive intervention in perceptual processing. In T. J. Knapp & L. C. Robertson (Eds.), *Approaches to cognition: Contrasts and controversies.* Hillsdale, NJ: Lawrence Erlbaum Associates.

Rock, I., & Anson, R. (1979). Illusory contours as the solution to a problem. *Perception, 8*, 665–681.

Rogers, B. J., & Graham, M. E. (1979). Motion parallax as an independent cue for depth perception, *Perception, 8*, 125–134.

Rosenbach, O. (1902). Zur lehre von den urtheilstaüschungen. *Zeitschrift für Psychologie, 29*, 434–448.

Rubin, E. (1915). *Synsoplevede figurer*. Copenhagen: Gyldendals.

Rubin, E. (1921). *Visuell wahrgenommene Figuren*. Copenhagen: Gyldendals.

Runeson, S. (1977). On the possibility of "smart" perceptual mechanisms. *Scandinavian Journal of Psychology, 18*, 172–179.

Sakurai, K., & Gyoba, J. (1985). Optimal occluder luminance for seeing stationary visual phantoms. *Vision Research, 25, 11*, 1735–1740.

Salapatek, P. (1975). Pattern perception in early infancy. In L. B. Cohen & P. Salapatek (Eds.), *Infant perception: From sensation to cognition, Vol. 1*. New York: Academic Press.

Salzman, B., & Halpern, D. F. (1982). Subjective towers: Depth relationships in multilevel subjective contours. *Perceptual and Motor Skills, 55*, 1247–1256.

Sambin, M. (1974a). Angular margins without gradient. *Italian Journal of Psychology, 1*, 355–361.

Sambin, M. (1974b). L'ambito di influenza delle tensioni terminali nella organizzazione di figure senza gradiente. [The influence of terminal tensions in the organization of subjective figures]. *Rivista di Psicologia*, 257–265.

Sambin, M. (1975). The role of terminal tensions in the organization of margins without gradient. *Italian Journal of Psychology, 2*, 239–257.

Sambin, M. (1978). Il contrasto di chiarezza nelle figure anomale [Brightness contrast in anomalous figures]. *Giornale Italiano di Psicologia, 3*, 543–564.

Sambin, M. (1979). Transphenomenal basis in the "moiré" effect explanation. *Italian Journal of Psychology, 6*, 185–201.

Sambin, M. (1980a). Figure anomale. Il contrasto di chiarezza come risultato delle disomogeneità indotte [Anomalous figures. Brightness contrast as a result of induced inhomogeneities]. *Giornale Italiano di Psicologia, 1*, 121–145.

Sambin, M. (1980b). *Le disomogeneità indotte nella formazione di margini e superfici anomale* [Induced inhomogeneties in the formation of anomalous contours and surfaces] pp. 1–31 (Report). Trieste, Italy: *Institute of Psychology, University of Trieste*.

Sambin, M. (1981a). *On the threshold measurement of anomalous figures* (Report No. 30), pp. 1–16.

Padova, Italy: Institute of Psychology, University of Padova.

Sambin, M. (1981b). Figure anomale. *La polarizzazione intrafigurale delle parti inducenti*. [Anomalous figures: the intrafigural polarization of inducing parts]. Giornale Italiano di Psicologia 8, 421–436.

Sambin, M. (1985). Figure anomale: La misura dell'ampiezza di una disomogeneità indotta [Anomalous figures: the measurement of an induced inhomogeneity], pp. 437–452. In W. Gerbino (Ed.), *Conoscenza e struttura*. Bologna:

Sambin, M. (1986). Concave vs. convex: A figure–ground problem from field theory point of view. *Paper presented at the annual meeting of Perceptual Psychologists*, Trieste, Italy.

Sambin, M., & Rocco, D. (in press). Punti di ancoramento nella formazione di figure anomale. [Anchor points in the a.f. organization]. *Giornale Italiano di Psicologia,*

Sampaio, A. C. (1943). *La translation des objects comme facteur de leur permanence phénoménale*. Louvain: Publications Universitaires de Louvain.

Schumann, F. (1900). Beitraege zur Analyse der Gesichtswahrnehmungen. Erste Abhandlung. Einige Beobachtungen über die Zusammenfassung von Gesichtseindruecken zu Einheiten (Contribution to the analysis of visual perception: First paper: Some observations on the combination of visual impressions into units]. *Zeitschrift für Psychologie und Physiologie der Sinnesorgane, 23*, 1–32. Reprinted (1904).

Schumann, F. (1904). Einige Beobachtungen Uber die Zusammenfassung von Gesichtseindruckern zu Binheiten *Psychologische Studien, 1*, 1–32.

Scrivener, S. (1983). Two for the price of one. *Perception, 12*, 769.

Sekuler, R., & Blake, R. (1985). *Perception*. New York: Alfred A. Knopf.

Sekuler, R., & Levinson, E. (1977). The perception of moving targets. *Scientific American, 236*(1), 60–73.

Shapley, R., & Enroth-Cugell, C. (1984). Visual adaptation and retinal gain controls. *Progress in Retinal Research, 3*, 263–346.

Shapley, R., & Gordon, J. (1983). A nonlinear mechanism for the perception of form. *Investigative Ophthalmology and Visual Science 24 (Supplement)*, 238.

Shapley, R., & Gordon, J. (1985). Nonlinearity in the perception of form. *Perception and Psychophysics, 37*, 84–88.

Shapley, R., & Perry, H. (1986). Cat and monkey retinal ganglion cells and their visual functional roles. *Trends in Neurosciences, 9*, 229–235.

Shimojo, S., Birch, E. E., Gwiazda, J., & Held, R.

(1986). Development of vernier acuity in infants. *Vision Research, 24,* 721–728.

Shipp, S., & Zeki, S. M. (1985). Segregation of pathways leading from area V2 to areas V4 and V5 of macaque monkey visual cortex. *Nature, 315,* 322–324.

Sigman, E., & Rock, I. (1974). Stroboscopic movement based on perceptual intelligence. *Perception, 3,* 9–28.

Sillito, A., Gregory, R. L., & Heard, P. (1982). Can cognitive contours con cat cortex? *Talk presented to the Experimental Psychology Meeting at St. Andrews.*

Skowbo, D. (1984). Are McCollough effects conditioned responses? *Psychological Bulletin, 96,* 215–216.

Sloboda, J. A. (1986). Reading: a paradigm of cognitive skill. In A. R. H. Gellatly (Ed.), *The skilful mind: An introduction to cognitive psychology.* Milton Keynes: Open University Press.

Smith, A. T., & Over, R. (1975). Tilt aftereffects with subjective contours. *Nature, 257,* 581–582.

Smith, A. T., & Over, R. (1976). Color-selective tilt aftereffects with subjective contours. *Perception and Psychophysics, 20,* 305–308.

Smith, A. T., & Over, R. (1977). Orientation masking and the tilt illusion with subjective contours. *Perception, 6,* 441–447.

Smith, A. T., & Over, R. (1979). Motion aftereffect with subjective contours. *Perception and Psychophysics, 25,* 95–98.

Smith, K. A. (1983). Evidence relating subjective contours and interpretations involving interposition. *Perception, 12,* 491–500.

Solo, D. X. (1982). *3-D and shaded alphabets.* New York: Dover Publications.

Soubitez, M. C. (1982). Perceptual development of the Ehrenstein illusion in children (Abstract). *Perception, 11,* A33.

Spillmann, L. (1975). Perceptual modification of the Ehrenstein illusion. In S. Ertel, L. Kemmler, & M. Stadler (Eds.), *Gestalt theorie in der modernen Psychologie* (pp. 210–218). Darmstadt: Steinkopff.

Spillman, L. Fuld, K., & Gerrits, H. J. M. (1976). Brightness contrast in the Ehrenstein illusion. *Vision Research, 16,* 713–719.

Spillman, L., Fuld, K., & Neumeyer, C. (1984). Brightness matching, brightness cancellation, and increment threshold in the Ehrenstein illusion. *Perception, 13,* 512–520.

Spillman, L., & Redies, C. (1981). Random-dot motion displaces Ehrenstein illusion. *Perception, 10,* 411–415.

Stadler, M., & Dieker, J. (1972). Untersuchungen zum Problem virtueller Konturen in der visuellen Wahrnehmung *Zeitschrift für Experimentelle und Angewandte Psychologie, 19,* 325–350.

Stevens, S. S., & Galanter, E. H. (1957). Ratio scales and category scales for a dozen perceptual continua. *Journal of Experimental Psychology, 54,* 377–409.

Streibel, M. J., Barnes, R. D., Julness, G. D., & Ebenholz, S. M. (1980). Determinants of the rod-and-frame effect: Role of organization and subjective contour. *Perception and Psychophysics, 27,* 136–140.

Teller, D. Y. (1984). Linking propositions. *Vision Research, 24,* 1233–1246.

Todd, J. T. (1982). Visual information about rigid and nonrigid motion: A geometric analysis. *Journal of Experimental Psychology: Human Perception and Performance, 8,* 238–252.

Treisman, A. (1983). The role of attention in object perception in physical and biological processing of images. O. J. Braddick & A. Sleigh (Eds.). Berlin: Springer-Verlag.

Treisman, A., & Gelade, G. (1980). A feature-integration theory of attention. *Cognitive Psychology, 12,* 97–136.

Tyler, C. W. (1977). Is the illusory triangle physical or imaginary? *Perception, 6,* 603–604.

Tynan, P., & Sekuler, R. (1975). Moving visual phantoms: A new completion effect. *Science, 188,* 951–952.

Ullman, S. (1976). Filling-in the gaps: the shape of subjective contours and a model for their generation. *Biological Cybernetics, 25,* 1–6.

Ullman, S. (1979). *The interpretation of visual motion.* Cambridge, MA: MIT Press.

Uttal, W. R. (1981). *A taxonomy of visual processes.* Hillsdale, NJ: Lawerence Erlbaum Associates.

Van Essen, J. S., & Novak, S. (1974). Detection thresholds within a display that manifests contour enhancement and brightness contrast. *Journal of the Optical Society of America, 64,* 726–729.

Van Essen, D. C. (1979). Visual areas of the mammalian cerebral cortex. *Annual Review of Neuroscience, 2,* 227–263.

Van Essen, D. C. (1985). Functional organization of primate visual cortex. In A. Peters & E. G. Jones (Eds.), *Cerebral cortex,* Vol. 3. New York: Plenum.

Van Tuijl, H. F. J. M. (1975). A new visual illusion: Neonlike color spreading and complementary color induction between subjective contours. *Acta Psychologia, 39,* 441–445.

Van Tuijl, H. F. J. M., & Leeuwenberg, E. L. J. (1979). Neon color spreading and structural information measures. *Perception and Psychophysics, 25,* 269–284.

Van Tuijl, H. F. J. M., & Leeuwenberg, E. L. J.

(1982). Peripheral and central determinants of subjective contour strength. In H. G. Geissler & P. Petzold (Eds.), *Psychological judgment and the process of perception*. Berlin: VEB Deutschen Verlag der Wissenschaften.

Varin, D. (1970). Fenomeni di constrasto e diffusione chromatica nell' organizzazione spaziale del campo percettivo, *Rivista di Psicolognia, 65*, 101–128.

Victor, J. D. (1985). Complex visual textures as a tool for studying the VEP. *Vision Research, 12*, 1811–1828.

Vitz, P. C., & Glimcher, A. B. (1984). *Modern art and modern science*. New York: Praeger.

von der Heydt, R., Peterhans, E., & Baumgartner, G. (1984). Illusory contours and cortical neuron responses. *Science, 224*, 1260–1261.

von Grünau, M. W. (1979). The involvement of illusory contours in stroboscopic motion. *Perception and Psychophysics, 25*, 205–208.

Vogels, R., & Orban, G. A. (1985). How finely can we judge the orientation of an illusory contour. *Archives Internationales de Physiologie et de Biochimie, 93*, P6–P7.

Wade, N. J. (1977). Distortions and disappearance of geometrical patterns. *Perception, 6*, 407–433.

Wade, N. (1982). *The art and science of visual illusions*. London: Routledge & Kegan Paul.

Wade, N. (1985). Literal pictures. *Words and Images, 1*, 242–272.

Wade, N. J., & Day, R. H. (1978). On the colours seen in achromatic patterns. *Perception and Psychophysics, 23*, 261–264.

Waldrop, M. M. (1984). Computer vision. *Science, 224*, 1225–1227.

Wallach, H., & O'Connell, D. (1953). The kinetic depth effect. *Journal of Experimental Psychology, 45*, 207–214.

Ward, F., & Tansley, B. W. (1974). Increment thresholds across minimally distinct borders. *Journal of the Optical Society of America, 64*, 760–762.

Ware, C. (1980). Coloured illusory triangles due to assimilation. *Perception, 9*, 103–107.

Ware, C. (1981). Subjective contours independent of brightness contrast. *Perception and Psychophysics, 29*, 500–504.

Ware, C., & Kennedy, J. M. (1977). Illusory line linking solid rods. *Perception, 6*, 601–602.

Ware, C., & Kennedy, J. M. (1978). Perception of subjective lines, surfaces and volumes in three-dimensional constructions. *Leonardo, 11*, 111–114.

Wassertein, J., Zappulla, R., Rosen, J., & Gerstman, L. (1987). In search of closure: subjective contour illusions, Gestalt completion tests, and implications. *Brain and Cognition, 6*, 1–14.

Watson, A. (1978). A Riemann geometric explanation of the visual illusions and figural aftereffects. In B. L. J. Leeuwenberg & H. J. M. Buffart (Eds.), *Formal theories of visual perception*. New York: Wiley.

Weimer, W. B. (1982). Hayek's approach to the problems of complex phenomena: An introduction to the theoretical psychology of The Sensory Order. In W. B. Weimer & D. S. Palermo (Eds.), *Cognition and the symbolic processes, Vol. 2* (pp. 241–285).

Weisstein, N. (1966). Backward masking and models of perceptual processing. *Journal of Experimental Psychology, 72*, 232–240.

Weisstein, N. (1970). Neural symbolic activity: A psychophysical measure. *Science, 168*, 1489–1499.

Weisstein, N., & Harris, C. S. (1974). Visual detection of line segments: An object superiority effect. *Science, 186*, 752–755.

Weisstein, N., & Maguire, W. (1978). Computing the next step: Psychophysical measures of representation and interpretation. In A. L. Hanson & E. M. Riseman (Eds.), *Computer Vision Systems*. New York: Academic Press.

Weisstein, N., Maguire, W., & Berbaum, K. (1977). A phantom-motion aftereffect. *Science, 189*, 955–958.

Weisstein, N., Maguire, W., & Williams, M. C. (1982). The effect of perceived depth on phantoms and the phantom motion aftereffect. In J. Beck (Ed.), *Organization and Representation in perception*. Hillsdale, NJ. Lawrence Erlbaum Associates.

Weisstein, N., Matthews, M., & Berbaum, K. (1974). Illusory contours can mask real contours. *Bulletin of the Psychonomic Society, 4*, 266, (abs.).

Werner, H. (1935). Studies on contour. *American Journal of Psychology, 47*, 40–64.

Werner, H., & Wapner, S. (1952). Toward a general theory of perception. *Psychological Review, 59*, 324–338.

Wheatstone, C. (1838). On some remarkable phenomena of binocular vision. *Philosophical Transactions, Royal Society of London, 128*, 371–394.

Wertheimer, M. (1923). Untersuchungen zur Lehre von der Gestalt. *Psychologische Forschung, 4*.

Wertheimer, M. (1945). *Productive thinking*. New York: Harper.

Wertheimer, M. (1958). Principles of perceptual organization. In D. C. Beardslee & M. Wertheimer (Eds.), *Readings in perception*. Princeton, NJ: Van Nostrand. (Originally published 1923).

Whitmore, J. M., Lawson, R. B., & Kozora, C. E. (1976). Subjective contours in stereoscopic space. *Perception and Psychophysics, 19*, 211–213.

Wildman, K. N. (1974). Visual sensitivity at an edge. *Vision Research, 14,* 749–755.

Wilkinson, F. (1986). Visual segmentation in cats. *Behavioural Brain Research, 19,* 71–82.

Williams, M. C., & Bologna, N. B. (1985). Perceptual grouping in good and poor readers. *Perception and Psychophysics, 38,* 367–374.

Witasek, S. Z. (1899). *Psychol. Physiol. Sinn, 19,* 81.

Wittebrood, J. E. M., Wansink, M. G., & de Weert, C. M. M. (1981). A versatile color stimulus generator. *Perception, 10,* 63–69.

Wolff, W. (1935). Induzierte Helligkeitsveranderung. *Psychologische Forschung, 20,* 159–194.

Wong, E., & Weisstein, N. (1982). A new perceptual context–superiority effect: Line segments are more visible against a figure than against a ground. *Science, 218,* 587–589.

Wong, E., & Weisstein, N. (1983). Sharp targets are detected better against a figure and blurred targets are detected better against a ground. *Journal of Experimental Psychology: Human Perception & Performance, 9,* 194–202.

Wong, E., & Weisstein, N. (1984). Flicker induces depth: Spatial and temporal factors in the perceptual segregation of flickering and nonflickering regions in depth. *Perception and Psychophysics, 35,* 229–236.

Woodworth, R. S. (1938). *Experimental psychology.* New York: Henry Holt.

Yarbus, A. L. (1967). *Eye movements and vision.* New York: Plenum Press.

Youniss, J., & Calvin, A. D. (1961). The enclosing contour effect. *Perceptual and Motor Skills, 13,* 75–81.

Zigler, M. J. (1920). An experimental analysis of visual form. *American Journal of Psychology, 31,* 273–300.

Author Index

Subject Index

Explanatory Note: Several terms such as "illusory contour" or "subjective contour" are not indexed as they appear on almost every page. Some entire chapters are referenced when the subject is a major concern of the contribution. Individuals are not indexed unless their name refers to an important macrolevel theory or specific figure, illusion, process, or effect.

DATE DUE